K.S. Breuer (Ed.)

Microscale Diagnostic Techniques

Kenneth S. Breuer (Ed.)

Microscale Diagnostic Techniques

With 117 Figures

Springer

Editor

Prof. Kenneth S. Breuer
Brown University
Division of Engineering, Box D
182 Hope Street
Providence, RI 02912
USA

ISBN 978-3-642-06202-5 e-ISBN 978-3-540-26449-1

Springer is a part of Springer Science+Business Media

springeronline.com

Final processing by PTP-Berlin Protago-TEX-Production GmbH, Germany
Cover-Design: design & production GmbH, Heidelberg
Printed on acid-free paper 62/3020Yu - 5 4 3 2 1 0

Preface

The fields of micro- and nanotechnology have emerged over the past decade as a major focus of modern scientific and engineering research and technology. Driven by advances in microfabrication, the investigation, manipulation and engineering of systems characterized by micrometer and, more recently, nanometer scales has become commonplace throughout all technical disciplines. With these developments, an entirely new collection of experimental diagnostic techniques have been developed to explore and characterize such systems. The purpose of this book is to highlight some of the most innovative and powerful developments in micron-scale diagnostics that have been presented over the past few years, and to provide a resource for researchers and scientists interested in learning about the techniques themselves – their capabilities and limitations.

As with any field at the leading edge of modern science, each day brings new ideas, and by the time these chapters were written and published, many new improvements have been suggested, implemented. Nevertheless we hope that the contributions here will continue to have some value to researchers in the new frontier of micron and nano-scale science and technology.

I must first and foremost thank the authors of each chapter who generously agreed to invest the considerable effort required to document their expertise. This effort started over two years ago and most of the contributions were submitted by the summer of 2003. It has taken this long to finish the formatting, assemble the various permissions and get the book to the printer. During this delay (which was due only to my own inefficiency busy schedule) , the chapter authors have been unreasonably patient, and I thank them for their good nature! Last, but not least, I must extend a special thanks to Shankar Devasenathipathy, who helped me with the final editing chores and gave that extra push to see the book out of the door.

Providence RI
June 2004

Kenny Breuer

Preface

[illegible]

Table of Contents

List of Contributors

Mehdi Asheghi
Department of Mechanical Engineering
Carnegie Mellon University
Pittsburgh, PA 15213

J. W. Bender
Department of Physics
North Carolina State University
Raleigh, NC 27695

Shankar Devasenathipathy
Department of Mechanical Engineering
Stanford University
Stanford, CA 94305

Margaret L. Gardel
Department of Physics
Harvard University
Cambridge, MA 02139

Jacqueline Krim
Department of Physics
North Carolina State University
Raleigh, NC 27695

Carl D. Meinhart
Department of Mechanical and Environmental Engineering
University of California, Santa Barbara
Santa Barbara, CA 93106-5070

Rodney S. Ruoff
Department of Mechanical Engineering
Northwestern University
Evanston, IL 60208

Juan G. Santiago
Department of Mechanical Engineering
Stanford University
Stanford, CA 94305

Megan T. Valentine
Department of Physics
Harvard University
Cambridge, MA 02139

David A. Weitz
Department of Physics
Harvard University
Cambridge, MA 02139

Steven T. Wereley
School of Mechanical Engineering
Purdue University
West Lafayette, IN 47907-1288

Y. Yang
Department of Mechanical Engineering
Carnegie Mellon University
Pittsburgh, PA 15213

Min-Feng Yu
Department of Mechanical and Industrial Engineering
University of Illinois at Urbana-Champaign
Urbana, IL 61801

1. Microrheology

M.L. Gardel, M.T. Valentine, and D.A. Weitz

1.1 Introduction

Rheology is the study of the deformation and flow of a material in response to applied stress. Simple solids store energy and provide a spring-like, elastic response, whereas simple liquids dissipate energy through viscous flow. For more complex viscoelastic materials, rheological measurements reveal both the solid- and fluid-like responses and generally depend on the time scale at which the sample is probed (Larson 1999). One way to characterize rheological response is to measure the shear modulus as a function of frequency. Traditionally, these measurements have been performed on several milliliters of material in a mechanical rheometer by applying a small amplitude oscillatory shear strain, $\gamma(t) = \gamma_o \sin(\omega t)$ where γ_o is the amplitude and ω is the frequency of oscillation, and measuring the resultant shear stress. Typically, commercial rheometers probe frequencies up to tens of Hz. The upper range is limited by the onset of inertial effects, when the oscillatory shear wave decays appreciably before propagating throughout the entire sample. If the shear strain amplitude is small, the structure is not significantly deformed and the material remains in equilibrium; in this case, the affine deformation of the material controls the measured stress. The time-dependent stress is linearly proportional to the strain, and is given by:

$$\sigma(t) = \gamma_o \left[G'(\omega)\sin(\omega t) + G''(\omega)\cos(\omega t) \right] \tag{1.1}$$

$G'(\omega)$ is the response in phase with the applied strain and is called the elastic or storage modulus, a measure of the storage of elastic energy by the sample. $G''(\omega)$ is the response out of phase with the applied strain, and in phase with the strain rate, and is called the viscous or loss modulus, a measure of viscous dissipation of energy. The complex shear modulus is defined as $G^* \equiv G' + iG''$. Alternatively, it is possible to apply stress and measure strain and obtain equivalent material properties.

Rheology measurements such as these have given valuable insight into the structural rearrangements and mechanical response of a wide range of materials. They are particularly valuable in characterizing soft materials or complex fluids, such as colloidal suspensions, polymer solutions and gels, emulsions, and surfactant mixtures (Ferry 1980, Macosko 1994, Larson 1999). However, conventional mechanical techniques are not always well-suited for all systems. Typically, milliliter sample volumes are required, precluding the study of rare or precious materials, including many biological samples that are difficult to obtain in large quantities. Moreover, conventional rheometers provide an average measurement ties. Moreover, conventional rheometers provide an average measurement of the bulk response, and do not allow for local measurements in inhomogeneous systems. To address these issues, a new class of microrheology measurement techniques has emerged. To probe the material response on micrometer length scales with microliter sample volumes. Microrheology methods typically use embedded micron-sized probes to locally deform a sample. There are two broad classes of micro-rheology techniques: those involving the active manipulation of probes by the local application of stress and those measuring the passive motions of particles due to thermal or Brownian fluctuations. In either case, when the embedded particles are much larger than any structural size of the material, particle motions measure the macroscopic stress relaxation; smaller particles measure the local mechanical response and also probe the effect of steric hindrances caused by local microstructure. The use of small colloidal particles theoretically extends the accessible frequency range by shifting the onset of inertial effects to the MHz regime; in practice, the measurable frequency range varies with the details of the experimental apparatus.

In this chapter, we will detail a variety of microrheology methods. In Section 1.2, we review the active manipulation techniques in which stress is locally applied to the material by use of electric or magnetic fields, or micromechanical forces. These active methods often require sophisticated instrumentation and have the advantage of applying large stresses to probe stiff materials and non-equilibrium response. Often single particle measurements are possible, allowing measurements of local material properties in inhomogeneous systems. In Section 1.3, we discuss the passive measurements of thermally excited probes, in which no external force is applied. For these methods, the mean squared displacement of the probe particle is measured using various experimental techniques and related to the macroscopic linear viscoelastic moduli of the material using a generalized Stokes-Einstein relationship. In Section 1.4, we discuss the practical application of microrheology techniques to number of systems, including heterogeneous materials. In heterogeneous systems, video-based multiple particle tracking methods are used to simultaneously measure the thermally-induced motions of dozens of particles in a single field of view. Single particle data is then used to map out the spatial variations in material mechanics and microstructure. In Section 1.5, we discuss two-particle microrheology, in which the correlated motions between pairs of particles are used to measure the coarse-grained macroscopic material properties. This allows the characterization of bulk material properties even in systems that are inhomogeneous on the length scale of the probe particle. We close the chapter with a brief summary and outlook. The experimental considerations of light scattering and particle tracking techniques are discussed in detail in the Appendix.

1.2 Active Microrheology Methods

One class of microrheology techniques involves the active manipulation of small probe particles by external forces, using magnetic fields, electric fields, or micromechanical forces. These measurements are analogous to conventional mechanical rheology techniques in which an external stress is applied to a sample, and the resultant strain is measured to obtain the shear moduli; however, in this case, micron-sized probes locally deform the material and probe the local viscoelastic response. Active measurements allow the possibility of applying large stresses to stiff materials in order obtain detectable strains. They can also be used to measure non-equilibrium behavior, as sufficiently large forces can be applied to strain the material beyond the linear regime.

1.2.1 Magnetic Manipulation Techniques

The oldest implementation of microrheology techniques involves the manipulation of magnetic particles or iron filings, which are embedded in a material, by an external magnetic field. This method was pioneered in the early 1920's and has been used to measure the mechanical properties of gelatin, cellular cytoplasm and mucus (Freundlich and Seifriz 1922, Heilbronn 1922, Crick and Hughes 1950, Yagi 1961, Hiramoto 1969, King and Macklem 1977). The visual observation of the particles' movements provided a qualitative measure of the viscoelastic response, but the irregularly shaped magnetic particles and simple detection schemes did not allow a precise measure of material properties. More recently, advances in colloidal engineering, video microscopy, and position sensitive detection have prompted the emergence of several high precision magnetic particle micro-rheological techniques.

One method called "magnetic bead microrheometry" or "magnetic tweezers" combines the use of strong magnets to manipulate embedded super-paramagnetic particles, with video microscopy to measure the displacement of the particles upon application of constant or time-dependent forces (Ziemann, et al. 1994, Amblard, et al. 1996, Schmidt, et al. 1996). In this case, strong magnetic fields are required to induce a magnetic dipole in the super-paramagnetic beads, and magnetic field gradients are applied to produce a force. The resultant particle displacements measure the rheological response of the surrounding material. Magnetic tweezers techniques have been used to measure the microscopic dynamics of a number of interesting materials that are not easily probed with traditional bulk techniques, including networks of filamentous actin (Ziemann, et al. 1994, Amblard, et al. 1996, Schmidt, et al. 1996, Keller, et al. 2001), living fibroblast (Bausch, et al. 1998), macrophage (Bausch, et al. 1999), endothelial (Bausch, et al. 2001) and dictyostelium cells (Feneberg, et al. 2001), and solutions of the semi-flexible filamentous bacteriophage fd (Schmidt, et al. 2000). In one experimental design, as shown in Fig. 1.1, the magnetic field is created by four pairs of soft ferromagnetic pole pieces arranged at right angles, where each pair is wound with a separate field coil (Amblard, et al. 1996).

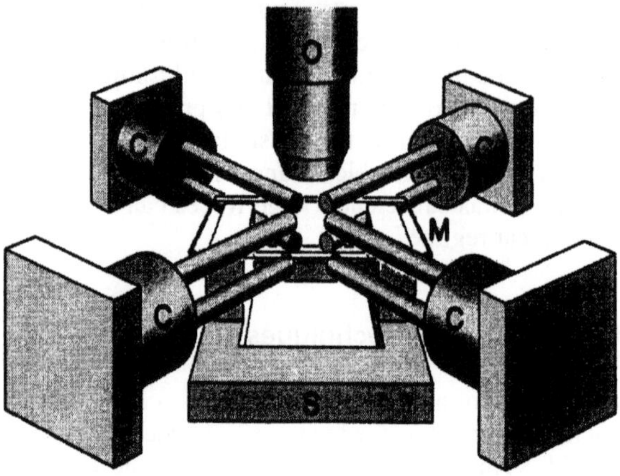

Fig. 1.1. A schematic of one experimental design of a magnetic bead microrheometer. The sample (M) is placed is the center of four coils (C) and magnetic pole pieces and supported by a sample holder (S) on an upright research microscope. The magnetic particles in the specimen plane are imaged using the objective lens (O) and particle displacements are measured with video-based detection. (Reprinted with permission from Amblard, et al. 1996).

Four attached Hall probes are used to measure the local magnetic field. Each pair of poles is precisely positioned in plane and the geometric center of the pair is at the optical focus of the microscope, ensuring a negligible vertical component to the magnetic field. This design creates a uniform magnetic field parallel to the focal plane and directed to one of the poles, and allows both translation and rotation of magnetic colloidal particles, which are typically 0.5 - 5 μm in diameter. In rotation mode, the field is uniform, with controlled angle relative to the orientation of the pole pieces, making it a potentially useful tool for measuring the local bending modulus of a material. In translation mode, a large magnetic field is generated at one attracting pole; field lines that originate from the attracting pole spread out to three opposing poles where smaller fields are generated. In order to generate forces, gradient fields are required, and are created by a precise balance of attracting flux and the total flux at the opposing poles. The force, $f(t)$, on the particle is given by:

$$f_x(t) = \vec{M}(t) \cdot \frac{\partial \vec{B}(t)}{\partial x} = \chi V \vec{B}(t) \cdot \frac{\partial \vec{B}(t)}{\partial x} \tag{1.2}$$

where $M(t)$ is the induced magnetic moment of the particle, $B(t)$ is the is the imposed magnetic field, χ is the susceptibility of the particle and V is the volume of the particle. Typically, for 0.1-0.2 T magnetic fields and 10-20 T/m gradients, applied forces are in the range of pN and torques are in the range of 10^{-14} N·m.

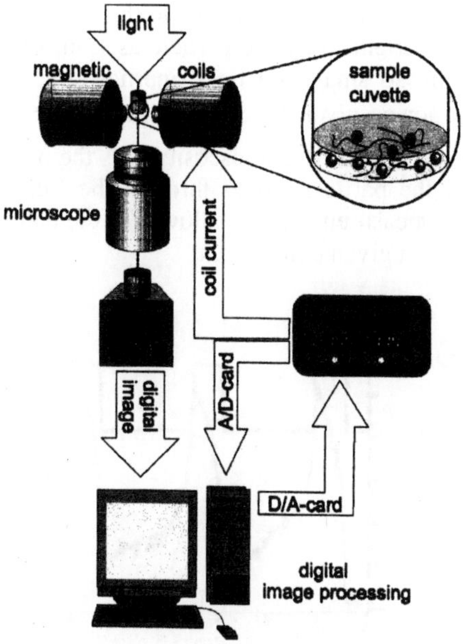

Fig. 1.2. A schematic view of one of the experimental designs of a magnetic bead microrheometer. The magnet consists of two coils with cylindrical soft iron cores. The sample and magnet are mounted on an inverted research microscope. A CCD camera is used to capture images of the particle and image analysis routines are used to measure particle displacements. The amplifier used to drive the magnet's power supply also delivers a signal to the computer to allow measurements of phase lag. (reprinted with permission from Keller, et al 2001).

A second design, shown in Fig. 1.2, uses one or two axisymmetrically arranged magnetic coils with soft iron cores that apply a field gradient to produce a force in the focal plane (Ziemann, et al. 1994, Schmidt, et al. 1996, Keller, et al. 2001). The force exerted depends on the details of the tip geometry, but is typically in the range of 10 pN to 10 nN. For higher forces, only one coil is used and the tip of the pole piece is positioned as close as 10 μm to the magnetic particle. Typically, the magnetic particles are separated by more than 50 μm and only single particle displacements are recorded to prevent neighboring spheres from creating induced dipolar fields. In both designs, video microscopy is used to detect the displacements of the particles under application of force. The instrumental precision depends on the details of the design and will be discussed in detail in Sec A.3; however, the spatial resolution is typically in the range of 10-20 nm and the temporal dynamic range is 0.01-100 Hz. Three modes of operation are available in any rheology measurement performed under applied force: a viscometry measurement obtained by applying constant force, a creep response measurement after the application of a pulse-like excitation, or a measurement of the frequency dependent viscoelastic moduli in response to an oscillatory stress. In constant force mode, the viscosity of a Newtonian fluid is measured by balancing the external driving force with the viscous drag force experienced by the particle as it moves through the fluid; because the particles are so small and light, inertial effects are typically ignored. The equation of motion is given by Stoke's Law, $f_o = 6\pi\eta a v$, where f_o is the constant external force, η is the fluid viscosity, a is the particle radius and v is the velocity with which the particle moves through the fluid. By using a fluid of known viscosity, this measurement also allows for the calibration of the force exerted on the particle by a given coil current.

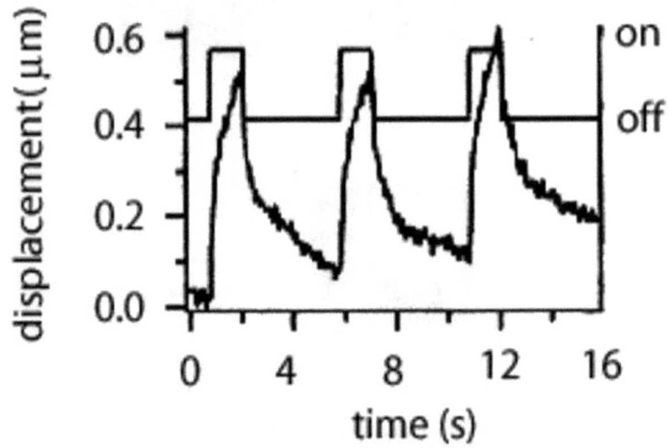

Fig. 1.3. A typical creep response and recovery curve from a magnetic particle measurement. The step pulses indicate the application of stress by turning on and off the external magnetic field. The resultant bead displacement consists of a fast elastic response at the initial onset of stress, followed by a slowing down and viscous flow regime. (reprinted with permission from Bausch, et. al. 1999).

In addition to constant force viscometry measurements, time-dependent forces can be applied to measure the frequency dependent viscoelastic response. In a creep-response measurement, a force pulse is applied to the particle and the particle deflection is measured as a function of time. Representative data curves are shown in Fig. 1.3. The time dependence of the bead deflection, $x_d(t)$ can be expressed as:

$$x_d(t) = J(t)\frac{f(t)}{6\pi a} \tag{1.3}$$

where $J(t)$ is the time-dependent creep compliance of the material in which the bead is embedded. In many cases, $J(t)$ can be interpreted with the use of mechanical equivalent circuits of springs, which represent elastic storage, and dashpots, which represent viscous loss, to model the local mechanical response (Ferry 1980, Bausch, et al. 1998). Alternatively, an oscillatory force can be applied to drive the particle at a controlled amplitude and frequency. The amplitude and phase shift of the particle's displacement with respect to the driving force are measured and are used to calculate the local frequency-dependent viscoelastic moduli. When an oscillatory force, $f(t) = f_0 \exp(i\omega t)$ is applied to the particles, the displacement can be expressed as $x(t) = x_0 \exp[i(\omega t - \varphi)]$ and the shear moduli are given by:

$$G'(\omega) = \frac{f_o}{6\pi a |x_o \omega|} \cdot \cos\varphi(\omega)$$

$$G''(\omega) = \frac{f_o}{6\pi a |x_o \omega|} \cdot \sin\varphi(\omega) \quad . \tag{1.4}$$

If the probe particles are larger than all length scales of the material, then the measured shear moduli report the macroscopic bulk response. If however, the particles are embedded in an inhomogeneous material, then each particle measures the dynamic microenvironment that surrounds it and the local material response. In materials that actively change in response to external stimuli, real-time measurements of the local dynamics are possible (Bausch, et al. 2001).

Local properties can be further probed by measuring the strain field around the each particle using mixtures of paramagnetic particles and non-magnetic latex spheres (Schmidt, et al. 1996, Bausch, et al. 1998). The magnetic particles are displaced by application of constant force and the resultant deformation field is visualized by measuring the movements of the surrounding latex particles. For a homogeneous elastic material, the deformation field is given by:

$$\vec{u} = \frac{1+\sigma}{8\pi E(1-\sigma)} \frac{(3-4\sigma)\vec{f} + \hat{r}(\hat{r}\cdot\vec{f})}{r} \tag{1.5}$$

where r is the distance from the point source, $\hat{r}$ is a unit vector in the direction of r, σ is the Poisson ratio, E is the Young's modulus (Landau and Lifshitz 1986). The elastic constants E and σ are measured, and from these the time-independent shear modulus is derived: $\mu = E/2(1+\sigma)$. Any deviations from the $1/r$ spatial decay in the strain field indicate the presence of local heterogeneities.

In addition to magnetic tweezers methods, a number of other magnetic particle techniques have been developed to measure material response. Twisting magnetometry measures the response of magnetic inclusions in a viscous or viscoelastic body to the brief application of a strong external magnetic field (Valberg 1984, Valberg and Albertini 1985, Valberg and Butler 1987, Valberg and Feldman 1987, Zaner and Valberg 1989). The strong field aligns the magnetic moments of the inclusions, which can be magnetic colloidal particles or polycrystalline iron oxide particles or aggregates. After the field is turned off, the aligned magnetic moments give rise to measurable magnetic field, the "remnant" field, which decays as the moments become randomized. In cases where rotational diffusion is the dominant randomizing agent, the decay can be interpreted in terms of the local viscosity. Viscoelastic response can also be measured by incorporating a weaker twisting field, in a direction perpendicular to the initial strong magnetic field (Zaner and Valberg 1989). When the twisting field is first applied, it lies in a direction perpendicular to the magnetic moments of the particles and the torque on the particles is maximal, causing the particles to rotate toward the direction of the weaker twisting field. The rate at which the particles align with the twisting field and the amount of recoil after the twisting field is turned off give a measure of local viscosity and elasticity. An in-line magnetometer allows the measurement of the angular strain and thus the local compliance, defined as a ratio of applied stress to strain.

A modification of the twisting magnetometry technique, called magnetic twisting cytometry, has been used to apply mechanical stresses directly to cell surface receptors using ligand coated magnetic colloidal particles that are deposited on the surface of a living cell (Wang, et al. 1993, Wang and Ingber 1994, Wang and Ingber 1995). The ferromagnetic particles are magnetized in one direction, and then twisted in a perpendicular direction to apply a controlled shear stress to the cell surface; as the particles re-orient, a magnetometer measures the change in remnant field, which is related to the angular strain. Alternatively, the twisting cytometry measurements can be mounted on a research microscope, and the particle displacements measured with video microscopy (Fabry, et al. 2001). When the twisting magnetic field is made to vary sinusoidally in time, bead displacement can be interpreted in terms of the local viscoelastic response (Fabry, et al. 2001). The frequency dependence of the material response can be obtained directly; however, in order to calculate the stress exerted on the cell surface by the particle and the absolute viscoelastic moduli, the details of the contact area and amount of particle embedding in the cell surface must be known.

Magnetic particle techniques allow measurements of bulk rheological response in homogeneous materials or local response in heterogeneous samples. Strain-field mapping identifies heterogeneities and allows the measurement of local microstructure and real-time measurements characterize dynamic changes in material response. Because such small sample volumes are required and non-invasive magnetic fields are used, these techniques are particularly useful for studying biological materials.

1.2.2 Optical Tweezers Measurements

Another active manipulation technique uses optical tweezers, also called optical traps or laser tweezers, that employ highly focused beams of light to capture and manipulate small dielectric particles (Ashkin 1992, Block 1992, Ashkin 1997, Ashkin 1998). Unlike magnetic tweezers, optical tweezers apply force very locally and the forces are typically limited to the pN range. The two main optical forces exerted on the illuminated particle are the scattering force, or radiation pressure, which acts along the direction of beam propagation, and the gradient force, which arises from induced dipole interactions with the electric field gradient and tends to pull particles toward the focus (Ashkin 1992, Ashkin 1997, Nemoto and Togo 1998, Neto and Nussenzveig 2000). Steep electric field gradients can be created using a high numerical aperture objective lens to focus a laser beam onto the sample; this allows the gradient force to dominate and forms a stable three-dimensional trap. Moving the focused laser beam forces the particle to move, apply local stress to the surrounding material, and probe the local rheological response.

The experimental design is typically based on an inverted optical microscope with a quality high numerical aperture oil-immersion objective lens (Fällman and Axner 1997, Visscher and Block 1998, Mio, et al. 2000, Mio and Marr 2000). The microscope allows for simultaneous imaging of the sample and facilitates placement of the beam in an inhomogeneous material. The illuminating laser beam is steered into the microscope with an external optical train, and is commonly introduced from the epi-fluorescence port and deflected into the optical path of the microscope by a dichroic mirror located below the objective lens. In order to achieve the most efficient and stable trapping, the beam is collimated at the back focal plane (BFP) of the objective and the objective entrance aperture is slightly overfilled. The external optical train allows the control of beam placement and movement, and even remote control of beam movement through the use of piezo-controlled mirror mounts or acousto-optic modulators. Steering mirrors are placed in a plane conjugate to the BFP of the objective to ensure that the intensity and strength of the laser trap does not fluctuate as the beam is moved (Fällman and Axner 1997). The slight tilting of a mirror in this plane will result in a corresponding change only in the direction of the laser beam at the BFP of the objective, maintaining a constant degree of overfilling at the entrance aperture and resulting only in the lateral movement of the optical trap in the specimen plane.

At the center of the optical trap, which is typically located slightly above the focal plane, the gradient and scattering forces balance and the net optical force is zero. At the trap center, the potential energy is given by:

$$U = \frac{-3V_p n_1}{c}\left(\frac{n_2^2 - n_1^2}{n_2^2 + 2n_1^2}\right) I_o e^{-r^2/R^2} \tag{1.6}$$

where V_p is the volume of the particle, n_2 is the index of refraction of the particle and n_1 is the index of refraction of the surrounding fluid, r is the radial distance from the center of the trap and R is the $1/e$ width of the Gaussian laser profile at the trap (Ou-Yang 1999). For stable trapping, $n_1 > n_2$ is required. The force on the particle as it moves from the trap center is given by:

$$\begin{aligned} F &= -\nabla U \\ &= -\frac{6rV_p n_1}{cR^2} I_o \left(\frac{n_2^2 - n_1^2}{n_2^2 + 2n_1^2}\right) e^{-r^2/R^2}\hat{r} \\ &\equiv k_{ot} r e^{-r^2/R^2}\hat{r} \end{aligned} \tag{1.7}$$

and for small displacements, the force is approximated by Hooke's law with an effective spring constant, k_{ot} (Ou-Yang 1999). Thus, if the laser beam center is offset from the center of the particle, the particle experiences a restoring force toward the center of the trap. By moving the trap with respect to the position of the bead, stress can be applied locally to the sample, and the resultant particle displacement reports the strain, from which rheological information can be obtained.

In order to apply a known force, the trap spring constant, k_{ot}, must be measured. There are several methods for calibration of k_{ot}, which is typically linearly dependent on the intensity of the incident laser beam. The escape force method measures the amount of force needed to remove a sphere from the trap. Although this method is simple and doesn't require a sophisticated detection scheme for measuring small displacements, it depends critically on the shape of the potential at large displacements where the trapping force response is likely non-linear. If high resolution position detection methods are available, the trap spring constant may be measured by slowly flowing a fluid of known viscosity past the trapped particle and measuring the displacement of the particle due to the viscous drag force. For small displacements, the viscous drag force can be balanced by the linear restoring force of the trap, and the trap spring constant can be determined. Alternatively, k_{ot} can be measured from the thermal fluctuations in the position of the trapped particle. The trap spring constant is calculated using the equipartition theorem:

$$\tfrac{1}{2}k_B T = \tfrac{1}{2}k_{ot}\left\langle x^2\right\rangle \tag{1.8}$$

where x is the particle position and $k_B T$ is the thermal energy.

For measurements of rheological properties, particle displacements in response to an applied force must be precisely detected. Position detection methods fall into two broad categories: direct imaging methods and laser-based detection schemes. Direct imaging can be achieved using video microscopy to record images of trapped particles in the specimen plane and centroid tracking algorithms to find the particle positions in each frame, typically with a spatial resolution of one-tenth of a pixel (Crocker and Grier 1996). The temporal resolution is limited by the capture rate of the camera, and is typically 30 frames per second. Alternatively, the shadow cast by the particle can be imaged onto a quadrant photodiode detector, which is aligned such that when the particle is in the center of the trap, the intensity of light on each of the four quadrants is equal (Ou-Yang 1999). As the particle moves from the trap center, the difference in light intensity on the four quadrants is recorded to measure the particle displacement. Although the direct imaging techniques are simple to implement and interpret, they do not provide the high spatial or temporal resolution of laser based detection schemes.

Interferometry detection is one laser-based detection scheme (Gittes, et al. 1997, Schnurr, et al. 1997, Visscher and Block 1998). In this design, a Wollaston prism, which is located behind the objective lens and used conventionally for Differential Interference Microscopy (DIC), splits the laser light into two orthogonally polarized beams. This produces two nearly overlapping, diffraction-limited spots in the specimen plane that act as a single optical tweezers. After passing through the sample, the beams are recombined behind the condenser lens by a second Wollaston prism; the recombined beam passes through a quarter wave plate. If the particle is centered or the optical trap is empty, then the recombined beam has the same linear polarization as the incoming beam and the final beam is circularly polarized; however, if the particle is slightly off-center there is a phase lag introduced between the two beams and final beam is elliptically polarized. The degree of ellipticity gives a measure of the particle displacement. The response is linear for displacements of up to 200 nm for 500 nm particles and larger particles have an extended linear range; larger displacements may be detected using a piezo-activated stage to realign the particle with the center of the laser beam. Data is typically acquired at rates of 50-60 kHz, with subnanometer resolution (Gittes, et al. 1997, Schnurr, et al. 1997). This interferometry design has the advantages of high sensitivity and inherent alignment; however, it gives only one-dimensional data along the shear axis of the Wollaston prism.

Alternatively, the forward deflected laser light can be projected onto a photodiode to detect the displacement of the trapped particle. A trapped bead acts as a mini-lens and deflects the illuminating laser light forward through the condenser lens, which relays the light onto the photodiode. In a single photodiode configuration, the detector is positioned so that roughly 50% of the optical power from the diverging cone of light is intercepted (Visscher and Block 1998). This configuration is qualitatively sensitive to both axial displacements, which change the diameter of the intercepted light cone and the intensity of light at the detector, and lateral displacements, which offset the cross-sectional area of the light cone from the active detector area. However, quantitative measurements of particle displacements are not straightforward with single photodiode detection since axial and lateral displacements are not easily decoupled and since no information about small movements in the focal plane is available. Alternatively, quantitative subnanometer displacements can be measured with a quadrant photodiode placed in the BFP of the condenser lens. Typically, the active area of the detector is larger than the area of the intercepted light cone, so axial displacements are not detected. The forward-scattered light is detected by the photodiode, where the photocurrent differences are amplified and converted into voltages to measure the relative displacement of the bead with respect to the trap center. The trajectory is obtained by sampling the voltages with an A/D converter at rates up to 50 kHz. The spatiotemporal resolution is 0.01 nm/Hz$^{1/2}$ above 500 Hz; at lower frequencies, the resolution decreases and degrades to 1 nm/Hz$^{1/2}$ at 20 Hz due to the mechanical resonance of the stage (Mason, et al. 2000). The maximal displacement that may be detected with this technique is approximately 200 nm.

To measure rheological properties, optical tweezers are used to apply a stress locally by moving the laser beam and dragging the trapped particle through the surrounding material; the resultant bead displacement is interpreted in terms of viscoelastic response. Elasticity measurements are possible by applying a constant force with the optical tweezers and measuring the resultant displacement of the particle. This approach has been used to measure the time-independent shear modulus of red blood cell membranes (Hénon, et al. 1999, Sleep, et al. 1999). Alternatively, local frequency-dependent rheological properties can be measured by oscillating the laser position with an external steerable mirror and measuring the amplitude of the bead motion and the phase shift with respect to the driving force (Valentine, et al. 1996, Ou-Yang 1999). The equation of motion for a colloidal particle in forced oscillation in a viscoelastic medium is given by:

$$m^*\ddot{x} + 6\pi\eta^* a\dot{x} + (k_{ot} + k)x = k_{ot} A\cos(\omega t) \tag{1.9}$$

where m^* is the effective mass, η^* is the effective frequency dependent viscosity of the medium, a is the particle radius, k_{ot} is the spring constant of the trap, k is the frequency dependent spring constant of the medium, A is the amplitude of the trap displacement and ω is the driving frequency (Ou-Yang 1999). The effective mass includes the bare mass of the particle and contribution of the inertia of the surrounding fluid entrained by the moving particle. The effective mass is given by:

$$m^* = m_o + \frac{2\pi}{3}a^3\rho + 3\pi a^2\sqrt{\frac{2\eta\rho}{\omega}} \tag{1.10}$$

where ρ is the mass density and η is the viscosity of the surrounding fluid. The effective viscosity also includes an inertial correction, and is given by:

$$\eta^* = \eta\left(1 + \sqrt{\frac{a^2\rho\omega}{2\eta}}\right). \tag{1.11}$$

The equation of motion can be solved by:

$$x(t) = D(\omega)\cos(\omega t - \delta(\omega)). \tag{1.12}$$

By detecting the forward-scattered light from a second weaker probing beam and using a lock-in amplifier, the relative displacement and phase are measured. With this dual beam approach, $D(\omega)$, the amplitude of the particle displacement given by:

$$D(\omega) = \frac{k_{ot}A}{\sqrt{(k_{ot} + k - m^*\omega^2)^2 + m^{*2}\beta^2\omega^2}} \tag{1.13}$$

The phase shift, $\delta(\omega)$, is given by:

$$\delta(\omega) = \tan^{-1}\frac{m^*\beta\omega}{k_{ot} + k - m^*\omega^2} \tag{1.14}$$

where $\beta = 6\pi\eta^* a / m^*$ and k_{ot} is now given by the sum of the spring constants of the two laser beams. The second probing beam is not required; the trapping beam can also be used to measure particle displacements with modified expressions for $D(\omega)$ and $\delta(\omega)$. The equations for displacement and phase are solved for the material viscosity, $\eta(\omega)$, and elasticity, $k(\omega)$, from which the frequency dependent viscoelastic moduli are derived:

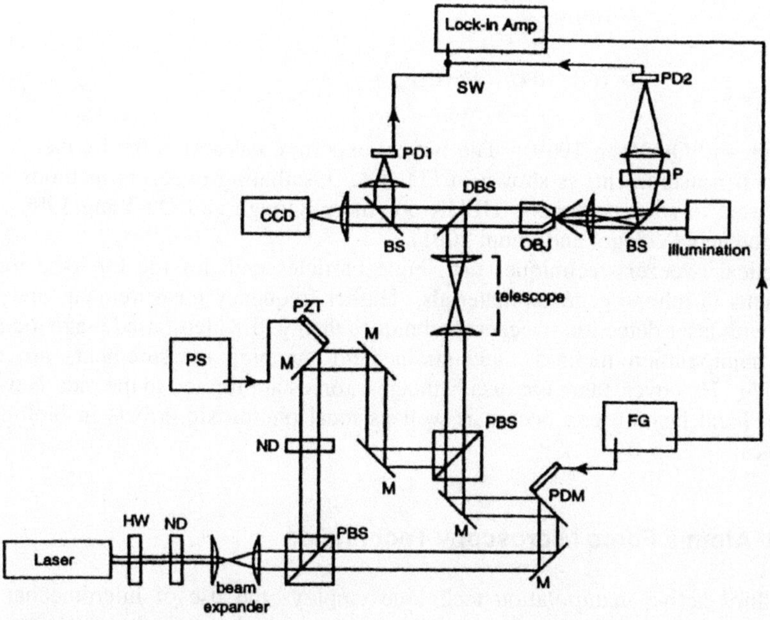

Fig. 1.4. A schematic of the experimental setup of the oscillating optical tweezers. The first polarizing beam splitter (PBS) splits the laser light into two separate beams, one stronger trapping beam and a second weaker probing beam. Both are independently aligned and steered by two piezoelectrically driven mirrors (PDM); rotation of the half-wave plate (HW) changes the relative intensity of the two beams. A function generator (FG) drives the PDM that moves the trapping beam and also delivers a signal to the lock-in amplifier, allowing the phase lag to be measured. PD1 and PD2 are quadrant photodiode detectors, and SW a switch to allow the signal from either PD1 or PD2 to reach the lock in amplifier. PD1 is used for direct imaging of the trapped particle while PD2 is used to measure the forward scattered laser light. The polarizer (P) placed before PD2 is used to select either the trapping or probing beam for position detection. ND is a neutral density filter, M a mirror, PS a power supply for the piezoelectric-driver (PZT), BS a beamsplitter, DBS a dichroic beam splitter which reflects the laser light and allows the broadband illumination light to pass. The sample chamber and trapped particle are located to the right of the high-numerical-aperture objective lens (OBJ) and are not shown. (reprinted with permission from Ou-Yang 1999).

$$G'(\omega) = \frac{k(\omega)}{2\pi a} \tag{1.15}$$

$$G''(\omega) = \omega(\eta(\omega) - \eta_{solvent}) \tag{1.16}$$

(Hough and Ou-Yang 1999). The typical experimental design for frequency dependent measurements is shown in Fig. 1.4. Oscillating tweezers methods have been used to study telechelic HEUR polymers (Hough and Ou-Yang 1999) and collagen gels (Velegol and Lanni 2001).

Optical tweezers techniques use single particles and provide for local measurements in inhomogeneous materials. Higher frequency measurements are possible with laser detection tweezers techniques than with video-based magnetic particle manipulation methods, and strain field mapping measurements are also possible. However, there are disadvantages: forces are limited to the pico-Newton range, local heating can occur, as well as local phototoxic effects in biological samples.

1.2.3 Atomic Force Microscopy Techniques

The third active manipulation technique employs the use of micromechanical forces created by an atomic force microscope to probe local mechanical response. The atomic force microscope (AFM), invented in 1986 (Binning, et al. 1986), has been widely used to study the structure of soft materials, and biological materials in particular, with sub-nanometer resolution (Drake, et al. 1989, Henderson, et al. 1992, Radmacher, et al. 1992, Bottomley, et al. 1996, Kasas, et al. 1997). In addition to imaging information about surface structure and topology, AFM techniques are sensitive to the force required to indent a surface and have been used to measure local elasticity and viscoelasticity of thin samples, including bone and bone marrow (Tao, et al. 1992), gelatin (Radmacher, et al. 1995, Domke and Radmacher 1998), polyacrylamide gels (Mahaffy, et al. 2000), platelets (Radmacher, et al. 1996), and living cells (Hoh and Schoenenberger 1994, Putman, et al. 1994, Shroff, et al. 1995, Goldman and Ezzell 1996, Rotsch, et al. 1997, A-Hassan, et al. 1998, Mahaffy, et al. 2000). Topographic images are obtained simultaneously with mechanical response, allowing elasticity to be correlated with local structure (Radmacher, et al. 1994). Local elasticity measurements have also provided information about the mechanical changes that accompany dynamic processes including cell division (Dvorak and Nagao 1998), activation of platelets (Radmacher, et al. 1996), exocytosis (Schneider, et al. 1997), and drug-induced changes in the cytoskeletal structure of living cells (Rotsch and Radmacher 2000).

Experimentally, a commercial AFM with soft cantilever is used in constant-force tapping mode for both imaging and elasticity measurements. The deflection of the cantilever is often measured with an optical "beam bounce" detection technique in which a laser beam bounces off the back of the cantilever onto a position sensitive photodetector. In constant force mode, the cantilever deflection is kept constant by a feedback circuit that changes the height of the piezo-electrically controlled scanner head in response to the local topography. In this mode, an image is generated from the scanner motion, and the scan speed is limited by the response time of the feedback circuit. In tapping mode, the tip of the cantilever is vibrated close to the sample surface, allowing the bottom of the tip to gently touch or "tap" the surface; the oscillation amplitude changes with tip-to-sample distance.

For each elasticity measurement, the deflection of the cantilever is measured as it approaches the sample. For small deflections, the loading force can be calculated using Hooke's law once the cantilever spring constant, k, has been calibrated (Butt and Jaschke 1995). For an extremely stiff sample, the deflection of the cantilever, d, is identical to the movement of the piezo scanner, z; however, for softer materials, the cantilever tip can indent the sample. The indentation, δ, reduces the total deflection, $d = z-\delta$, and the loading force is now given by $F = kd = k(z-\delta)$. A modified Hertz model is used to describe the elastic deformation of the sample by relating the indentation and loading force (Hertz 1881, Sneddon 1965). For a conical tip pushing onto a flat sample, the force is given by:

$$F = \frac{2}{\pi}\tan(\alpha)\frac{E}{1-\nu^2}\delta^2 \tag{1.17}$$

where α is the half-opening angle of the AFM cone-tip, E is the Young's modulus, and ν is the Poisson ratio of the sample. By combining the above equations we obtain:

$$z - z_o = d - d_o + \sqrt{\frac{k(d-d_o)}{(2/\pi)[E/(1-\nu^2)]\tan(\alpha)}} \tag{1.18}$$

where d_o is the zero deflection position and is determined from the non-contact part of the force-curve, and z_o is the contact point. Typically, ν is assumed or measured independently and the force curve is fit to determine E and z_o. There are two common sources of measurement error. For very soft samples, it is difficult to determine the exact point of contact, leading to uncertainty in the measurement of E. Also, for very thin or soft materials, the elastic response of the underlying hard substrate that supports the soft sample can contribute; in this case, the measured value of E should be taken as an upper bound. The contribution of the rigid substrate is greater for higher forces and indentations, and can be reduced by attaching a colloidal particle to the conical tip. With a spherical tip, the contact area is increased, allowing the same stress to be applied to the sample with a smaller force. Moreover, using a range of sizes of colloidal particles, the applied stress can be varied in a controlled manner; the applied stress is typically 100 – 10000 Pa for colloids of ranging in size from less than 1 μm to 12 μm in diameter (Mahaffy et. al. 2000). For a spherical tip of radius R, the modified Hertz model predicts:

$$F = \frac{4E\sqrt{R}}{3(1-\nu)}\delta^{3/2} \tag{1.19}$$

Another related technique, called Force Integration to Equal Limits (FIEL), allows the mapping of relative micro-elastic response in systems with spatial inhomogeneities or dynamic re-arrangements (A-Hassan, et al. 1998). This technique has several advantages over traditional analysis since the relative elastic map is independent of the tip-sample contact point and the cantilever spring constant. In FIEL, a pair of force-curves is collected at two different positions in the sample in constant force mode, imposing the condition that $F_1 = F_2$ where the subscript distinguishes the two measurements. For a spherical tip geometry, the force balance gives:

$$\frac{4}{3}\frac{\sqrt{R}}{\pi k_1}\delta_1^{3/2} = \frac{4}{3}\frac{\sqrt{R}}{\pi k_2}\delta_2^{3/2} \tag{1.20}$$

where k is the local spring constant of the sample is the defined as: $k = 1 - \nu / \pi E$. This equation reduces to:

$$\left(\frac{\delta_1}{\delta_2}\right)^{3/2} = \frac{k_1}{k_2} \tag{1.21}$$

The work done by the AFM cantilever during indentation can be calculated by integrating the force-curve over the indentation depth:

$$w_i = \int_0^{\delta_i} \frac{4}{3}\frac{\sqrt{R}}{\pi k_i}\delta_i^{3/2} d\delta = \frac{8}{15}\frac{\sqrt{R}}{\pi k_i}\delta_i^{5/2} \tag{1.22}$$

where the index i indicates a single force-curve measurement. The relative work done is given by the ratio of work done in each measurement:

$$\frac{w_1}{w_2} = \left(\frac{\delta_1}{\delta_2}\right)^{5/2} \frac{k_2}{k_1}. \tag{1.23}$$

Combining the two above equations, we obtain an expression for the relative local elasticity, given by:

$$\frac{w_1}{w_2} = \left(\frac{k_1}{k_2}\right)^{2/3}. \tag{1.24}$$

This approach works for other tip geometries as well, with a change only in the scaling exponent; the exponent is 2/3 for a spherical or parabolic tip, 1/2 for a conical tip, and one for a flat-end cylinder. By comparing many force curves obtained at many different locations in the sample, a map of relative microelasticity across the surface is obtained. If the same probe is used in all measurements, the result is independent of the exact probe size, cantilever spring constant, and deflection drift. This method is independent of sample topography and does not require absolute height measurements. FIEL mapping is most useful for measuring relative changes in elasticity in dynamic systems and is not appropriate for measuring absolute moduli. In order to obtain absolute measures of elasticity and to compare FIEL maps obtained with different cantilevers, additional calibration procedures are necessary.

In viscoelastic samples, AFM techniques can be modified to measure viscosity and the frequency dependent response. Qualitative measures of the viscosity are possible by measuring the relaxation of the tip into the sample or the hysteresis of the force-curves. For more precise and frequency-dependent measurements, an oscillating cantilever tip can be used (A-Hassan, et al. 1998, Mahaffy, et al. 2000). A small amplitude sinusoidal signal, $\tilde{\delta}$, typically 5-20 nm, is applied normal to the surface around the initial indentation, δ_o, at frequencies in the range of 20-400 Hz. A lock-in amplifier is used to measure the phase and amplitude of the response with respect to the driving force. The modified Hertz model must now include a frequency dependent response term, and for small oscillations the force is given by:

$$f_{bead} \approx \frac{4}{3}\sqrt{R}\left(\bar{E}_o \delta^{3/2} + \frac{3}{2}\bar{E}^* \sqrt{\delta_o}\,\tilde{\delta}\right) \tag{1.25}$$

where $\bar{E}^*$ is analogous to the complex shear modulus, G^*, and is defined as the frequency-dependent part of the constant ratio $E/(1-\nu^2)$:

$$\bar{E}^* \equiv \frac{E}{1-\nu^2} = \frac{2(1+\nu)}{(1-\nu^2)G^*} \tag{1.26}$$

and $\bar{E}_o$ refers to the zero-frequency value of $\bar{E}^*$ defined as:

$$\bar{E}_o \equiv \frac{2(1+\nu)}{(1-\nu^2)G'(0)} \tag{1.27}$$

where $G'(0)$ is the real part of the complex shear modulus, the elastic modulus, at zero frequency. The second term in the modified Hertz model describes the time-dependent response and includes contributions of both the viscous drag force on the cantilever as it oscillates in the surrounding fluid and the viscoelastic response of the substrate. The viscous force on the cantilever is dependent on the frequency of oscillation and is given by:

$$f_{drag} = i\omega\alpha\tilde{\delta} \tag{1.28}$$

where ω is oscillation frequency, and α is a constant that includes the driving amplitude, the viscosity of the fluid, and the geometry of the cantilever. This contribution must be subtracted from the time-dependent response in order to measure the frequency dependent viscoelastic moduli, which depend only on the material properties of the soft substrate.

AFM techniques allow measurements of elastic or viscoelastic response of thin samples and surfaces. Images are often obtained simultaneously, allowing mechanical properties to be correlated with local topography and microstructure. Relative elastic mapping and fast AFM scans allow measurements of the dynamic changes in mechanics or structure. As in all active manipulation techniques, the strain amplitude and driving frequency can be varied and out-of-equilibrium measurements are possible.

1.3 Passive Microrheology Methods

A second class of microrheology techniques uses the Brownian dynamics of embedded colloids to measure the rheology and structure of a material. Unlike *active* microrheology techniques that measure the response of a probe particle to an external driving force, *passive* measurements use only the thermal energy of embedded colloids, determined by k_BT, to measure rheological properties. For passive measurements, materials must be sufficiently soft in order for embedded colloids to move detectably with only k_BT of energy. The thermal motion of the probe in a homogeneous elastic medium depends on the stiffness of the local microenvironment. Equating the thermal energy density of a bead of radius a to the elastic energy needed to deform a material with an elastic modulus G' a length L yields:

$$\frac{k_BT}{a^3} = \frac{G'L^2}{a^2}. \tag{1.29}$$

For most soft materials, the temperature cannot be changed significantly. Thus, the upper limit of elastic modulus we are able to measure with passive techniques depends on both the size of the embedded probe and on our ability to resolve small particle displacements of order L. The resolution of detecting particle centers depends on the particular detection scheme used and typically ranges from 1 Å to 10 nm, allowing measurements with micron-sized particles of samples with an elastic modulus up to 10 to 500 Pa. This range is smaller than that accessible by active measurements, but is sufficient to study many soft materials. Moreover, passive measurements share the distinct advantage that results are always within the linear viscoelastic regime because there is no external stress applied.

To understand how the stochastic thermal energy of embedded micron-sized particles is used to probe the frequency dependent rheology of the surrounding viscoelastic material, it is useful to first consider the motion of spheres in a purely viscous fluid then generalize to account for elasticity. Micron-sized spheres in a purely viscous medium undergo simple diffusion, or Brownian motion. The dynamics of particle motions are revealed in the time dependent position correlation function of individual tracers. This correlation function, also known as the mean squared displacement (MSD), is defined as:

$$\left\langle \Delta\vec{x}^2(\tau)\right\rangle = \left\langle \left|\vec{x}(t+\tau)-\vec{x}(t)\right|^2\right\rangle_t \tag{1.30}$$

where $\vec{x}$ is the d-dimensional particle position, τ is the lag time and the brackets indicate an average over all times t. The time-average assumes the fluid is in always in thermal equilibrium and the material properties do not evolve in time. The diffusion coefficient, D, of the Brownian particles is obtained from the diffusion equation:

$$\left\langle \Delta\vec{x}^2(\tau)\right\rangle = 2dD\tau \tag{1.31}$$

From this, the viscosity η of the fluid surrounding the beads of radius a is obtained using the Stokes-Einstein equation: $D = k_BT/6\pi\eta a$ (Reif 1965).

Many materials are more complex, exhibiting both viscous and elastic behavior. Additionally, the responses are typically frequency dependent and depend on the time and length scale probed by the measurement. For such materials, the thermally driven motion of embedded spheres reflects both the viscous and elastic contributions, which are revealed in the MSDs of the tracers (Mason and Weitz 1995). Unlike a simple fluid where the MSDs of embedded tracers evolve linearly with time, the MSDs of tracers in a complex material may scale differently with τ,

$$\left\langle \Delta\vec{x}^2(\tau)\right\rangle \sim \tau^{\alpha} \tag{1.32}$$

where $\alpha<1$ and is called the diffusive exponent. The particles may exhibit subdiffusive motion ($0<\alpha<1$) or become locally constrained ($\alpha=0$) at long times.

In the case of a pure elastic homogenous material, a plateau in the MSD occurs when the thermal energy density of the bead equals the elastic energy density of the network that is deformed by the displacement of the bead:

$$\left\langle \Delta x^2(\tau\rightarrow\infty)\right\rangle = \frac{k_BT}{\pi G'a} \tag{1.33}$$

Analogous to a harmonic oscillator, the elastic energy of deformation of a material can be understood as the energy of a spring with a spring constant proportional to $G'a$. The energy of the spring is simply the thermal energy, k_BT. A viscoelastic material can be modeled as an elastic network that is viscously coupled to and embedded in an incompressible Newtonian fluid (Levine and Lubensky 2000). A natural way to incorporate the elastic response is to generalize the standard Stokes-Einstein equation for a simple, purely viscous fluid with a complex shear modulus $G(\omega)= i\omega\eta$ to materials that also have a real component of the shear modulus. A generalized Langevin equation is used to describe the forces on a small thermal particle of mass m and velocity $v(t)$ in a complex material:

$$m\dot{v}(t) = f_R(t) - \int_0^t \zeta(t-\tau)v(\tau)d\tau \tag{1.34}$$

where $f_R(t)$ represents all the forces acting on the particle, including both the interparticle forces and stochastic Brownian forces. The integral represents the viscous damping of the fluid with a time dependent memory function $\zeta(t)$ to account for the elasticity in the network. By taking the unilateral Laplace transform of the generalized Langevin equation and using the equipartition theorem, the viscoelastic memory function can be related to the velocity autocorrelation function (Mason, et al. 1997):

$$\langle v(s)v(0)\rangle = \frac{k_B T}{ms - \zeta(s)} \tag{1.35}$$

where s represents frequency in the Laplace domain. The inertial term is negligible except at very high (~ MHz) frequencies (Levine and Lubensky 2000). When the velocity autocorrelation is written in terms of the Laplace transform of MSD, the expression for the memory function in Laplace space becomes

$$\tilde{\zeta}(s) = \frac{6k_B T}{s^2 \langle \Delta\tilde{r}^2(s)\rangle}. \tag{1.36}$$

To relate the microscopic memory function to the bulk viscoelasticity, the Stokes law is generalized to include a frequency dependent complex viscosity (Mason and Weitz 1995). In the Laplace domain, this relates the complex shear modulus $\tilde{G}(s)$ to the memory function $\tilde{\zeta}(s)$ as

$$\tilde{G}(s) = \frac{s\tilde{\zeta}(s)}{6\pi a}. \tag{1.37}$$

By combining these two equations, we obtain a relationship that directly relates the mean-squared displacement of the tracers to the bulk modulus of the material:

$$\tilde{G}(s) = \frac{k_B T}{\pi a s \langle \Delta\tilde{r}^2(s)\rangle}. \tag{1.38}$$

This equation is a generalized, frequency-dependent form of the Stokes-Einstein equation for complex fluids. In the limit of a freely diffusing particle in a purely viscous solution,

$$\langle \Delta \tilde{r}^2(s) \rangle = 6D / s^2 \quad , \tag{1.39}$$

and the generalized Stokes-Einstein relation (GSER) recovers the frequency independent viscosity, $\eta_0 = k_B T / 6\pi a D$, where D is the diffusion coefficient of the particle in the fluid. This result of the generalized Stokes-Einstein equation is remarkable: simply by observing the time-evolution of the MSD of thermal tracers, we obtain the linear, frequency dependent viscoelastic response.

To compare with bulk rheology measurements, $\tilde{G}(s)$ is transformed into the Fourier domain to obtain $G^*(\omega)$. $G^*(\omega)$ is the complex shear modulus and is the same quantity measured with a conventional mechanical rheometer. $G^*(\omega)$ can be written as the sum of real and imaginary components: $G^*(\omega) = G'(\omega) + iG''(\omega)$. Since $G'(\omega)$ and $G''(\omega)$ are not independent and obey Kramers-Kronig relations, it is possible to determine both from the single, real function $\tilde{G}(s)$. This can be done, in principle, by calculating the inverse unilateral Laplace transform and then taking the Fourier transform (Schnurr, et al. 1997).

Equivalently, an alternative expression for the GSER can be written in the Fourier domain as:

$$G^*(\omega) = \frac{k_B T}{\pi a i \omega \Im_u \langle \Delta r^2(t) \rangle} \tag{1.40}$$

A unilateral Fourier transform, $\Im_u$, is effectively a Laplace transform generalized for a complex frequency $s=i\omega$. In practice, the numerical implementation of this process for discretely sampled data of $< \Delta r^2(t) >$ over a limited range of times can cause significant errors in $G^*(\omega)$ near the frequency extremes. Alternatively, a local power law expansion of $< \Delta r^2(t) >$ can be used to derive algebraic estimates for $\tilde{G}(s)$ and $G^*(\omega)$ (Mason, et al. 1997, Dasgupta, et al. 2001). This approximation is discussed in the Appendix.

To use the generalized Stokes-Einstein relation to obtain the macroscopic viscoelastic shear moduli of a material, it is necessary that the medium around the sphere may be treated as a continuum material. This requires that the size of bead be larger than any structural length scales of the material. For example, in a polymer network, the size of the bead should be significantly larger than the characteristic mesh size.

Recent theoretical work has shown that the GSER describes the thermal response of a bead embedded in a viscoelastic medium within a certain frequency range, $\omega_B < \omega < \omega^*$ (Levine and Lubensky 2000). The lower limit, ω_B, is the time scale at which longitudinal, or compressional, modes become significant compared to the shear modes that are excited in the system. In bulk rheology, the applied strain has only a shear component, but the thermally driven probe particle responds to all of the thermally excited modes of the system including the longitudinal modes of the elastic network. At frequencies lower than ω_B, the network compresses and the surrounding fluid drains from denser parts of the network. Above ω_B, the elastic network is coupled with the incompressible fluid and longitudinal modes of the network are suppressed. In this regime, the probe motion is entirely due to excited shear modes of the material (Schnurr, et al. 1997). An estimate of the lower crossover frequency, ω_B, can be determined by balancing local viscous and elastic forces. The viscous force per volume exerted by the solvent on the network is $\sim \eta v / \xi^2$, where v is the velocity of the fluid relative to the network, η is the viscosity of the fluid and ξ is the characteristic length scale of the elastic network. The local elastic force per volume exerted by the network is $G'\nabla^2 u \sim G'u / a^2$ at the bead surface where u is the network displacement field and a is the radius of the bead. Viscous coupling will then dominate above a crossover frequency

$$\omega_B \geq \frac{G'\xi^2}{\eta a^2}. \tag{1.41}$$

For a typical soft material with an elastic modulus of 1 Pa, viscosity of 0.001 Pa*sec and a mesh size one-tenth the radius of embedded probe, this crossover frequency ω_B is approximately 10 Hz.

The upper frequency limit, ω^*, exists due to the onset of inertial effects of the material at the length scale of the bead. Shear waves propagated by the motion of the tracer decay exponentially from the surface of the bead through the surrounding medium. The characteristic length scale of decay is called the viscous penetration depth and is proportional to $\sqrt{G^* / \rho\omega^2}$ where ρ is the density of the surrounding fluid and ω is the frequency of the shear wave (Ferry 1980). The viscous penetration depth sets a length scale for how far information is propagated in the medium when probed with a shear strain at a certain frequency ω. When the magnitude of the viscous penetration depth equals the size of the bead, inertial terms cannot be neglected. For a typical soft material, inertial effects can be expected to be significant only for frequencies larger than 1MHz (Schnurr, et al. 1997).

From these analyses, we find in typical experiments there is a very large frequency range 10 Hz $< \omega <$ 100 kHz where the generalized Stokes-Einstein equation is accurate and valid. Note that this is much higher than traditional mechanical measurements where inertial effects begin to become significant around 50 Hz. Additionally, models have been proposed for the frequency regimes where the GSER does not hold (Levine and Lubensky 2000).

To take full advantage of the range of frequencies and complex moduli accessible in a passive microrheology experiment, it is necessary to use techniques that measure the mean-squared displacement (MSD) of embedded spheres with excellent temporal and spatial resolution. The MSD can be calculated from methods that directly track the particle position as a function of time or can be obtained from ensemble-averaged light scattering experiments. Methods of particle detection vary significantly in temporal and spatial resolution, affecting the types of measurement possible with each technique. Additionally, techniques differ significantly in their ability to provide statistical accuracy over an ensemble of probes.

Particle tracking methods have been developed to directly image the position of a colloidal sphere as a function of time. Because the entire particle trajectory is directly obtained, these techniques allow further analysis of individual trajectories beyond an ensemble averaged MSD. These analyses often provide further insight into the local structures and rheology of the surrounding medium. Methods of particle tracking differ in the spatial and temporal resolution of the particle trajectories. The temporal resolution is determined by the frequency at which particle positions can be recorded. The spatial resolution is determined by how precisely differences in the particle position are measured. This, in turn, is used to determine an upper bound on the elastic modulus that can be detected using thermal motion with a given experimental technique.

The motion of individual tracers can be measured with laser detection schemes nearly identical to the optical tweezers setup described in Section 1.2.2 (Mason, et al. 1997, Schnurr, et al. 1997). Unlike optical tweezers, the laser power used in laser deflection particle tracking is quite low so that the optical forces are very small (< 5%) compared to the thermally driven forces of the bead. The thermally driven motion will cause the bead to move off the beam's axis and deflection of the laser beam can be measured. From this deflection, the displacement of the single bead is detected from which the MSD (Mason, et al. 1997) or the power spectral density (Schnurr, et al. 1997), the position correlation function in frequency space, can be calculated. The power spectral density of the beads is interpreted as the viscoelastic response of the material in a similar manner as the MSD (Schnurr, et al. 1997). This detection scheme has excellent spatiotemporal resolution; individual particles are tracked with subnanometer precision at frequencies up to 50 kHz. The enhanced frequency regime allows study of rheology of polymer networks at time scales where single filament properties often dominate the rheological response. However, this technique is limited in its statistical accuracy in two ways. First, it is somewhat difficult to obtain particle trajectories for a large ensemble of beads as this requires many consecutive measurements of individual beads. Secondly, in practice, it is difficult to track a single bead with this technique for longer than a few minutes because freely moving particles can diffuse out of the beam. While this track length is more than sufficient for the higher end of the frequency sweep, the low frequency statistics are limited. This strength of this technique resides in its ability to detect extremely small displacements of individual beads at high frequencies inaccessible to other video-based methods. Laser Deflection Particle Tracking has been used to study the rheology of F-Actin networks (Gittes, et al. 1997, McGrath, et al. 2000, Tseng and Wirtz 2001) and living cells (Yamada, et al. 2000).

Alternatively, it is possible to directly image the embedded beads using a simple video microscopy setup. Video microscopy of single beads is often used in active measurements as well, in particular with the magnetic bead microrheology experiments discussed in Section 1.2.1. Techniques in image processing have been developed to automate the process of accurate particle center location to simultaneously track hundreds of embedded probes in a single field of view of the microscope with submicron precision. While video microscopy is limited to frequencies available to the camera, the strength of the technique is in its ability to obtain good statistics on ensembles of beads.

Embedded spheres are imaged with a conventional light microscope using either fluorescence or bright field microscopy. Using bright field microscopy, spheres larger than a few hundred nanometers can be observed but the diffraction limited resolving power of the microscope precludes the study of smaller probes. Fluorescent labeling offers the ability to observe smaller probes, which now act as point sources of light, as well as the opportunity to perform colocalization studies with differently dyed beads. Fluorescently labeled colloidal spheres are commercially available from 20 nm up to several microns.

In a typical video based experiment, a time series of microscope images is obtained with a CCD camera and recorded in analog format onto a S-VHS cassette using commercially available video tape recorders. Video images are digitized using a computer equipped with a frame grabber card. Until recently, it was not possible to write a full frame image of 480 x 640 pixels directly to the hard drive at the standard video rates of 30 Hz due to limitations in the speed at which information can be transferred. With advances in computer technology, it is now possible to write full frame images directly to the hard drive at 30 Hz (Keller, Schilling et al. 2001); nonetheless, capturing movies to videotape affords the ability to store large amounts of data conveniently.

Of some concern is that the frequency ranges for video microscopy are around 10 Hz, earlier estimated as the lower frequency limit of the generalized Stokes-Einstein relation (GSER). This frequency limit is simply an estimate for when compressibility effects may become significant in a viscoelastic medium and preclude the use of the GSER. However, this lower frequency limit varies widely in different samples. Some materials, like simple fluids, are known to be incompressible at all frequencies. Additionally, in Section 1.5, formalism will be introduced to test for and even quantify compressibility effects using particle tracking with a video microscopy apparatus.

In a homogeneous, isotropic material, it is sufficient to examine the projection of the particle trajectory along a single axis. In heterogeneous materials, it may be useful to be able to obtain two- or three-dimensional particle trajectory. In video microscopy, the motion of the particle is projected into the plane of the focus and a two dimensional trajectory is obtained for further analysis. Techniques have been developed to track particles in the direction perpendicular to the plane of focus either by modifying the optics in a conventional microscope (Kao and Verkman 1994) or by carefully examining the structure of the Airy disk created by circular particles in bright field microscopy (Kao and Verkman 1994, Ovryn 2000,

Ovryn and Izen 2000). However, confocal microscopy is currently most widely used to follow the three dimensional motion of fluorescently tagged colloids (Weeks, et al. 2000, Dinsmore, et al. 2001).

The power in using video microscopy for microrheology lies in the potential of following the motions of roughly a hundred colloidal particles simultaneously and the ability to obtain the ensemble averaged mean-squared displacement (MSD) while still retaining each of the individual particle trajectories. The ability to accurately and precisely find the centers of the two-dimensional colloidal images in each frame of video is crucial. Algorithms have been developed to automate the process of finding particle centers and accurately find particles to roughly 1/10 of a pixel, and are described in the Appendix (Crocker and Grier 1996). For a typical magnification, this is a resolution of 10 nm. Once colloidal particles are located in a sequence of video images, particle positions in each image are correlated with positions in later images to produce trajectories. To track more than one particle, care is required to uniquely identify each particle in each frame (Crocker and Grier 1996).

Multiparticle tracking is particularly well suited to study materials that are heterogeneous at the length scales of the bead; for these systems, single bead measurements are not sufficient to describe a bulk response, but particle movements do reveal details of the local mechanics and microstructure. Measurements on heterogeneous materials will be discussed in Section 1.4. In the case of homogeneous materials, each thermally activated particle measures the same continuum viscoelastic response; as a result, measurements on ensembles of particles are often preferable to single bead measurements by providing better statistical accuracy in calculating the MSD and moduli. Ensemble averaged behaviors can be obtained by averaging many single particle motions that are simultaneously obtained with video microscopy; however, light scattering techniques are often preferable. Light scattering methods inherently average over a large ensemble of particles, and are not appropriate for samples that may exhibit local heterogeneity; however, for homogeneous samples, light scattering has the advantage of better averaging and statistical accuracy and a larger accessible frequency range than any macroscopic measurement or video-based microrheology technique.

In a typical dynamic light scattering measurement, a laser beam impinges on a sample and is scattered by the particles into a detector placed at an angle, θ, with respect to the incoming beam (Berne and Pecora 2000). As the particles diffuse and rearrange in the sample, the intensity of light that reaches the detector fluctuates in time. In the simplest case, each photon is scattered only once within the illumination volume directly into the detector. The intensity fluctuations are measured as a function of time, $I(t)$, and the normalized intensity correlation function, $g_2(\tau)$, is calculated:

$$g_2(\tau) = \frac{\langle I(t)I(t+\tau)\rangle}{\langle I(t)\rangle^2} \tag{1.42}$$

where the brackets indicate an average over time. The measured g_2, can be related to the calculated field correlation function, g_1, which is given by:

$$g_1(\tau) = \frac{\langle E(t)E^*(t+\tau)\rangle}{\langle |E(t)|\rangle^2} \tag{1.43}$$

where E is the scattered electric field, using the Siegert relation:

$$g_2(\tau) = 1 + \beta |g_1|^2 \tag{1.44}$$

where β is determined by the coherence of the detection scheme. For measurements of a single coherence area, or speckle, $\beta \approx 1$. If all particles are statistically independent, and moving randomly due to thermal impulses only, then:

$$g_1(\tau) = \exp[-q^2 \langle \Delta r^2(\tau) \rangle / 6] \tag{1.45}$$

where $\langle \Delta r^2(\tau) \rangle$ is the ensemble averaged three-dimensional MSD, and q is the scattering wave vector given by:

$$q = \frac{4\pi n}{\lambda} \sin\left(\frac{\theta}{2}\right) \tag{1.46}$$

where n is the index of refraction of the sample and λ is the wavelength of the laser *in vacuuo*. The correlation function decays as the scatters move a distance $1/q$. For some elastic samples, particles may be locally constrained and unable to move $1/q$ during the measurement, leading to "non-ergodic" behavior. In order to extract the ensemble average of the field correlation function from the measured time-averaged intensity fluctuations, a different method of analysis is required (Pusey and van Megen, 1989, Joosten et. al. 1990, van Megen et. al. 1991, Xue et. al. 1992). Once the MSD is obtained, the generalized Stokes-Einstein formalism can be applied to extract the frequency dependent viscoelastic moduli. Single light scattering techniques are typically sensitive to frequencies in the range of 0.01 – 10 Hz, similar to the frequency range available with a conventional macroscopic rheometer.

A second light scattering technique, Diffusing Wave Spectroscopy (DWS), allows measurements of multiple scattering media and extends the accessible frequency range to much higher frequencies (Pine, et al. 1988, Weitz and Pine 1993). The experimental set-up is similar to that of the single-scattering experiment; however, in this case, a laser beam impinges on an opaque sample and the light is scattered multiple times before exiting. The diffusion equation is used to describe the propagation of light through the sample. All q-dependent information is lost as the photons average over all possible angles, resulting in only two experimental geometries: transmission and backscattering. Like single scattering experiments, the intensity of a single coherence area is detected; fluctuations in intensity reflect the dynamics of the scattering medium and the mean squared displacement of the particles can be obtained. The field correlation function can be expressed as:

$$g_1(\tau) \propto \int_0^{\infty} P(s) \exp\left[-\frac{k_o^2 s \left\langle \Delta r^2(\tau) \right\rangle}{3l^*} \right] ds \tag{1.47}$$

where $P(s)$ is the probability of light traveling a path length s, and is determined by solving the diffusion equation with the experimental boundary conditions, $k_o = 2\pi n/\lambda$ where n is the index of refraction of the solution, λ is the wavelength of light *in vacuuo*, and l^* is transport mean free path and is defined as the distance the light must travel before its direction is completely randomized. The mean free path is determined in an independent measurement of the transmitted intensity and is typically much smaller than the thickness of the sample chamber. The correlation function decays when the total path length of the light through the sample changes by roughly the wavelength of the incident beam. To achieve this, each particle in the path of the light needs to move only a fraction of a wavelength; as a result, DWS is sensitive to motions on much smaller length scales and faster time scales than single scattering measurements. Analytic inversion is used to obtain the MSD from $g_1(\tau)$. The typical frequency range in a DWS measurement is $10 - 10^5$ Hz, allowing direct measurements of the high-frequency response of polymer solutions and other materials that are impossible with traditional mechanical measurements. The microrheology of flexible and semi-flexible polymer solutions has been measured using light scattering techniques (Mason, et al. 1996, Mason, et al. 1997, Gisler and Weitz 1998, Gisler and Weitz 1999, Palmer, et al. 1999, Mason, et al. 2000, Dasgupta, et al. 2001).

As seen in Fig. 1.5, Dasgupta et al. have demonstrated excellent agreement between moduli obtained for a flexible polymer solution, polyethylene oxide (PEO), using DWS and single light scattering microrheology and mechanical rheometry.

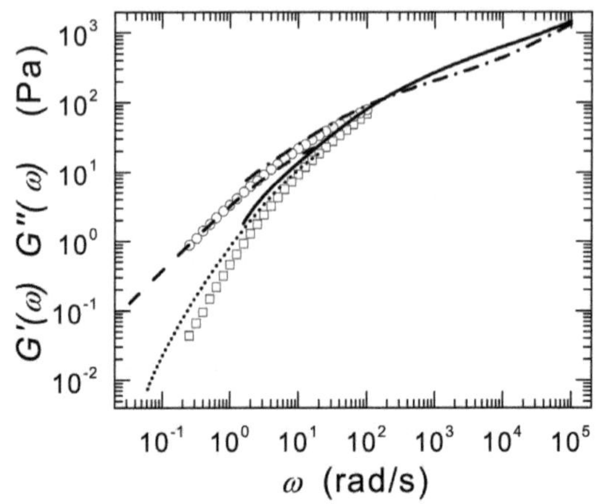

Fig. 1.5. The storage and loss moduli obtained by Dasgupta et al. (Dasgupta, et. al. 2001) for a 4% by weight 900 kDa PEO solution comparing moduli obtained with a conventional strain controlled rheometer (G' – open square, G" – open circle) to those obtained by both DWS (G' – solid line, G" – dash-dot) and single scattering at 20o (G'- dot, G" – dash). The beads used in both light scattering techniques are 0.65 micron spheres. Using the three techniques, it is possible to obtain data over ~6 decades in frequency. Additionally, the moduli obtained via light scattering are in excellent agreement with bulk measurement. Similar agreement between DWS and bulk rheology was found for other concentrations of PEO as well. (reprinted with permission from Dasgupta et al. 2001).

1.4 Practical Applications of One-Particle Microrheology

Because the techniques discussed in Sections 1.2 and 1.3 interpret the dynamics of individual probe particles as a viscoelastic response, these techniques have come to be known as one-particle microrheology. One-particle microrheology is a powerful tool to study the rheological properties of samples with extremely small sample volumes at frequencies inaccessible to bulk measurements. The development of microrheological techniques is currently an active field and the full range of possibilities, and limitations, of microrheology tools has yet to be completely understood. Here we discuss important issues to consider before interpreting the individual bead motion as a bulk rheological response of the material.

One-particle microrheology assumes the local environment of the bead reflects that of the bulk. If the surface chemistry of the bead modifies the structure of the material around the bead, the one-particle response will be a reflection of the local microenvironment rather than bulk rheology. Interactions between the embedded probe and sample are of much interest and are highly system dependent. In studies with polyethylene oxide, an uncross-linked flexible polymer solution, there is no effect of bead chemistry (Dasgupta, et al. 2001). However, surface chemistry seems to have significant effects with biopolymer networks (McGrath, et al. 2000). The charge groups used to stabilize commercially available colloids are reactive with many proteins, leading to unspecific binding. In a careful study with F-actin networks, the bead chemistry was changed to either inhibit or to encourage binding of actin to the bead surface (McGrath, et al. 2000). The beads that prevented actin binding were insensitive to changes in the mechanical properties of the network. By contrast, beads that bound to actin filaments reflected the bulk properties of the networks more accurately. However, it is often difficult to precisely control protein adsorption onto the beads. Moreover, although in some cases binding helps one-particle microrheology probe bulk properties, there may be other consequences. In the worst-case scenario, there is significant aggregation of the probes and the macroscopic gel-like structures are significantly altered. In less extreme cases, the presence of the bead affects only the surrounding local network but the bulk properties are unchanged. In this case, it is possible to obtain a modulus from one-particle microrheology but it is unclear whether the measured local modulus reports the bulk response.

In general, it is advisable to test for probe surface chemistry effects in a new system. In Section 1.5, two-particle microrheology will be discussed. Unlike one-particle microrheology that measures individual bead response to the surrounding microenvironment, two-particle microrheology is independent of bead surface chemistry.

One-particle microrheology has the additional feature that bulk response is measured only if the probe size is larger than the length scale of heterogeneity in the sample. These length scales are often unknown prior to a microrheology experiment. When the particle diameter is comparable to or smaller than the length scale of structures in the medium, the tracers can move within small cavities and their motions are not only a measure of the viscoelastic response, but also of the effect of steric hindrances caused by the cavity walls (Valentine, et al. 2001). A material like agarose is a prime example. Agarose is known to be structurally heterogeneous and consists of a network of fibrous molecules. The elastic modulus of agarose, as measured in a bulk rheometer, is roughly 2700 Pa and too high to measure with a passive microrheological technique. However, while agarose contains large elastic structures that span the sample and bear macroscopic stress, these structures do not form a homogeneous elastic medium. Instead, agarose is characterized by many smaller voids, or pores, through which smaller particles may move. By observing the dynamics of smaller particles within the pores, one is actually characterizing the structural and mechanical properties of the weaker pores rather than the bulk continuum properties.

In a particle tracking experiment, a plateau in the ensemble averaged mean-squared displacement at long lag times, $<\Delta x^2(\tau \rightarrow \infty)>$, indicates that the particles are constrained by the material, but it is necessary to examine how this plateau varies with particle radius, a, to determine the nature of the constraint. If the plateau is a measure of local elasticity G then $<\Delta x^2(\tau \rightarrow \infty)> = kT / \pi G a$, so $<\Delta x^2(\tau \rightarrow \infty)>$ scales with $1/a$. If the plateau is a measure of a pore size d then $d=a+h$ where h is the size of the fluid filled gap between the particle and the pore wall and can be approximated by $h = <\Delta x^2(\tau \to \infty)>^{1/2}$. Thus, if the particle is measuring a purely steric boundary then $a + <\Delta x^2(\tau \to \infty)>^{1/2}$ remains roughly constant. It is important to test trends in mean-squared displacement as a function of bead size to determine the nature of the constraints felt by the bead. The technique of two-particle microrheology is able to distinguish between measurement of a steric boundary and a local modulus.

In heterogeneous materials, individual particles movements must be considered since different particles may be exploring different microenvironments. Statistical techniques have been developed to compare the individual particles and map spatial and temporal variation in mechanical response (Valentine et al. 2001). Furthermore, particles in similar microenvironments can be grouped together into a meaningful ensemble and average rheological and structural properties can be obtained.

1.5 Two-Particle Microrheology

One-particle microrheology is very sensitive to the local environment of the embedded bead. If the tracers locally modify the structure of the medium or sample only the weak pores in a heterogeneous material, then one-particle microrheology determines the structure and mechanics of the local microenvironment rather than bulk rheology. The recently developed technique of two-particle microrheology (Crocker, et al. 2000) eliminates motion due to purely local structure and mechanics by measuring the cross-correlated motion of pairs of tracer particles within the sample. The correlated motion of the particles is not affected by the size, or even shape, of the tracer particles and is independent of the specific coupling between the probe and the medium. Furthermore, the length scale being probed is not the individual bead radius, *a*, but is the distance, *r*, between the tracers which is typically 10-100 microns rather than 1 micron. This increase in length scale means that the technique is insensitive to short wavelength heterogeneities in the sample smaller than the bead separation distance and thus may probe bulk rheology even if individual particles do not. Additionally, probing longer length scales lowers the frequency limit, ω_B, of the generalized Stokes-Einstein equation by replacing *a* by *r* in Eqn. 1.40.

Two-particle microrheology directly maps the long-range deformation or flow of the material due to a single tracer's motion. Since one tracer's strain field will entrain a second particle, the cross-correlated motion of two tracers' movements is a direct map of the strain field in the material. In a medium that is homogeneous at long length scales and characterized by a bulk viscoelasticity, the strain field is proportional to the tracer motion and decays like *a/r* where *r* is the distance from the tracer. Local heterogeneities either intrinsic to the material or created by the presence of the probe will affect individual particle motions but the movements will be uncorrelated at large distances.

With modifications, a two-particle measurement is possible with most of the active and passive techniques previously discussed. Video based multiparticle tracking is particularly well suited to examine cross-correlated motion because several hundred tracers can be imaged simultaneously (Crocker, et al. 2000). In a typical two-particle measurement, roughly one hundred tracers are observed for several hundred seconds at video rate to gather sufficient statistics. Vector displacements of individual tracers are calculated as a function of lag time, τ, and absolute time, t: $\Delta r_\alpha(t,\tau) = r_\alpha(t+\tau) - r_\alpha(t)$. Then the ensemble averaged tensor product of the vector displacements is calculated:

$$D_{\alpha\beta}(r,\tau) = \left\langle \Delta r_\alpha^i(t,\tau)\Delta r_\beta^j(t,\tau)\delta\left[r - R^{ij}(t)\right]\right\rangle_{i\neq j,t} \tag{1.48}$$

where i and j label two particles, α and β are coordinate axes and R^{ij} is the distance between particles i and j. The average is taken over the only the distinct terms ($i \neq j$); the "self" term yields the one-particle mean-squared displacement, $<\Delta r^2(\tau)>$.

The two-particle correlation for particles in an incompressible continuum is calculated by treating each thermal particle as a point stress source and mapping its expected strain field (Landau and Lifshitz 1986). In the limit where the particle separation, r, is much greater than the particle radius a ($r >> a$), this is calculated by multiplying the one-particle mean-squared displacement predicted by conventional generalized Stokes-Einstein relation in (1.38) by a/r, to obtain:

$$\tilde{D}_{rr}(r,s) = \frac{k_B T}{2\pi r s \tilde{G}(s)}$$

$$D_{\theta\theta} = D_{\phi\phi} = \frac{1}{2}D_{rr} \tag{1.49}$$

where $\tilde{D}_{rr}(r,s)$ is the Laplace transform of $D_{rr}(r,t)$ and the off-diagonal terms vanish. While this result has been obtained for an incompressible medium, compressible materials can be treated by using a modifed Stokes-Einstein relation and strain field (Landau and Lifshitz 1986). The Brownian motion of a single probe is the superposition of all modes with wavelengths greater than the particle radius, a. The correlated motion of two tracers a separation r apart is driven only by modes with wavelengths greater than the separation distance. Therefore, two tracers that are separated by more than the coarse-grained length scale in an inhomogeneous medium will depend on the coarse-grained, macroscopic complex modulus. In an experiment, it is necessary to confirm that $\tilde{D}_{rr}(r,s) \sim 1/r$ by examining the correlated motion of at least several pairs of probes with different pairwise separations. If the strain field follows $1/r$ within a certain range of interparticle distances, the material can be treated as a homogeneous continuum at those length scales.

Comparing the longitudinal two-point correlation to the generalized Stokes-Einstein equation used in one-particle microrheology suggests defining a new quantity: the distinct mean-squared displacement, $<\Delta r^2(\tau)>_D$, as

$$\left\langle \Delta r^2(\tau) \right\rangle_D = \frac{2r}{a} \tilde{D}_{rr}(r,s) \tag{1.50}$$

This is the thermal motion obtained by extrapolating the long-wavelength thermal undulations of the medium to the bead radius. In a homogenous material where the GSER is valid, the distinct mean-squared displacement matches the conventional one-particle mean-squared displacement. In inhomogeneous materials, differences between $< \Delta r^2(\tau) >_D$ and $< \Delta r^2(\tau) >$ provide insight into the local microenvironment experienced by the tracers. In this case, $< \Delta r^2(\tau) >$ may be understood as a superposition of a long-wavelength motion described by $< \Delta r^2(\tau) >_D$ plus a local motion in a cavity. Fig. 1.6a shows the comparison between the self and distinct mean squared displacements of 0.20 μm beads in a 0.25% guar solution. Guar is a naturally occurring neutral polysaccharide extracted from guar gum bean. A small concentration of guar in water dramatically changes the viscoelastic properties because of the formation of high-molecular weight, mesoscopic aggregates (Gittings, et al. 2000). Two-particle microrheology results are obtained by substituting $< \Delta r^2(\tau) >_D$ into the generalized Stokes-Einstein equation in place of $< \Delta r^2(\tau) >$. The self and distinct mean squared displacements results for the guar solution do not correspond, but disagree by a factor of two. In Fig. 1.6b, the data are converted into $G'(\omega)$ and $G''(\omega)$, and compared to results obtained from a macroscopic strain-controlled mechanical rheometer. As shown, the moduli calculated from the two-point correlation function are in good agreement with the results obtained with the rheometer. Single-particle microrheology provides qualitatively different moduli and completely fails to detect the crossover frequency. Unlike one-particle microrheology, two-particle microrheology is successful in determining the bulk rheological behavior of an inhomogeneous medium. This allows measurements in a larger range of materials than previously accessible with one-particle microrheology.

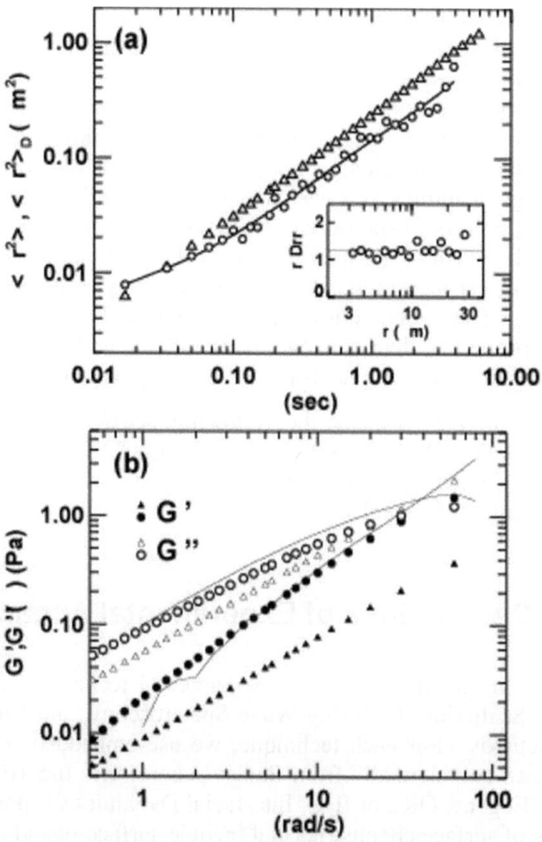

Fig. 1.6. The comparison of one- and two-particle microrheology to bulk measurements in a guar solution seen by Crocker et al. (Crocker, et al. 2000) (a) Comparison of the one-particle MSD (triangles) and distinct MSD (circles) of 0.20 μm diameter beads in 0.25% weight guar solution. Due to the heterogeneous nature of the medium, the curves differ by a factor of two. The solid line is a smooth fit to the data used for calculating rheology. (b) The elastic (filled circles) and loss (open circles) moduli calculated using the distinct MSD showing a crossover at high frequencies are in good agreement with the mechanical bulk measurement (solid curves). The moduli calculated using the one-particle MSD (triangles) do not agree. (reprinted with permission from Crocker, et al. 2000).

1.6 Summary

Microrheological techniques are powerful methods to characterize the mechanics and structure of novel and complex materials on length scales much shorter than those measured with bulk techniques. In an incompressible, homogeneous material the response of an individual probe due to external forcing or thermal fluctuations is a reflection of the bulk, viscoelastic properties of the surrounding medium. In heterogeneous materials, the motion of individual beads allows characterization of local mechanics while macroscopic rheological response is obtained by calculating the cross-correlated motion of the tracers from the same data. By combining the local and macroscopic measurements, a new understanding of how structure and mechanical response at the micron length scale relates to the bulk material properties emerges. Only microliter sample volumes are required, allowing the application of rheological techniques to materials too costly or difficult to synthesize in large quantities, or systems that are inherently small like living cells. Furthermore, viscoelastic response can be measured at frequencies ranging from 0.01 Hz to 10^5 Hz, much larger than the range of traditional mechanical measurements, allowing direct measurements of high frequency response in a wide range of soft materials. These techniques allow the study of both new systems and different material properties than conventional methods, and open new possibilities for understanding the microscopic properties of complex materials.

The authors would like to thank the following people for useful discussions: F. Amblard, A. Bailey, A.R. Bausch, L. Cipelletti, J.C. Crocker, B.R. Dasgupta, B. Frisken, P.D. Kaplan, A. Levine, F. MacKintosh, T. Mason, H.D. Ou-Yang, V. Trappe, C. Schmidt, E. Weeks.

Appendix: Descriptions of Experimental Apparati

Here we discuss in detail the various experimental techniques used in our lab: Dynamic Light Scattering, Diffusing Wave Spectroscopy, and Video-based particle tracking methods. For each technique, we use embedded colloidal particles that are purchased commercially from Bangs Laboratories Inc. (Fishers, IN), Molecular Probes (Eugene, OR), or IDC, Interfacial Dynamics Corporation (Portland, OR). A variety of surface chemistries that include surface-bound carboxyl, amine, or sulfate groups, sizes that range from approximately 20 nm to several microns, and different fluorescent dyes are available.

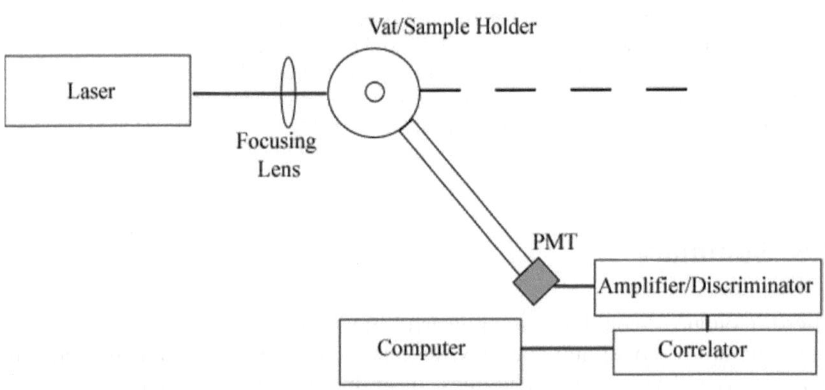

Fig. A.1. A standard dynamic light scattering setup.

A.1 Dynamic Light Scattering

The typical dynamic light scattering apparatus includes a light source, a goniometer that contains the sample and defines the scattering geometry, a detector, and a digital correlator that calculates the intensity autocorrelation function in real time, as shown in Fig. A.1 (Berne and Pecora 2000; Pecora 1985; Johnson and Gabriel 1981). The common light source is a continuous wave laser, a coherent, monochromatic source of light with an emission wavelength in the range of 400-700 nm. For single light scattering measurements, our lab employs a Coherent Innova 300-series Argon-Ion Laser (Santa Clara, CA), which is operated at a wavelength of 514.5 nm; the laser power at the sample is typically in the range of 50-300 mW. The operational wavelength is not critical, although the absorbance lines for a sample are avoided to prevent local heating, convection, and thermal lensing effects. The excitation wavelengths for fluorescent samples are also rejected. In cases where the excitation spectrum is wide, and it is not possible to eliminate fluorescence, filters are used to prevent any small emitted signal from reaching the detector. Plane-polarized light is required, as fluctuations in polarization give rise to undesired fluctuations in the intensity of the scattered light. To reduce mechanical vibrations, the experiment is often placed on an air-cushioned optical table, and to prevent relative movement of the laser and the sample, all optical elements are placed on the same plate.

The goniometer holds the sample and defines the scattering geometry. Several commercial goniometers are available; our lab uses models manufactured by Brookhaven Instruments (Holtzville, NY) and ALV (Langen, Germany). An entrance lens is used to focus the laser to a beam diameter of 50-100 microns, which increases the intensity of each coherence area, or speckle. Sample cells made from optical quality glass are used to reduce scattering and unwanted reflections from irregularities on the surface. Cylindrical vials are used for measurements at multiple scattering angles and are positioned such that the laser beam passes through the center of the vial; square cells are also useful for measurements at a fixed scattering angle of 90 degrees. Often the vial is placed in a vat filled with a fluid such as decalin or toluene with an index of refraction nearly equal to that of glass, in order to reduce the refraction and scattering at the vial surface. A window along the circumference of the vat allows the scattered light to reach the detector, which is placed on an arm that rotates about the center of the vial and collects the light at various angles. Typically, scattering angles ranging from 15 to 150 degrees are accessible, corresponding to q-vectors in the range of approximately 4-30 μm^{-1} (using Eqn. 1.46). At smaller angles, flare or scattering from large dust particles can dominate the signal and prevent good measurements of the particle mean-squared displacements (MSD). Using multiply filtered solutions may reduce the amount of dust present in the sample.

Detection optics, which include a series of lenses and pinholes or a fiber optic cable, define the scattering volume and collect the scattered light. A bright speckle occurs when light interferes constructively at the detector and the angular extent of a each speckle is given by: $\Delta\theta = \lambda / l$, where λ is the wavelength of the incoming light and l is the size of the beam in the scattering volume. For a beam of 50 microns in diameter that passes through a vial of 5 mm in diameter, the speckle size will be roughly 25 microns in width and 2.5 mm in height at a distance of 0.5 m from the center of the beam. The detector is typically positioned at a specific distance from the scattering volume to ensure that the collection area is limited to 1-2 speckles. When larger numbers of speckles are collected with traditional pin-hole optics systems, their fluctuations tend to cancel and reduce the overall signal; however, this effect is not observed in fiber coupled systems (Gisler et. al., 1995). The detector typically consists of a photomultiplier tube (PMT), which is mounted on the goniometer arm and collects the incoming photons at a specific angle. Within the PMT, each photon strikes the cathode and emits an electron that is accelerated and collides with a dynode, which in turn emits several electrons. The current passes through a series of additional dynodes, amplifying a single electron roughly 10^6 times (Pecora 1985). Once one photon strikes the cathode of the PMT, there is a time delay before another photon may be detected. This "dead time" is due to the electron transit time and is typically in the range of tens of nanoseconds, setting a lower limit on the temporal resolution of this device. For most DLS measurements, this transit time is much shorter than any time scale of interest.

The amplified signal from the PMT is passed to a pulse amplifier discriminator circuit (PAD) that converts the small incoming voltage pulses into standard logic pulses of defined duration and height, which are then passed to the correlator. Typically PADs that are designed specifically for spectroscopy applications are used. The amplifier discriminator sets a threshold level for the incoming pulses in order to reject the low voltage signals that arise from spurious electrons, which are inadvertently amplified through the cascade circuit. In addition to these rogue electrons, positive ions are occasionally generated at some point in the electron cascade and return to the cathode or an early dynode to initiate a second cascade. In this case, a second pulse follows the first by several hundred nanoseconds and results in a peak in the correlation function at short delay times. The shortest delay times used experimentally are usually in the microsecond range, and this "afterpulsing" peak is not observed.

In cases where the short time dynamics are of interest, the scattered light is directed by a beam splitter onto two independent PMTs, which are processed by two amplifier discriminator circuits and the output of both is passed to the correlator. A pseudo-cross-correlated signal is then obtained, $\langle I_A(t)I_B(t+\tau)\rangle$ where the indices *A* and *B* distinguish the signals received by the two PMTs. The cross-correlation also reduces dead time effects (Weitz and Pine 1993).

After processing by the amplifier-discriminator, the signal is then transmitted to a digital correlator that calculates the intensity autocorrelation function in real time. The correlator is typically available as a PCI or ISA compatible card with a software interface. A range of delay times is available, and the shortest time is approximately 10 - 25 nanoseconds. Through the software interface, the number of channels, or delay times that are calculated, is selected and the spacing of the channels is also specified. Often the last few channels are shifted out to very long times to allow an independent measure of the baseline intensity, which is used to normalize the correlation function.

In order to calculate the mean squared displacement of the particles reliably, the intensity auto correlation function must be calculated with good statistical accuracy. There are two issues that reduce the signal to noise ratio: the finite intensity of the incoming light, and the limited duration of the experiment. The output signal from the PAD is typically in the range of one hundred thousand of photons per second, expressed as a count rate of 100 kHz. The photon counting statistics are Poisson whereby the errors are given roughly by $N^{1/2}$, where N is the number of independent measurements. For a count rate of 100 kHz, the counting error would be roughly 0.3%; however, for a count rate of only 100 Hz, the counting error would be much larger, of order 10%. Additionally, for such low count rates the amount of noise present in the data becomes significant. The noise level is primarily due to the "dark current" of the PMT and is roughly 50 Hz, although the level varies depending on the details of the detector. This dark current arises from thermally excited electrons that produce an anode current even in the absence of any incoming light. In rare cases where the signal is so small that the dark current noise is appreciable, the PMT may be cooled to reduce the contribution of these thermal electrons. Alternatively, when the scattering signal is very large, some attenuation may be required; in general, count rates of greater than 1 MHz cause a nonlinear response, and count rates greater than 20 MHz damage the photosensitive PMT.

The second consideration in the statistical accuracy of the correlation function is the duration of the experiment. For simple fluids, the field correlation function, given in Eqn. 1.45 can be re-written as:

$$g_1(\tau) = \exp\left[-q^2 D\tau\right] \tag{1.51}$$

by substituting $\langle\Delta r^2(\tau)\rangle = 6D\tau$. The decay time is thus given by $1/q^2D$. Although viscoelastic materials will display a different dependence on τ, an estimate of the decay time can similarly obtained. The square root of the ratio of the decay time to the duration of the experiment gives a rough estimate of the statistical uncertainty in the MSD. For errors to be of order 3%, the duration must be is at least one thousand times longer than any decay time, a criterion that is easy to meet at large angles but more challenging at smaller angles due to the q^{-2} dependence on wave-vector. We collect data for roughly an hour at each angle to ensure sufficient statistical accuracy. Long experiments are not possible in time-evolving systems that may sediment or undergo chemical reactions during the course of the measurement. In this case, many consecutive short runs may be averaged together to obtain the MSD. Another disadvantage of long collection times is the increased likelihood of measuring contributions from stray dust particles or other contaminants that are present in solution; careful sample preparation will reduce this possibility.

For DLS measurements, only samples that are nearly transparent may be used in order to insure that each incoming photon is scattered only once before reaching the detector. For fluids or low contrast polymer solutions, a small amount of colloidal particles are added to a final volume fraction of 10^{-5} – 10^{-6}. Typically, the scattering signal from the colloidal particles is significantly larger than the scattering from the solvent. For cloudy and opaque samples, single light scattering measurements are not possible, and the Diffusing Wave Spectroscopy (DWS) method should be used.

A.2 Diffusing Wave Spectroscopy

The Diffusing Wave Spectroscopy (DWS) apparatus is similar to that of the single light scattering experiment, and consists of a laser source, a simple optical train and sample holder, a detector, and digital correlator (Pine, et. al., 1988). The optical train allows for two boundary conditions, in which either a collimated or focused beam impinges on the sample cell. There are two experimental geometries: forward and backscattering. Our lab typically employs the forward scattering geometry, as shown in Fig. A.2. Higher laser powers are required for DWS measurements than for single scattering experiments and the laser power at the sample is roughly 100mW. Additionally, the coherence length of the laser is critical in DWS and must be larger than the longest paths of the scattered light through the sample, to insure that these paths are not discarded. The coherence length is increased by the addition of an intercavity etalon in our Coherent Innova 300 series Argon-ion laser (Santa Clara, CA) that insures operation in a single longitudinal mode. Photons that are multiply scattered report an angular average and lose their q-dependence; thus, a goniometer is not required. Multiply scattered light is depolarized and signals of equal intensity are found with polarization parallel or perpendicular to the incident beam. However, because each polarization is independent, this reduces the signal to noise ratio and causes the intercept of the intensity correlation function to fall to 0.5. To prevent this, a polarization analyzer is placed before the detector to restrict the scattered light to a single polarization.
Often in DWS experiments, the timescales of interest are extremely short and are comparable to the dead time of the PMT. In order to measure the dynamics of the sample on these timescales, a pseudo-cross-correlated signal is used. Cross-correlation also reduces afterpulsing effects, which occur at timelags of roughly 100 nanoseconds. For DWS experiments, the volume fraction of the embedded colloidal spheres is large, roughly 10^{-2}, in order to insure that the transport mean path, l^* is a small fraction of the length of the sample chamber, l. The ratio of l/l^* is typically greater than five. The mean free path is determined by comparing the transmitted intensity of a reference sample, whose transport mean path is known, to the experimental sample (Dasgupta, et. al. 2001).

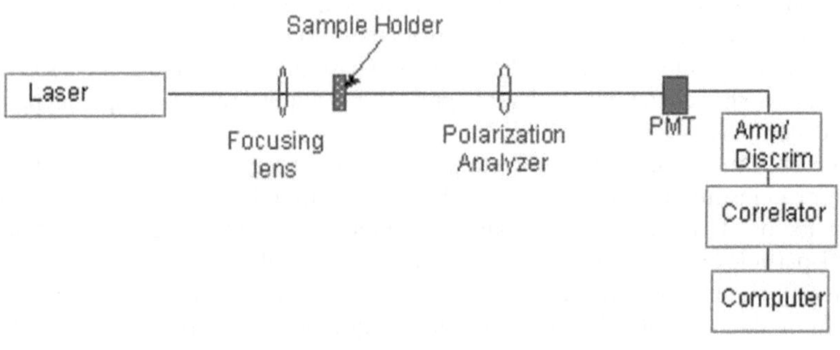

Fig. A.2. Diffusing Wave Spectroscopy setup.

A.3 Video Microscopy

Several of the microrheological techniques rely on accurately tracking the time evolved positions of individual probe particles. Laser Deflection Particle Tracking (Mason, et al. 1997, Schnurr, et al. 1997) measures the motion of individual beads with subnanometer precision at frequencies up to 50 kHz. This technique has excellent spatiotemporal resolution but is not designed to observe the dynamics of large ensembles of beads easily. Our lab uses video microscopy to follow the dynamics of ~100 beads simultaneously with a spatial resolution of 10 nm and temporal resolution of ~30 Hz. The time and spatial resolution of a particle tracking experiment with video microscopy relies on both the hardware used to capture images and the software algorithms used to detect particle centers. In the simplest setup an analog CCD camera (COHU, San Diego, CA) is attached to the side port of an optical microscope (Leica, Bannockburn, IL) and 480 x 640 pixel images are captured with a S-VHS video cassette recorder at a rate of 30 images per second. For most experiments, an eight bit analog, uncooled monochrome CCD camera with a variable shutter speed is sufficient. Monochrome CCD cameras are preferable to color cameras because they are more sensitive to subtle brightness variations, and are significantly cheaper. A larger dynamic range may be necessary for experiments with very dim or low contrast particles. The videotape of particle dynamics is then digitized by a computer equipped with a frame grabber card; digital images are analyzed to determine the particle positions in each frame.

For one micron spheres, images are typically obtained with bright field microscopy using a 40x air objective at a magnification of 250 nm/CCD pixel. In order for particle tracking algorithms to accurately determine particle centers, the number of pixels subtended by the image of each particle must be four or more CCD pixels. The image magnifications necessary to achieve this diameter will change based on the size of the embedded probe and if particles are imaged with bright field or fluorescence microscopy.

Colloidal particles are commercially available in sizes between 20 nm and several microns in diameter. The diffraction limited resolution, d, of a microscope is $d = 0.61 * \lambda / N.A.$ where $N.A.$ is the numerical aperture of the objective used and λ is the wavelength of light. For light microscopy, this resolution limit is a few hundred nanometers. Colloidal spheres larger than this resolution limit can be observed directly with bright field microscopy. For smaller sizes, it is possible to use fluorescence microscopy to image dyed colloids. In either method, the colloidal particle position is observed as a circularly symmetric Gaussian image intensity profile centered at its geometrical center. In general, particle tracking routines are able to locate particle positions with subpixel accuracy by iterating an initial position, which is determined as the brightest pixel in a local region, with the offsets in position, determined by calculating the brightness-weighted centroid of the surrounding region, to refine the location of the peak in brightness within a single pixel. At a magnification of 100x (10 pixels/micron), subpixel accuracy corresponds to a spatial resolution of 10 nm, an order of magnitude better than diffraction limited resolution! Because these particle tracking routines depend on variations of brightness over distances larger than the diffraction limited resolution, the numerical aperture of the objective does not affect the accuracy of detecting centers. However, a lower numerical aperture increases the depth of focus and projection error of particle motion perpendicular to the field of view increases.

The shutter speed of the CCD camera sets the exposure time, τ_e, of a single image. If the exposure time is long enough to allow significant particle motion, the microscope image of the particle will not be circularly symmetric which results in a decreased ability of finding an accurate center. The shutter speed is set so a probe of radius a embedded in a fluid of viscosity η diffuses less than the spatial resolution, 10 nm, in τ_e. We calculate the one dimensional root mean-squared displacement, $<\Delta x^2(\tau_e)>^{1/2}=(2D\tau_e)^{1/2} \leq 10$ nm, where the diffusion constant, D, is determined by the Einstein relation, $D = k_B T / 6\pi\eta a$. For a typical experiment with a one micron probe embedded in a medium with a viscosity of 0.001 Pa*sec, a shutter speed of 1 msec is sufficient.

Typically, a single CCD image is captured with alternate rows of pixels captured every 1/60 of a second. This allows the temporal resolution of video microscopy to be extended to 60 Hz by extracting the even and odd rows of the image to give two 240 x 640 images captured every 1/60 of a second (Crocker and Grier 1996). Without extracting the separate fields, the full 480 x 640 image is a superposition of two vertically interlaced half frame images, or fields, taken 1/60 second apart. If the particle moves significantly during that time, it is impossible to resolve an accurate particle center. A 100 nm particle in water (η=0.001 Pa*sec) imaged at a magnification of 10 pixels/μm (100x oil immersion objective) moves 100 nm, or one pixel, in 1/60 sec. Without a field analysis, the particle tracking resolution decreases by an order of magnitude and the particle dynamics at the shortest lag times near 1/30 sec, are seriously affected. Unless the particle motion between captured fields is beneath the noise floor of the particle tracking routines, the short time dynamics analyzed with an interlaced image will be affected by image averaging error. The resolution with a field analysis is significantly improved for the horizontal direction, but in the vertical direction the resolution is often adversely affected because of the number of pixels subtended by the image in that direction is halved.

The CCD camera BNC output is directly connected to a television for viewing and a high quality S-VHS cassette recorder (Sanyo, Chatsworth, CA) to record time series of images at video rate. A computer equipped with a frame grabber card is interfaced with the video cassette recorder to digitize images at rates accessible to the available RAM of the computer by capturing images for a short time and then pausing the movie while images are written to a file. In most cases, the limitation to writing images directly to the hard drive at video rates is that it takes longer than 1/30 second to write an image from RAM to the disk. With a special configuration of the hardware of a personal computer and custom software, it is now possible to write full frame images directly to the hard drive at video rates in standard movie file format (Keller, Schilling et al. 2001). Commercially available software (Universal Imaging Corporation, Downingtown, PA; Scion, Frederick, MA) to control frame grabbing hardware is also available.

Digital cameras (Hamamatsu, Bridgewater, NJ) now offer an alternative to traditional CCD cameras and allow control over pixel resolution, integration time, size and capture rate of the images. This enables us to optimize image quality for very dim particles or achieve capture rates faster than a traditional CCD camera by decreasing resolution and frame size. Digital movies are converted to a three-dimensional tiff stack of images and software is used to locate colloidal features in each image. We use particle tracking routines developed by John Crocker and David Grier (Crocker and Grier 1996). An online tutorial of this method with software routines written in IDL is maintained by John Crocker and Eric Weeks and is available at http://glinda.lrsm.upenn.edu/~weeks/idl/. The particle tracking algorithms are comprised of three steps: identification of appropriate parameters to detect the position of desired particles appearing in a single image, using a macro to automate the identification for every tiff image in a 3D tiff array and linking the positions found in each frame to form particle trajectories. The particle identification software detects bright 'spots' against a dark, zero intensity background pixel map. A 'spot', or feature, is a region of locally higher intensity with a circularly symmetric Gaussian brightness profile across its diameter. Because our tracking programs are dependent on variations in brightness; the image contrast should be maximized without saturating the image so there is a unique maximum in the brightness profile across the bead image.

To identify features, the tiff image is smoothed using a spatial bandpass filter with the lower bound of allowed wavelengths set to retain subtle variations in brightness (usually one pixel) and the upper bound set to the average diameter of the features. After smoothing the image, the average background intensity is subtracted so the final image is a low intensity background with sharply peaked circular 'spots' where the original particle images are. After locating the brightest pixels in a given region, a circular Gaussian mask with a diameter greater than or equal to the upper bound of the spatial bandpass is iterated around this guess to refine the located center of these circular peaks in the image brightness. Given a smoothed image and diameter of a Gaussian mask, our feature finding program will return a five dimensional array with the x-centriod, y-centroid, integrated brightness, radius of gyration and eccentricity for each feature found. To obtain subpixel accuracy, we choose the diameter of the mask to be slightly larger than that subtended by the particle image. This ensures the algorithm is able to find the unique maximum of the feature upon iteration.

This feature finding routine is very sensitive and will detect many possible particles. To separate the actual particles from false identifications, we further discriminate the found features based on their integrated brightness, eccentricity and radius of gyration. Colloidal features will fall into a broad cluster around certain values of radius of gyration and brightness. For any given image, false particle identifications will tend to lie outside this target cluster and can be clipped. Eccentricity, a geometrical measure of how circular an ellipse is, ranges from zero for circles and one for lines. Since we track circular features, we can set an upper bound on the eccentricity of 0.2 to allow for slight deviations from circular symmetry. We find the parameters that successfully eliminate rogue particle identifications for a single image and use identical bounds for subsequent images. It is often useful to overlay the located particle positions with the original microscope image to visually check particle identifications.

Once colloidal particles are located in a sequence of video images, particle positions in each image are correlated with positions in later images to produce trajectories. To track more than one particle, care is required to uniquely identify each particle in each frame (Crocker and Grier 1996). In practice, the typical distance a particle moves between images must be significantly smaller than the typical interparticle spacing. Otherwise, particle positions will be confused between snapshots. Particles that are a few hundred nanometers in diameter typically diffuse a distance smaller than their diameters between frames and, therefore, relatively high concentrations of particles can be used.

Because particles can move in and out of the focused field of view, it is useful to include a memory function in the tracking algorithm that allows gaps in a trajectory where a feature is not found. The last known locations of missing particles are retained in case unassigned particles reappear sufficiently nearby to resume the trajectory. Using a memory function allows the length of individual tracks to be maximized, therefore greatly increasing the statistics for the mean-squared displacement (MSD). Trajectories are identified for every feature in the field of view and saved as an array. In a typical multiparticle tracking experiment, millions of positions are assigned to thousands of particle trajectories. We usually require 1000 independent events to calculate the MSD at a given lag time. The number of events, or independent particle displacements, increases with both the number of particles in a field of view and the length of particle tracks (Valentine, et. al. 2001). For an experiment tracking forty beads with a diameter of one micron in a viscous medium of 0.001 Pa*sec, around ten minutes of video is required to calculate the MSD to lag times of one minute.

A.4 Obtaining $G^*(\omega)$ from $\left\langle \Delta\vec{r}^2(t) \right\rangle$

In all the methods discussed, we desire to obtain knowledge of the complex shear modulus from the bead dynamics. In order to relate the mean-squared displacement of embedded Brownian probes, $\left\langle \Delta\vec{r}^2(t) \right\rangle$, to a frequency dependent complex modulus, $G^*(\omega)$, using the generalized Stokes-Einstein relation, it is necessary to calculate the numerical Laplace transform of $\left\langle \Delta\vec{r}^2(t) \right\rangle$ to obtain $\tilde{G}(s)$ using Eqn. 1.37. We then fit $\tilde{G}(s)$ to a continuous functional form in the real variable s and substitute $s=i\omega$ into $\tilde{G}(s)$ to obtain $G^*(\omega) = G'(\omega) + iG''(\omega)$. While direct, this method of transforming the mean-squared displacement can introduce significant errors in the moduli obtained. The numerical Laplace transform is typically implemented by selecting a frequency s, multiplying $\left\langle \Delta\vec{r}^2(t) \right\rangle$ by a decaying exponential and integrating using the trapezoid rule. While this method is very accurate within frequency extremes, it introduces errors near frequency extremes due to truncation of the data set. These errors are usually significant for data within a decade of either extrema. Additionally, the analytic continuation of $\tilde{G}(s)$ requires finding an appropriate functional form of discrete data. Without an accurate functional form of the discrete data, significant errors can result in the elastic and loss complex moduli.

To overcome these errors, Mason, et. al. (Mason 2001) developed a method to estimate the transforms algebraically by using a local power law around a frequency of interest, ω, and retaining the leading term:

$$\left\langle \Delta\vec{r}^{\,2}(t)\right\rangle \approx \left\langle \Delta\vec{r}^{\,2}(1/\omega)\right\rangle (\omega t)^{\alpha(\omega)} \tag{1.52}$$

where $\left\langle \Delta\vec{r}^{\,2}(1/\omega)\right\rangle$ is the magnitude of at $t=1/\omega$ and

$$\alpha(\omega) \equiv \left.\frac{d\ln\left\langle \Delta\vec{r}^{\,2}(t)\right\rangle}{d\ln t}\right|_{t=1/\omega} \tag{1.53}$$

is the power law exponent describing the logarithmic slope of $\left\langle \Delta\vec{r}^{\,2}(t)\right\rangle$ at $t=1/\omega$.

The Fourier transform, $\Im\left\langle \Delta\vec{r}^{\,2}(t)\right\rangle$, of the power law is directly evaluated:

$$i\omega\Im\left\langle \Delta r^2(t)\right\rangle \approx \left\langle \Delta r^2(1/\omega)\right\rangle \Gamma[1+\alpha(\omega)]\,i^{-\alpha(\omega)} \tag{1.54}$$

where Γ is the gamma function. Using a local power law approximation implicitly assumes that contributions to the transform integral from the behavior of $<\Delta r^2(t)>$ at times different than *1/ω* can be neglected. By substitution into the Fourier representation of the GSER and the use of Euler's equation, we obtain:

$$\begin{aligned} G'(\omega) &= |G^*(\omega)|\cos(\pi\alpha(\omega)/2) \\ G''(\omega) &= |G^*(\omega)|\sin(\pi\alpha(\omega)/2) \end{aligned} \tag{1.55}$$

where

$$|G^*(\omega)| \approx \frac{k_B T}{\pi a\left\langle \Delta r^2(1/\omega)\right\rangle \Gamma[1+\alpha(\omega)]} \tag{1.56}$$

These relations provide a direct physical intuition of how the elastic and loss moduli depend on $<\Delta r^2(t)>$. In a pure viscous medium, the sphere diffuses and $\alpha \approx 1$ resulting in a dominant loss modulus. Constrained in a pure elastic medium, the α approaches zero and the elastic modulus dominates.

While this estimation method is convenient and intuitive to use, it can fail to give an accurate estimation of the moduli when the mean-squared displacement is sharply curved with a rapidly changing slope. These regions can be of particular interest because such changes reflect significant relaxation times of the sample. To account for these issues, modifications (Dasgupta et. al. 2002) have been made to Eqn. 1.56 to better account for curvature in the mean-squared displacement and give improved estimates of the moduli in these regions.

References

A-Hassan E, Heinz WF, Antonik MD, D'Costa NP, Nageswaran S (1998) Relative microelastic mapping of living cells by atomic force microscopy. Biophysical Journal 74:1564-1578

Amblard F, Maggs AC, Yurke B, Pargellis AN, Leibler S (1996) Subdiffusion and anomalous local viscoelasticity in actin networks. Physical Review Letters 77:4470-4473

Amblard F, Yurke B, Pargellis A, Leibler S (1996) A magnetic manipulator for studying local rheology and micromechanical properties of biological systems. Review of Scientific Instruments 67:818-827

Ashkin A (1992) Forces of a single-beam gradient laser trap on a dielectric sphere in the ray optics regime. Biophysical Journal 61:569-582

Ashkin A (1997) Optical trapping and manipulation of neutral particles using lasers. Proceedings of the National Academy of Sciences of the United States of America 94:4853-4860

Ashkin A (1998) Forces of a single-beam gradient laser trap on a dielectric sphere in the ray optics regime. Methods in Cell Biology 55:1-27

Bausch AR, Hellerer U, Essler M, Aepfelbacher M, Sackmann E (2001) Rapid stiffening of integrin receptor-actin linkages in endothelial cells stimulated with thrombin: A magnetic bead microrheometry study. Biophysical Journal 80:2649-2657

Bausch AR, Möller W, Sackmann E (1999) Measurement of local viscoelasticity and forces in living cells by magnetic tweezers. Biophysical Journal 76:573-579

Bausch AR, Ziemann F, Boulbitch AA, Jacobson K, Sackmann E (1998) Local measurements of viscoelastic parameters of adherent cell surfaces by magnetic bead microrheometry. Biophysical Journal 75:2038-2049

Berne BJ, Pecora R (2000) Dynamic Light Scattering with applications to chemistry, biology, and physics. Dover, Mineola

Binning G, Quate CF, Gerber C (1986) Atomic Force Microscope. Physical Review Letters 56:930-933

Block SM (1992) Making light work with optical tweezers. Nature 360:493-495

Bottomley LA, Coury JE, First PN (1996) Scanning probe microscopy. Biophysical Journal 74:1564-1578

Butt H-J, Jaschke M (1995) Thermal noise in atomic force microscopy. Nanotechnology 6:1-7

Crick F, Hughes A (1950) The physical properties of the cytoplasm. Experimental Cell Research 1:37-80

Crocker JC, Grier DG (1996) Methods of digital video microscopy. Journal of Colloid and Interface Science 179:298-310

Crocker JC, Valentine MT, Weeks ER, Gisler T, Kaplan PD, Yodh AG, Weitz DA (2000) Two-point microrheology of inhomogeneous soft materials. Physical Review Letters 85:888-891

Dasgupta BR, Tee S-Y, Crocker JC, Frisken BJ, Weitz DA (2001) Microrheology of polyethylene oxide using diffusing wave spectroscopy and single scattering. Physical Review E 65:051505

Dinsmore AD, Weeks ER, Prasad V, Levitt AC, Weitz DA (2001) Three-dimensional confocal microscopy of colloids. Applied Optics 40:4152-4159

Domke J, Radmacher M (1998) Measuring the elastic properties of thin polymer films with the AFM. Langmuir 14:3320-3325

Drake B, Prater CB, Weisenhorn AL, Gould SAC, Albrecht TR, Quate CF, Channell DS, Hansma HG, Hansma PK (1989) Imaging crystals, polymers, and biological processes in water with AFM. Science 243:1586-1589

Dvorak JA, Nagao E (1998) Kinetic analysis of the mitotic cycle of living vertebrate cells by atomic force microscopy. Experimental Cell Research 242:69-74

Fabry B, Maksym GN, Butler JP, Glogauer M, Navajas D, Fredberg JJ (2001) Scaling the microrheology of living cells. Physical Review Letters 87:148102(4)

Fällman E, Axner O (1997) Design for fully steerable dual-trap optical tweezers. Applied Optics 36:2107-2113

Feneberg W, Westphal M, Sackmann E (2001) Dictyostelium cells' cytoplasm as an active viscoplastic body. European Biophysical Journal 30:284-294

Ferry J (1980) Viscoelastic properties of polymers. Wiley, New York

Ford NC (1985) Light Scattering Apparatus. In: Pecora R (ed) Dynamic light scattering: Applications of photon correlation spectroscopy. Plenum, London pp. 7-58

Freundlich H, Seifriz W (1922) Ueber die elastizität von solen und gelen. Zeitschrift fur physikalische chemie 104:233

Gisler T, Weitz DA (1998) Tracer microrheology in complex fluids. Current Opinion in Colloid and Interface Science 3:586-592

Gisler T, Weitz DA (1999) Scaling of the microrheology of semidilute F-actin solutions. Physical Review Letters 82:1606-1609

Gisler T, Ruger H, Egelhaaf SU, Tschumi J, Schurtenberger P, Ricka J (1995) Mode-selective dynamic light scattering: theory versus experimental realization. Applied Optics 34:3546-3553

Gittes F, Schnurr B, Olmsted PD, MacKintosh FC, Schmidt CF (1997) Microscopic viscoelasticity: shear moduli of soft materials determined from thermal fluctuations. Physical Review Letters 79:3286-3289

Gittings MR, Cipelletti L, Trappe V, Weitz DA, In M, Marques C (2000) Structure of guar in solutions of H_20 and D_20: An ultra-small-angle light scattering study. Journal of Physical Chemistry B 104:4381-4386

Goldman WH, Ezzell RM (1996) Viscoelasticity in wild-type and vinculin-deficient mouse F9 embryonic carcinoma cells examined by atomic force microscopy. Experimental Cell Research 226:234-237

Heilbronn A (1922) Eine neue methode zur bestimmung der viskosität lebender protoplasten. Jahrbuch der Wissenschaftlichen Botanik 61:284-338

Henderson E, Haydon PG, Sakaguchi DS (1992) Actin filament dynamics in living glial cells imaged by atomic force microcopy. Science 257:1944-1946

Hénon S, Lenormand G, Richert A, Gallet F (1999) A new determination of the shear modulus of the human erythrocyte membrane using optical tweezers. Biophysical Journal 76:1145-1151

Hertz H (1881) Über die berührung fester elastischer körper. J. Reine Agnew. Mathematik 92:156-171

Hiramoto Y (1969) Mechanical properties of the protoplasm of the sea urchin egg. Experimental Cell Research 56:201-218

Hoh JH, Schoenenberger CA (1994) Surface morphology and mechanical properties of MDCK monolayers by atomic force microscopy. Journal of Cell Science 107:1105-1114

Hough LA, Ou-Yang HD (1999) A new probe for mechanical testing of nanostructures in soft materials. Journal of Nanoparticle Research 1:495-499

Johnson CS, Gabriel DA (1995) Laser Light Scattering. Dover, New York.

Joosten JGH, Gelade ETF, Pusey PN (1990) Dynamic light scattering by non-ergodic media: Brownian particles trapped in polyacrylamide gels Physical Review A 42:2161-2175

Kao HP, Verkman AS (1994) Tracking of single fluorescent particles in three dimensions: the use of cylindrical optics to encode particle position. Biophysical Journal 67:1291-1300

Kasas S, Thomson NH, Smith BL, Hansma PK, Mikossy J, Hansma HG (1997) Biological applications of the AFM: from single molecules to organs. International Journal of Imaging Systems and Technology 8:151-161

Keller M, Schilling J, Sackmann E (2001) Oscillatory magnetic bead rheometer for complex fluid microrheometry. Review of Scientific Instruments 72:3626-3624

King M, Macklem PT (1977) Rheological properties of microliter quantities of normal mucus. Journal of Applied Physiology 42:797-802

Landau LD, Lifshitz EM (1986) Theory of Elasticity. Pergamon Press, Oxford

Larson RG (1999) The structure and rheology of complex fluids. Oxford University Press, New York

Levine AJ, Lubensky TC (2000) One- and two-particle microrhelogy. Physical Review Letters 85:1774-1777

Macosko CW (1994) Rheology: principles, measurements, and applications. VCH, New York

Mahaffy RE, Shih CK, MacKintosh FC, Käs J (2000) Scanning probe-based frequency-dependent microrheology of polymer gels and biological cells. Physical Review Letters 85:880-883

Mason TG (2000) Estimating the viscoelastic moduli of complex fluids using the generalized Stokes-Einstein equation. Rheologica Acta 39: 371-378

Mason TG, Ganesan K, Van Zanten JH, Wirtz D, Kuo SC (1997) Particle tracking microrheology of complex fluids. Physical Review Letters 79:3282-3285

Mason TG, Gang H, Weitz DA (1996) Rheology of complex fluids measured by dynamic light scattering. Journal of Molecular Structure 383:81-90

Mason TG, Gang H, Weitz DA (1997) Diffusing-wave spectroscopy measurements of viscoelasticity of complex fluids. Journal of the Optical Society of America 14:139-149

Mason TG, Gisler T, Kroy K, Frey E, Weitz DA (2000) Rheology of F-actin solutions determined from thermally driven tracer motion. Journal of Rheology 44:917-928

Mason TG, Weitz DA (1995) Optical measurements of the frequency-dependent linear viscoelastic moduli of complex fluids. Physical Review Letters 74:1250-1253

McGrath JL, Hartwig JH, Kuo SC (2000) The mechanics of F-actin microenvironments depend on the chemistry of probing surfaces. Biophysical Journal 79:3258-3266

Mio C, Gong T, Terray A, Marr DWM (2000) Design of a scanning laser optical trap for multiparticle manipulation. Review of Scientific Instruments 71:2196-2200

Mio C, Marr DWM (2000) Optical Trapping for the Manipulation of Colloidal Particles. Advanced Materials 12:917-920

Nemoto S, Togo H (1998) Axial force acting on a dielectric sphere in a focused laser beam. Applied Optics 37:6386-6394

Neto PAM, Nussenzveig HM (2000) Theory of optical tweezers. Europhysics Letters 50:702-708

Ou-Yang HD, (1999) Design and applications of oscillating optical tweezers for direct measurements of colloidal forces. In: Farinato RS and Dubin PL (eds) Colloid-Polymer Interactions: From Fundamentals to Practice. Wiley, New York, pp 385-405

Ovryn B (2000) Three-dimensional forward scattering particle image velocimetry applied to a microscopic field of view. Experiments in Fluids 29:S175-S184

Ovryn B, Izen SH (2000) Imaging of transparent spheres through a planar interface using a high numerical-aperture optical microscope. Journal of the Optical Society of America, A 17:1202-1213

Palmer A, Mason TG, Xu J, Kuo SC, Wirtz D (1999) Diffusing wave spectroscopy microrheology of actin filament networks. Biophysical Journal 76:1063-1071

Pine DJ, Weitz DA, Chaikin PM, Herbolzheimer E (1988) Diffusing Wave Spectroscopy. Physical Review Letters 60:1134-1137

Pusey PN, van Megen W (1989) Dynamic Light Scattering by non-ergodic media. Physica A 157:705-741

Putman CA, Werf KOVD, Grooth BGD, Hulst NFV, Greve J (1994) Viscoelasticity of living cells allows high resolution imaging by tapping mode atomic force microscopy. Biophysical Journal 67:1749-1753

Radmacher M, Cleveland JP, Fritz M, Hansma HG, Hansma PK (1994) Mapping interaction forces with the atomic force microscope. Biophysical Journal 66:2159-2165

Radmacher M, Fritz M, Hansma PK (1995) Imaging soft samples with the atomic force microscope: gelatin in water and propanol. Biophysical Journal 69:264-270

Radmacher M, Fritz M, Kasher CM, Cleveland JP, Hansma PK (1996) Measuring the viscoelastic properties of human platelets with the atomic force microscope. Biophysical Journal 70:556-567

Radmacher M, Tillmann RW, Fritz M, Gaub HE (1992) From molecules to cells - imaging soft samples with AFM. Science 257:1900-1905

Reif F (1965) Fundamentals of statistical and thermal physics. McGraw-Hill, Inc., New York

Rotsch C, Braet F, Wisse E, Radmacher M (1997) AFM imaging and elasticity measurements of living rat liver macrophages. Cell Biology International 21:685-696

Rotsch C, Radmacher M (2000) Drug-induced changes of cytoskeletal structure and mechanics in fibroblasts: an atomic force microscopy study. Biophysical Journal 78:520-535

Schmidt FG, Hinner B, Sackmann E, Tang JX (2000) Viscoelastic properties of semiflexible filamentous bacteriophage fd. Physical Review E 62:5509-5517

Schmidt FG, Ziemann F, Sackmann E (1996) Shear field mapping in actin networks by using magnetic tweezers. European Biophysics Journal 24:348-353

Schneider SW, Sritharan SW, Geibel JP, Oberleithner H, Jena B (1997) Surface dynamics in living acinar cells imaged by atomic force microscopy: identification of plasma membrane structures involved in exocytosis. Proceedings of the National Academy of Sciences of the United States of America 94:316-321

Schnurr B, Gittes F, MacKintosh FC, Schmidt CF (1997) Determining microscopic viscoelasticity in flexible and semiflexible polymer networks from thermal fluctuations. Macromolecules 30:7781-7792

Shroff SG, Saner DR, Lal R (1995) Dynamic micromechanical properties of cultured rat atrial myocytes measured by atomic force microscopy. American Journal of Physiology 269:C286-C289

Sleep J, Wilson D, Simmons R, Gratzer W (1999) Elasticity of the red cell membrane and its relation to hemolytic disorders: an optical tweezers study. Biophysical Journal 77:3085-3095

Sneddon IN (1965) The relation between load and penetration in the axisymmetric Boussinesq problem for a punch of arbitrary profile. International Journal of Engineering Science 3:47-57

Tao NJ, Lindsay SM, Lees S (1992) Measuring the microelastic properties of biological material. Biophysical Journal 63:1165-1169

Tseng Y, Wirtz D (2001) Mechanics and multiple particle tracking microheterogeneity of α-actinin-crosslinked actin filament networks. Biophysical Journal 81:1643-1656

Valberg PA (1984) Magnetometry of ingested particles in pulmonary macrophages. Science 224:513-516

Valberg PA, Albertini DF (1985) Cytoplasmic motions, rheology, and structure probed by a novel magnetic particle method. Journal of Cell Biology 101:130-140

Valberg PA, Butler JP (1987) Magnetic particle motions within living cells: Physical theory and techniques. Biophysical Journal 52:537-550

Valberg PA, Feldman HA (1987) Magnetic particle motions within living cells: Measurement of cytoplasmic viscosity and motile activity. Biophysical Journal 52:551-561

Valentine MT, Dewalt LE, Ou-Yang HD (1996) Forces on a colloidal particle in a polymer solution: a study using optical tweezers. Journal of Physics: Condensed Matter (U.K.) 8:9477-9482

Valentine MT, Kaplan PD, Thota D, Crocker JC, Gisler T, Prud'homme RK, Beck M, Weitz DA (2001) Investigating the microenvironments of inhomogeneous soft materials with multiple particle tracking. Physical Review E 64:061506

van Megen W, Underwood SM, Pusey PN (1991) Nonergodicity parameters of colloidal glasses. Physical Review Letters 67:1586-1589

Velegol D, Lanni F (2001) Cell Traction Forces on Soft Biomaterials. I. Microrheology of Type I Collagen Gels. Biophysical Journal 81:1786-1792

Visscher K, Block SM (1998) Versatile optical traps with feedback control. Methods in Enzymology 298:460-479

Wang N, Butler JP, Ingber DE (1993) Mechanotransduction across the cell surface and through the cytoskeleton. Science 260:1124-1127

Wang N, Ingber DE (1994) Control of cytoskeletal mechanics by extracellular matrix, cell shape, and mechanical tension. Biophysical Journal 66:1281-1289

Wang N, Ingber DE (1995) Probing transmembrane mechanical coupling and cytomechanics using magnetic twisting cytometry. Biochemistry and Cell Biology 73:327-335

Weeks ER, Crocker JC, Levitt AC, Schofield A, Weitz DA (2000) Three-dimensional imaging of structural relaxation near the colloidal glass transition. Science 287:627-631

Weitz DA, Pine DJ, (1993) Diffusing-wave spectroscopy. In: Brown W (ed) Dynamic Light Scattering. Oxford University Press, Oxford, pp 652-721

Xue JZ, Pine DJ, Milner ST, Wu XL, Chaikin PM (1992) Non-ergodicity and light scattering from polymer gels. Physical Review A 46:6550-6563

Yagi K (1961) The mechanical and colloidal properties of Amoeba protoplasm and their relations to the mechanism of amoeboid movement. Comparative Biochemistry and Physiology 3:73-91

Yamada S, Wirtz D, Kuo SC (2000) Mechanics of living cells measured by laser tracking microrheology. Biophysical Journal 78:1736-1747

Zaner KS, Valberg PA (1989) Viscoelasticity of F-actin measured with magnetic particles. Journal of Cell Biology 109:2233-2243

Ziemann F, Rädler J, Sackmann E (1994) Local measurements of viscoelastic moduli of entangled actin networks using an oscillating magnetic bead micro-rheometer. Biophysical Journal 66:2210-2216

2. Micron-Resolution Particle Image Velocimetry

S.T. Wereley and C.D. Meinhart

Abstract

During the past five years, significant progress has been made in the development and application of micron-resolution Particle Image Velocimetry (μPIV). Developments of the technique have extended typical spatial resolutions of PIV from order 1-mm to order 1-μm. These advances have been obtained as a result of novel improvements in instrument hardware and post processing software.

Theories describing the limits of in-plane and out-of-plane spatial resolution are presented. The basis of the theory for in-plane spatial resolution extends the original work of Adrian & Yao (1985). The theory for out-of-plane spatial resolution closely follows the recent work of Olsen & Adrian (2000).

The desire for high spatial resolution dictates that the flow tracing particles typically range between 200 – 700 nm in diameter. The effect of Brownian forces on particle motion is discussed in detail. Guidelines are given to determine optimal particle size and to estimate particle flow following fidelity.

Advances in post processing algorithms provide improvements in velocity accuracy and spatial resolution. The correlation-averaging algorithm increases the effective particle concentration, while maintaining sufficiently low particle concentration in the working fluid. Central difference interrogation provides second order accurate estimates of velocity, which becomes important in regions containing high spatial variations in velocity. These post-processing techniques are particularly useful in challenging micro length scales, and can also be extended to macroscopic flows.

The utility of μPIV is demonstrated by applying it to flows in microchannels, micronozzles, BioMEMS, and flow around cells. While the technique was initially developed for microscale velocity measurements, it has been extended to measure wall positions with tens of nanometers resolution, the deformation of hydrogels, micro-particle thermometry, and infrared-PIV.

2.1 Introduction

Micron-resolution Particle Image Velocimetry (μPIV) refers to the application of PIV to measure velocity fields of fluid motion with length scales of order 100 microns, and with spatial resolution of individual velocity measurements of order 1 - 10 microns. The PIV technique is well established for macroscopic flows. However, it has been limited to maximal spatial resolutions of 0.2 – 1.0 millimeters

(Urushihara, Meinhart & Adrian; 1993) because of fundamental physical limitations as well as practical implementation difficulties. In μPIV, emphasis is placed on the ability to accurately and reliably measure fluid velocity with micron spatial resolution. In order to achieve microscale velocity measurements, novel developments in PIV image recording hardware, flow-tracing particles, system design, and analysis software is required. The theoretical underpinnings of μPIV are rooted in the interactions between the flow fluid and the seed particles which occur at nanometer length scales. μPIV can be thought of as a practical application of nanotechnology to perform science and engineering at micrometer length scales.

Over the past five to ten years there has been an increasing interest in understanding fluid phenomena at the micrometer and nanometer length scales. This has been evident in both basic and applied fluid mechanics research. The application of microscale fluid mechanics to MEMS and BioMEMS represents one of the most significant practical applications. A MEMS market study published by System Planning Corporation (Detlefs, 1999) projected that by 2003 the worldwide sales of microfluidic devices would range between $3 – 4.5 Billion. This projection includes inkjet printer heads, lab-on-a-chip devices, and mass flow sensors. According to the study, microfluidic devices will account for 25% - 35% of the total MEMS market.

Until the development of pointwise measurement techniques, such as micron-resolution PIV, most of the experiments conducted in microscale geometries consisted of bulk flow measurements, such as flow rate, pressure drop, thrust, etc. For a comprehensive review see Gad-el-Hak M (1999) and Ho & Tai (1998). Most bulk measurements are conducted outside the microdevice. An exception is the work by Pong, et al. (1994) who obtained nonlinear pressure drop measurements inside a uniform microchannel. This was achieved by microfabricating pressure sensors directly adjacent to the microchannel.

The earliest published work of using flow-tracing particles to estimate velocities in microscale geometries was reported by Brody, et al. (1996). He used a mercury arc lamp to continuously illuminate 0.9 μm dia. fluorescent particles in an epi-fluorescent microscope. He used the length of the particle streaks to estimate the local velocity. The resolution of his measurements were on the order of 10 microns.

The technique was extended further by Santiago, et al. (1998) by using a mercury arc lamp to continuously illuminate 300 nm fluorescent particles. Discrete particle images were recorded by an intensified CCD camera, by using the intensifier as the shuttering mechanism. Correlation analysis was then applied to the particle-image field, producing regularly-spaced velocity fields of the Hele-Shaw flow. In order to record particle images with continuous light sources, ten's of milliseconds are required for exposure. This limits the magnitude of velocity that can be practically measured using μPIV using sub-micron flow-tracing particles to order 100 μm/s.

Meinhart et al. (1999b) used a pulsed Nd:YAG laser to illuminate 200 nm dia. polystyrene beads. The pulsed illumination source allowed for exposure times down to the pulse duration of the laser, ~5ns. The pulsed illumination allows for much higher velocities to be measured (~ 10 mm/s) and smaller particles to be recorded. Meinhart et al. (1999b) achieved a spatial resolution of 0.9 µm.

The first µPIV measurement in circular tubes was obtained by Koutsiaris et al. (1999). They used a 20 W Halogen lamp to illuminate a glycerol suspension of 10 µm dia. glass spheres flowing through ~200 µm dia. glass capillaries. The large 10 µm dia. particle size allowed for relatively short exposure times with continuous illumination. The spatial resolution of these measurements was approximately 26 µm. The µPIV technique has been applied to a variety of flow regimes. A few of these examples range from fundamental studies of fluid motion (Tretheway & Meinhart 2002), to practical applications such as commercial inkjet printheads (Meinhart & Zhang, 2000), and BioMEMS devices like electrokinetic-based devices (Santiago, 2001). More details of the applications of µPIV will be given in Section 2.6

2.2 Theory of µPIV

2.2.1 In-Plane Spatial Resolution Limits

The overall goal of µPIV is to obtain reliable two-dimensional velocity fields in microfluidic devices with high accuracy and high spatial resolution. In this section, we will discuss the theoretical requirements for achieving both of these outcomes, and address the relative tradeoffs between velocity accuracy and spatial resolution.

The most common mode of PIV is to record two successive images of flow-tracing particles that are introduced into the working fluid, and which accurately follow the local motion of the fluid. The two particle images are separated by a known time delay, Δt. Typically, the two particle image fields are divided into uniformly spaced interrogation regions, which are cross correlated to determine the most probable local displacement of the particles. A first-order estimate of the local velocity of the fluid, $\boldsymbol{u}$, is then obtained by dividing the measured displacement, $\boldsymbol{\Delta x}$, by the time delay

$$\boldsymbol{u} = \frac{\boldsymbol{\Delta x}}{\Delta t} \tag{2.1}$$

High spatial resolution is achieved by recording the images of flow-tracing particles with sufficiently small diameters, d_p, so that they faithfully follow the flow in microfluidic devices, which often exhibit high velocity gradients near flow boundaries. The particle should be imaged with high numerical aperture diffraction-limited optics and with sufficiently high magnification so that the particles are resolved with at least 3–4 pixels per particle diameter. Following Adrian (1991), the diffraction-limited spot size of a point source of light, d_s, imaged through a circular aperture is given by

$$d_s = 2.44(M+1)f^{\#}\lambda, \tag{2.2}$$

where M is the magnification, $f^{\#}$ is the *f-number* of the lens, and λ is the wavelength of light. For infinity-corrected microscope objective lenses, $f^{\#} \approx 1/2\left[(n/NA)^2 - 1\right]^{1/2}$. The numerical aperture, *NA*, is defined as $NA \equiv n\sin\theta$, where n is the index of refraction of the recording medium, and θ is the half-angle subtend by the aperture of the recording lens. The actual recorded image can be estimated as the convolution of point-spread function with the geometric image. Approximating both these images as Gaussian functions, the effective image diameter, d_e, can be written as (Adrian & Yao, 1985).

$$d_e = \left[d_s^2 + M^2 d_p^2\right]^{1/2}. \tag{2.3}$$

The most common microscope objective lenses range from diffraction-limited oil-immersion lenses with M = 60, NA = 1.4 to air lenses with M = 10, NA = 0.1. Table 2.1 gives effective particle image diameters recorded through a circular aperture and then projected back into the flow, d_e/M. Using conventional microscopic optics, particle-image resolutions of d_e/M ~ 0.3 μm can be obtained using oil-immersion lenses with numerical apertures NA = 1.4, and particle diameters $d_p \le 0.2\ \mu\text{m}$. For particle diameters $d_p \ge 0.3\ \mu\text{m}$, the geometric component of the image decreases the resolution of the particle image. The M = 10, NA = 0.25 lens is diffraction-limited for particle diameters $d_p \le 1.0\ \mu\text{m}$.

Table 2.1. Effective particle image diameters when projected back into the flow, d_e/M (μm).

Particle Size d_p	Microscope Objective Lens Characteristics				
	M = 60 NA = 1.4	M = 40 NA = 0.75	M = 40 NA = 0.6	M = 20 NA = 0.5	M = 10 NA = 0.25
0.01 μm	0.29	0.62	0.93	1.24	2.91
0.10 μm	0.30	0.63	0.94	1.25	2.91
0.20 μm	0.35	0.65	0.95	1.26	2.92
0.30 μm	0.42	0.69	0.98	1.28	2.93
0.50 μm	0.58	0.79	1.06	1.34	2.95
0.70 μm	0.76	0.93	1.17	1.43	2.99
1.00 μm	1.04	1.18	1.37	1.59	3.08
3.00 μm	3.01	3.06	3.14	3.25	4.18

The effective particle image diameter places a bound on the spatial resolution that can be obtained by μPIV. Assuming that the particle images are sufficiently resolved by the CCD array, such that a particle diameter is resolved by 3 – 4 pixels, the location of the correlation peak can be sufficiently resolved to within 1/10th the particle image diameter (Prasad et al., 1993). Therefore, the uncertainty of the correlation peak location for a d_p = 0.2 μm diameter particle recorded with a NA = 1.4 lens is $\delta x \sim d_e / 10M = 35$ nm.

The measurement error due to detectability, ε_d, can be written as the ratio of the uncertainty in the correlation peak location, δx, to the particle displacement, Δx

$$\varepsilon_d = \frac{\delta x}{\Delta x}. \tag{2.4}$$

For an error of ε_d = 2%, the required particle displacement is Δx = 1.8 μm, for the highest resolved case. For a low-resolution case, with a d_p = 3.0 μm diameter particle, recorded by a M = 10, NA = 0.25 recording lens, the required particle displacement would be Δx = 21 μm. From Equation 4, there is clearly a tradeoff between spatial resolution and accuracy of the velocity measurements.

2.2.2 Out-of-Plane Spatial Resolution

It is common practice in PIV to use a sheet of light to illuminate the flow tracing particles. In principle, the light sheet illuminates only particles contained within the depth of focus of the recording lens. This provides reasonably high quality in-focus particle images to be recorded with low levels of background noise being emitted from the out-of-focus particles. The out-of-plane spatial resolution of the velocity measurements is defined clearly by the thickness of the illuminating light sheet.

Due to the small length scales associated with μPIV, it is difficult if not impossible to form a light sheet that is only a few microns thick, and even more difficult to align a light sheet with the object plane of an objective lens. Consequently, it is common practice in μPIV to illuminate the test section with a volume of light, and rely on the depth of field of the lens to define the out-of-plane thickness of the measurement plane (see Fig. 2.1).

Following the analysis of Olsen & Adrian (2000), using $f^{\#} \approx 1/2\left[(n/NA)^2 - 1\right]^{1/2}$, the effective image diameter of a particle displaced a distance z from the objective plane can be approximated by combining Equations (2.2) and (2.3), and adding a third term to account for the geometric spreading of a slightly out of focus particle

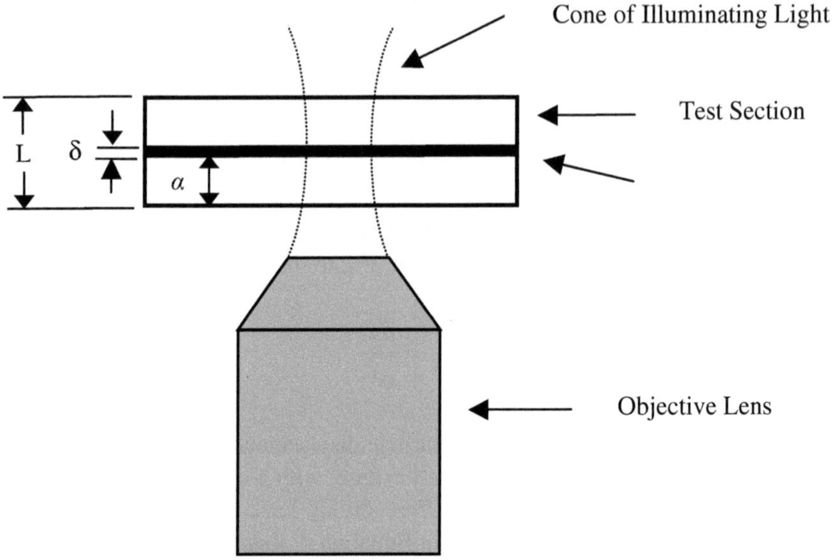

Fig. 2.1. Schematic showing the geometry for volume illumination particle image velocimetry. In the epi-fluorescent mode, the objective lens is used to deliver the illumination light and record the particle images. The particles located within δ/2 of the object plane are sufficiently in focus to produce visible images.

$$d_e = \left[M^2 d_p^2 + 1.49 (M+1)^2 \lambda^2 \left[(n/NA)^2 - 1 \right] + \frac{M^2 D_a^2 z^2}{(s_o + z)^2} \right]^{1/2}, \quad (2.5)$$

where s_o is the object distance, D_a is the diameter of the recording lens aperture.

The out-of-plane spatial resolution can be determined in terms of the depth of correlation. The depth of correlation is defined as the axial distance, z_{corr}, from the object plane in which a particle becomes sufficiently out of focus so that it no longer contributes significantly to the signal peak in the particle-image correlation function. The relative contribution, ε, of a particle displaced a distance z from the object plane, compared to a similar particle located at the object plane can be expressed in terms of the ratio of the effective particle image diameters raised to the fourth power

$$\varepsilon = \frac{d_e^4(0)}{d_e^4(z_{corr})}. \quad (2.6)$$

Using $D_a^2/(s_o+z)^2 \approx D_a^2/s_o^2 = 4\left[(n/NA)^2 - 1\right]^{-1}$, combining Equations (2.5) & (2.6) and solving for z_{corr} yields an expression for the depth of correlation

$$z_{corr} = \left[\left(\frac{1-\sqrt{\varepsilon}}{\sqrt{\varepsilon}} \right) \left[\frac{d_p^2 \left[(n/NA)^2 - 1 \right]}{4} + \frac{1.49(M+1)^2 \lambda^2 \left[(n/NA)^2 - 1 \right]^2}{4M^2} \right] \right]^{1/2} \tag{2.7}$$

where ε is chosen as 0.1.

The depth of correlation, z_{corr}, is strongly dependent on numerical aperture, NA, and particle size, d_p, and is weakly dependent upon magnification, M. Table 2.2 gives the thickness of the measurement plane, 2 z_{corr}, for various microscope objective lenses and particle sizes. The highest out of plane resolution for these parameters is 2 z_{corr} = 0.36 μm for a NA = 1.4, M = 60 lens and particle sizes d_p < 0.1 μm. For these calculations, it is important to note that the effective numerical aperture of an oil immersion lens is reduced when imaging particles suspended in fluids such as water, where the refractive index is less than that of the immersion oil.

Table 2.2. Thickness of the measurement plane for typical experimental parameters, $2z_{corr}$ (μm).

Particle Size d_p	Microscope Objective Lens Characteristics				
	M = 60 NA = 1.4	M = 40 NA = 0.75	M = 40 NA = 0.6	M = 20 NA = 0.5	M = 10 NA = 0.25
0.01 μm	0.36	1.6	3.7	6.5	34
0.10 μm	0.38	1.6	3.8	6.5	34
0.20 μm	0.43	1.7	3.8	6.5	34
0.30 μm	0.52	1.8	3.9	6.6	34
0.50 μm	0.72	2.1	4.2	7.0	34
0.70 μm	0.94	2.5	4.7	7.4	35
1.00 μm	1.3	3.1	5.5	8.3	36
3.00 μm	3.7	8.1	13	17	49

2.2.3 Particle Visibility

The ability to obtain highly reliable velocity data depends significantly upon the quality of the recorded particle images. In macroscopic PIV experiments, it is customary to use a sheet of light to illuminate only those particles that are within the depth of field of the recording lens. This minimizes background noise resulting from light emitted by out of focus particles. However, in μPIV, small measurement length scales and poor optical access necessitates the use of volume illumination.

Experiments using the μPIV technique must be designed so that in-focus particle images can be observed over the background light produced by out of focus particles and the test section surfaces. The background light from test section surfaces can be removed by using fluorescent techniques to filter out elastically scattered light (Santiago, et al., 1998).

Background light is not so easily removed, but can be lowered to acceptable levels by choosing judiciously proper experimental parameters. Olsen & Adrian (2000) present a theory to estimate peak particle visibility, defined as the ratio of the intensity of an in-focus particle image to the average intensity of the background light produced by the out of focus particles.

Assuming light is emitted uniformly from the particle, the light from a single particle reaching the image plane can be written as

$$J(z) = \frac{J_p D_a^2}{16(s_o + z)^2}, \tag{2.8}$$

where J_p is total light flux emitted by a single particle. Approximating the intensity of an in-focus particle image as Gaussian,

$$I(r) = I_0 \exp\left(\frac{-4\beta^2 r^2}{d_e^2}\right), \tag{2.9}$$

where the unspecified parameter, β, is chosen to determine the cutoff level that defines the edge of the particle image. Approximating the Airy distribution by a Gaussian distribution, with the area of the two axisymmetric functions being equal, the first zero in the Airy distribution corresponds to $I/I_0 = \exp(-\beta^2 = -3.67)$ (Adrian & Yao, 1985). Since the total light flux reaching the image plane is $J = \int I(r)\,dA$, Equations (2.8) and (2.9) can be combined yielding (Olsen & Adrian, 2000)

$$I(r,z) = \frac{J_p D_a^2 \beta^2}{4\pi d_e^2 (s_o + z)^2} \exp\left(\frac{-4\beta^2 r^2}{d_e^2}\right). \tag{2.10}$$

Idealizing particles that are located a distance $|z| > \delta/2$ from the object plane as being out of focus and contributing uniformly to background intensity, while particles located within a distance $|z| < \delta/2$ as being completely in-focus, the total flux of background light, J_B, can be approximated by

$$J_B = A_v C \left\{ \int_{-a}^{-\delta/2} J(z)\,dz + \int_{\delta/2}^{L-a} J(z)\,dz \right\}, \tag{2.11}$$

where C is the number of particles per unit volume of fluid, L is the depth of the device, and A_v is the average cross sectional area contained within the field of view. Combining Equations (2.8) & (2.11), correcting for the effect of magnification, and assuming $s_o >> \delta/2$, the intensity of the background glow can be expressed as (Olsen & Adrian, 2000)

$$I_B = \frac{C J_p L D_a^2}{16 M^2 (s_o - a)(s_o - a + L)}. \tag{2.12}$$

Following Olsen & Adrian (2000), the visibility of an in-focus particle, V, can be obtained by combining Equations (2.5) & (2.10) dividing by Equation (2.12), and setting $r = 0$ and $z = 0$,

$$V = \frac{I(0,0)}{I_B} = \frac{4 M^2 \beta^2 (s_o - a)(s_o - a + L)}{\pi C L s_o^2 \left(M^2 d_p^2 + 1.49 (M+1)^2 \lambda^2 \left[\left(n/NA \right)^2 - 1 \right] \right)}. \tag{2.13}$$

For a given set of recording optics, particle visibility can be increased by decreasing particle concentration, C, or by decreasing test section thickness, L. For a fixed particle concentration, the visibility can be increased by decreasing the particle diameter, or by increasing the numerical aperture of the recording lens. Visibility depends only weakly on magnification and object distance, s_o.

An expression for the volume fraction, V_{fr}, of particles in solution that produce a specific particle visibility can be obtained by rearranging Equation (2.13) and multiplying by the volume occupied by a spherical particle

$$V_{fr} = \frac{2 d_p^3 M^2 \beta^2 (s_o - a)(s_o - a + L)}{3 V L s_o^2 \left(M^2 d_p^2 + 1.49 (M+1)^2 \lambda^2 \left[\left(n/NA \right)^2 - 1 \right] \right)} \times 100\%. \tag{2.14}$$

Reasonably high quality particle-image fields require visibilities of, say, $V \sim 1.5$. For the purpose of illustration, assume that we are interested in measuring the flow at the centerline, $a = L/2$, of a microfluidic device with a characteristic depth, $L =$ 100 μm. It is also important to seed the flow so that the volume fraction of seed particles is kept below a suitable level. Table 2.3 shows the maximum volume fraction of particles that can be in the fluid, while maintaining an in-focus particle visibility $V = 1.5$, for various experimental parameters. Here, the object distance, s_o, is estimated by adding the working distance of the lens to the designed cover-slip thickness.

Table 2.3. Maximum volume fraction of particles, V_{fr}, (in percent) while maintaining an in-focus visibility, $V = 1.5$, for imaging the center of an $L = 100$ μm deep device.

Particle Size d_p	Microscope Objective Lens Characteristics				
	$M = 60$ $NA = 1.4$ s_o=0.38 mm	$M = 40$ $NA = 0.75$ s_o=0.89 mm	$M = 40$ $NA = 0.6$ s_o=3 mm	$M = 20$ $NA = 0.5$ s_o=7 mm	$M = 10$ $NA = 0.25$ s_o=10.5 mm
0.01 μm	2.0E-5	4.3E-6	1.9E-6	1.1E-6	1.9E-7
0.10 μm	1.7E-2	4.2E-3	1.9E-3	1.1E-3	1.9E-4
0.20 μm	1.1E-1	3.1E-2	1.4E-2	8.2E-3	1.5E-3
0.30 μm	2.5E-1	9.3E-2	4.6E-2	2.7E-2	5.1E-3
0.50 μm	6.0E-1	3.2E-1	1.8E-1	1.1E-1	2.3E-2
0.70 μm	9.6E-1	6.4E-1	4.1E-1	2.8E-1	6.2E-2
1.00 μm	1.5E+0	1.2E+0	8.7E-1	6.4E-1	1.7E-1
3.00 μm	4.8E+0	4.7E+0	4.5E+0	4.2E+0	2.5E+0

2.3 Particle/Fluid Dynamics

In order to obtain accurate PIV measurements, the seed particles must follow the flow faithfully. If we precisely measure the particle motion to within 1% but the particle speed differs from the flow speed by 5%, the results will contain more than 5% error. Consequently, when performing PIV experiments, one must verify that the particles are following the flow according to a theoretical analysis. It is important to analyze the measured velocity fields and look for evidence of unexpected forces that may cause the particles not to follow the flow. In microfluidic experiments, the effects of Brownian motion and surface forces must be taken into consideration, while they may usually be neglected in macroscopic experiments.

An accurate equation for predicting the interacting of a dilute concentration of spherical particles with a fluid velocity field is needed. Many such equations of motion have been developed. Maxey and Riley (1983) developed a general-purpose equation for the force balance on a dilute suspension of rigid spherical particles in a fluid. They derive a dimensional equation of motion

$$m_p \frac{dV_i}{dt} = m_F \left.\frac{Du_i}{Dt}\right|_{\mathbf{Y}(t)} - \frac{1}{2} m_F \frac{d}{dt}\left\{ V_i(t) - u_i\left[\mathbf{Y}(t),t\right] - \frac{1}{10} a^2 \nabla^2 u_i\Big|_{\mathbf{Y}(t)} \right\}$$
$$+\left(m_p - m_F\right) g_i + f_i - 6\pi a \mu \left\{ V_i(t) - u_i\left[\mathbf{Y}(t),t\right] - \frac{1}{6} a^2 \nabla^2 u_i\Big|_{\mathbf{Y}(t)} \right\}, \quad (2.15)$$
$$-6\pi a^2 \mu \int_0^t d\tau \left(\frac{d/d\tau \left\{ V_i(\tau) - u_i\left[\mathbf{Y}(\tau),\tau\right] - (1/6) a^2 \nabla^2 u_i\Big|_{\mathbf{Y}(\tau)} \right\}}{\left[\pi \nu (t-\tau)\right]^{1/2}} \right)$$

where m_p is the mass of a particle, m_F is the mass of fluid displaced by a particle, $\mathbf{Y}(t)$ is the location of a particle, $V_i(t)$ is the velocity of a particle, $u_i(x,t)$ is the velocity field of fluid, a is the radius of a particle, μ is the dynamic viscosity of the fluid, ν is the kinematic viscosity of the fluid. The terms in Equation (2.15) represent, from left to right, the particle inertia, the pressure-viscous force, the added mass force, the buoyancy force, an arbitrary external force applied to the particle, the Stokes drag force, and the Basset history force.

Equation (2.15) was derived by making some basic assumptions about the particles and the surrounding flow. Each particle that is examined is assumed to be far from any neighboring particles and also far from any boundaries of the flow. In practice this restriction translates to the distance from the nearest boundary or neighboring particle being very much larger than the particle's diameter. Effects due to nonzero relative Reynolds number are also ignored. These effects, for the case of steady relative motion, are specifically the Oseen correction to Stokes drag, the modified drag due to particle rotation, and Saffman effect—a lateral force due to shear in the undisturbed flow. All of these effects are small compared to the remaining Stokes drag term with the assumption of low Reynolds number. The overriding criteria that must be satisfied for Equation (2.15) to accurately model the dynamics of a particle suspended in a flow are that the relative particle Reynolds number, aW_0/ν, be much less than unity and that the quantity $(a^2/\nu)(U_0/L)$ also be very much less than unity. In these parameters W_0 is a measure of the particle velocity relative to the flow and U_0/L is a scale for the velocity gradients in the problem.

For the small-sized particles typically used in μPIV, Equation (2.15) can be simplified to the Stokes drag law plus the arbitrary force f_i, which can assume any form or value depending on the particular experiment being conducted. For example, f_i could represent an electrostatic force acting on the particles, as in electrophoresis, or it could represent a magnetic body force. The arbitrary force f_i could be a quantity being measured or it could be a quantity degrading the accuracy of the fluid velocity measurements.

For μPIV, three phenomena primarily act to prevent the seed particles from following the flow. These are:

- Saffman effect—which can become large in the case of particles very near a boundary
- Brownian motion—the random thermal vibrations of the seed particles
- Arbitrary external forces

Two of these phenomena, the Saffman effect and Brownian motion, are of particular importance when measuring fluid velocities and will be discussed in greater detail here. The influence of arbitrary external forces cannot be considered in detail here because of its dependence on intrinsic conditions of each experiment.

2.3.1 Brownian Motion

In stark contrast to many macroscale fluid mechanics experiments, the hydrodynamic size of a particle (a measure of its ability to follow the flow based on the ratio of inertial to drag forces) is usually not a concern in microfluidic applications because of the large surface to volume ratios at small length scales. A simple model for the response time of a particle subjected to a step change in local fluid velocity can be used to gauge particle behavior. Based on a simple first-order inertial response to a constant flow acceleration (assuming Stokes flow for the particle drag), the response time τ_p of a particle is

$$\tau_p = d_p^2\, \rho_p/(18\mu_f) \tag{2.16}$$

where d_p and ρ_p are the diameter and density of the particle, respectively, and μ_f is the dynamic viscosity of the fluid. Considering typical μPIV experimental parameters of 300 nm diameter polystyrene latex spheres immersed in water, the particle response time is approximately 10^{-9} sec. This response time is much smaller than the time scales of any realistic liquid or low-speed gas flow field.

In the case of high-speed gas flows, the particle response time may be an important consideration when designing a system for microflow measurements. For example, a 400 nm particle seeded into an air micronozzle that expands from the sonic at the throat to Mach 2 over a 1 mm distance may experience a particle-to-gas relative flow velocity of more than 5% (assuming a constant acceleration and a stagnation temperature of 300 K). Particle response to flow through a normal shock would be significantly worse. For the case of the slip flow regime ($10^{-3} < Kn_p < 0.1$), it is possible to use corrections to the Stokes drag relation to quantify particle dynamics (Beskok, et al., 1996). For example, a correction offered by Melling (1986) suggests the following relation for the particle response time:

$$\tau_p = (1 + 2.76\, Kn_p)\, d_p^2\, \rho_p/(18\mu_f) \tag{2.17}$$

Once the response time of the particle is established, further consideration of the phenomenon causing Brownian motion is necessary. Brownian motion is the random thermal motion of a particle suspended in a fluid (Probstein, 1994). The motion results from collisions between fluid molecules and suspended particles. For time intervals Δt much larger than the particle inertial response time, the dynamics of Brownian motion are independent of inertial parameters such as particle and fluid density. The mean square distance of diffusion is proportional to $D\Delta t$, where D is the diffusion coefficient of the particle. For a spherical particle subject to Stokes drag law, the diffusion coefficient D was first given by Einstein (1905) as

$$D = \frac{\kappa T}{3\pi\mu d_p} \tag{2.18}$$

where d_p is the particle diameter, κ is Boltzmann's constant, T is the absolute temperature of the fluid, and μ is the dynamic viscosity of the fluid. The random particle displacements measured with respect to the moving fluid can be described by the following three-dimensional (Gaussian) probability density function

$$p(x,y,z) = \frac{\exp\left[-\left(x^2+y^2+z^2\right)/4D\Delta t\right]}{(2\pi)^{3/2}\left(2D\Delta t\right)^{3/2}}, \tag{2.19}$$

where the displacements in the x, y, and z directions can be considered statistically independent random variables (Devasenathipathy, et al. 2003).

In all of the μPIV techniques developed to date and discussed here, particle displacements are determined by tracking the two-dimensional projections of particles located within some measurement depth. Therefore, the probability density function of the imaged particle displacements with respect to the moving fluid can be described by integrating Equation (2.19) along the optical axis (z) to get

$$p(x,y) = \int_{-\infty}^{\infty} p(x,y,z)dz = \frac{\exp\left[-\left(x^2+y^2\right)/4D\Delta t\right]}{4\pi D\Delta t}, \tag{2.20}$$

where the coordinates x, y, and z are taken to be displacements with respect to the moving fluid, assumed constant throughout the region over which the Brownian particle diffuses—the diffusing particles are assumed to sample a region of low velocity gradient. In practice, Equation (2.20) is an approximation to the imaged particle displacement distribution since particles may leave the measurement volume altogether during the interval Δt due to diffusion or convection in the z-direction. Therefore, the two-point probability density function described by Equation (2.20) can be interpreted as being valid for cases where $\Delta z = w\,\Delta t < \delta z_m$, where w is the z-component of velocity. This limitation is not especially restrictive in microflows because of the absence of turbulence and the relatively large depth of correlation.

The random Brownian displacements cause particle trajectories to fluctuate about the deterministic pathlines of the fluid flow field. Assuming the flow field is steady over the time of measurement and the local velocity gradient is small, the imaged Brownian particle motion can be considered a fluctuation about a streamline that passes through the particle's initial location. An ideal, non-Brownian (i.e. deterministic) particle following a particular streamline for a time period Δt has x- and y-displacements of

$$\Delta x = u \, \Delta t \tag{2.21a}$$

$$\Delta y = v \, \Delta t \tag{2.21b}$$

where u and v are the x- and y- components of the time-averaged, local fluid velocity. The relative errors, ε_x and ε_y, incurred as a result of imaging the Brownian particle displacements in a two-dimensional measurement of the x- and y-components of particle velocity is given as

$$\varepsilon_x = \frac{\sigma_x}{\Delta x} = \frac{1}{u}\sqrt{\frac{2D}{\Delta t}} \tag{2.22a}$$

$$\varepsilon_y = \frac{\sigma_y}{\Delta y} = \frac{1}{v}\sqrt{\frac{2D}{\Delta t}} \tag{2.22b}$$

This Brownian error establishes a lower limit on the measurement time interval Δt since, for shorter times, the measurements are dominated by uncorrelated Brownian motion. These quantities (ratios of the root mean square fluctuation-to-average velocity) describe the relative magnitudes of the Brownian motion and will be referred to here as Brownian intensities. The errors estimated by Equations (2.22a,b) show that the relative Brownian intensity error decreases as the time of measurement increases. Larger time intervals produce flow displacements proportional to Δt while the root mean square of the Brownian particle displacements grow as $\Delta t^{1/2}$. In practice, Brownian motion is an important consideration when tracing 50 to 500 nm particles in flow field experiments with flow velocities of less than about 1 mm/s. For a velocity on the order of 0.5 mm/s and a 500 nm seed particle, the lower limit for the time spacing is approximately 100 μs for a 20% error due to Brownian motion. This error can be reduced by both averaging over several particles in a single interrogation spot and by ensemble averaging over several realizations. The diffusive uncertainty decreases as $1/\sqrt{N}$, where N is the total number of particles in the average (Bendat and Piersol, 1986).

Equations (2.22a,b) demonstrates that the effect of Brownian motion is relatively less important for faster flows. However, for a given measurement, when u increases, Δt will generally be decreased. Equation (2.22a,b) also demonstrates that when all conditions but the Δt are fixed, going to larger Δt will decrease the relative error introduced by Brownian motion. Unfortunately, longer Δt will decrease the accuracy of the results because the PIV measurements are based on a first order accurate approximation to the velocity. Using a second order accurate technique called Central Difference Interrogation (CDI) allows for longer Δt to be used without increasing this error.

2.3.2 Saffman Effect

For flow in a long channel, the deterministic effects of shear-induced migration will compete with the random effects of Brownian motion. Many authors have considered the case of particle migration in a shear flow. Poiseuille (1836) is generally acknowledged to be the first modern scientist who recorded evidence of particle migration with his observations that blood cells flowing through capillaries tended to stay away from the walls of the capillaries. Taylor (1955) scanned the cross-section of a tube carrying a suspension and noticed areas of reduced cell concentration not only near the walls, but also near the center of the channel. Segré and Silberberg (1962) systematically performed experiments that confirmed both observations—migration away from the walls *and* migration away from the center of the channel and determined that migration rate was proportional to the square of the mean velocity in the channel as well as the fourth power of the particle radius. Saffman (1965) analytically considered the case of a rigid sphere translating in a linear unbounded shear field. He used matched asymptotic expansions to find an equation for the particle migration velocity that is correct to lowest order. Consider a rigid sphere of radius a in an unbounded shear flow of fluid density ρ and kinematic viscosity ν. The velocity field depends linearly on one spatial coordinate such that the velocity gradient is G. The particle is initially sitting at the origin (at which point the fluid velocity is identically zero). The particle is assumed to move relative to the fluid at a speed $-V_s$ and rotate with an angular velocity Ω. The pertinent Reynolds numbers in this situation are

$$\mathrm{Re}_G = \frac{4a^2G}{\nu}, \mathrm{Re}_s = \frac{2aV_s}{\nu}, \mathrm{Re}_\Omega = \frac{4a^2\Omega}{\nu} \tag{2.23}$$

where the quantity Re_s can be referred to as the slip Reynolds number. As long as these Reynolds numbers are small compared to unity, Saffman's analysis holds.

His analysis states that the migration velocity V_m should be given by

$$\frac{V_m}{V_s} = 0.343a\sqrt{\frac{G}{\nu}}. \tag{2.24}$$

When the quotient V_m/V_s is small compare to unity, the particle migration across streamlines caused by the velocity gradient will have a negligible effect on the velocity measurements.

2.4 Typical Micro-PIV Hardware Implementation

Figure 2.2 is a schematic of a typical μPIV system, originally described by Meinhart et al. (1999b). It is common to use a pulsed monochromatic light source, such as a pulsed Nd:YAG laser system, which are available from NewWave Research, Inc., 47613 Warm Springs Blvd., Fremont, CA 94539. The laser system is specifically designed for PIV applications, and consists of two Nd:YAG laser cavities, beam combining optics, and a frequency doubling crystal. The laser emits two pulses of light at $\lambda = 532$ nm. The duration of each pulse is on the order of 5 ns and the time delay between light pulses can vary from order hundreds of nanoseconds to a few seconds. The illumination light is delivered to the microscope through beam-forming optics, which can consist of a variety of optical elements that will sufficiently modify the light so that it will fill the back of the objective lens, and thereby broadly illuminate the microfluidic device. The beam-forming optics can consist of a liquid-filled optical fiber to direct the light into the microscope. The illumination light is reflected upward towards the objective lens by an antireflective coated mirror (designed to reflect wavelength 532 nm and transmit 560 nm).

A number of researchers have used continuous chromatic light sources, such as a mercury arc lamp or halogen lamp, to provide illumination light (see Santiago et al., 1998). In this situation, an excitation filter must be used to allow only a narrow wavelength band of light to illuminate the test section. If a continuous light source is used, then a mechanical or electro-optical shutter must be used to gate the light before reaching the image recording device, so that discrete particle images are formed.

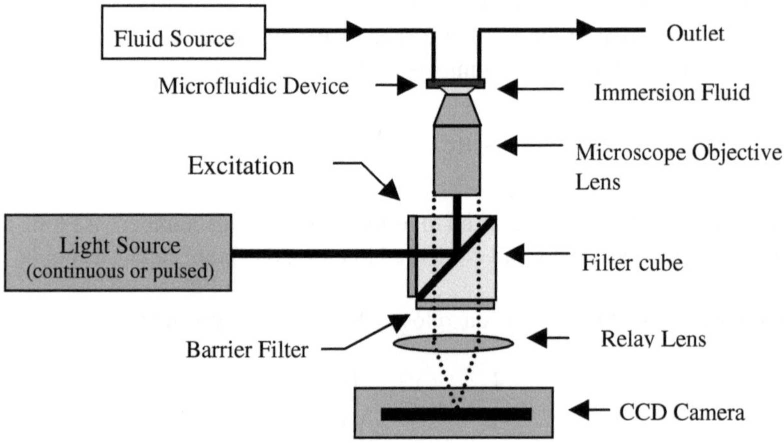

Fig. 2.2. Schematic of a μPIV system using either a continuous or pulsed illumination light source.

For high resolution measurements, the microscope lens can be an oil immersion, high numerical aperture (NA = 1.4), high magnification (M = 60, or M = 100), low distortion, *CFI Plan Apochromat* lens. Lower resolution and lower magnification microscope lenses, such as an air immersion lens with a numerical aperture NA = 0.6 and magnification M = 40, can be used, but with decreased measurement resolution. Commonly used lens configurations are shown in Tables 2.1–2.3.

Typically, the working fluid is directed through the microfluidic device by pressure or induced electrokinetically. The working fluid can be any visibly transparent fluid, such as water. Liquids are most commonly used. It is conceivable to use gaseous fluids, such as air, but μPIV experiments using air have not been demonstrated successfully to date. The working fluid should be seeded with fluorescent particles which can be manufactured from of a variety of materials, such as polystyrene. It is important that the particles have a specific gravity closely matched to the working fluid, and are less than, say, one micron, preferably 200 – 700 nm. Smaller particles are subject to Brownian motion, and are difficult to image. Larger particles can be used, but with decreased measurement resolution and accuracy. The particles must be coated with a fluorescent dye with an excitation wavelength closely matched to light source, and an emission wavelength closely matched to barrier filter. Suitable particles can be purchased from a variety of manufactures, such as *Molecular Probes, Inc.*, Eugene, Oregon, *Duke Scientific Corporation*, Palo Alto, California, *Bangs Laboratory*, Fishers, Indiana, and *EM Industries, Inc*., Hawthorne, New York.

The microfluidic test section must have at least one optically transparent wall, so that it can be viewed through the microscope lens. A barrier filter is positioned between the mirror and the relay lens. The barrier filter is usually a long pass filter that filters out the illumination light that is reflected by the surface of the test section or scattered by the particles.

A sensitive large-format interline-transfer CCD camera is commonly used to record the particle image fields. Suitable cameras are available from most PIV system manufacturers. A large-format CCD array is desirable because it allows for more particle images to be recorded, and increases the spatial dynamic range of the measurements. The interline transfer feature of the CCD camera allows for two particle image frames to be recorded back-to-back to within a 500 nm time delay.

2.5 Algorithms and Processing for μPIV

The fundamental physical differences between μPIV and macroscopic PIV necessitates the changes in the hardware (discussed above) as well as changes in the method of interrogating the images—algorithmic and processing changes. Several authors have reported developing specialized μPIV software (Wereley and Meinhart, 1998; Han, et al., 2004; Gui and Wereley, 2001). As of the time of the writing of this chapter, a demonstration version of one of these software packages is being distributed on the internet at
http://www.ecn.purdue.edu/microfluidics

2.5.1 Processing Methods Most Suitable for μPIV

When evaluating digital PIV recordings with conventional correlation-based algorithms or image-pattern tracking algorithms, a sufficient number of particle images are required in the interrogation window or the tracked image pattern to ensure reliable and accurate measurement results. However, in many cases, especially in μPIV measurements, the particle image density in the PIV recordings is usually not high enough (e.g. Fig. 2.3a). These PIV recordings are called low image density (LID) recordings and are usually evaluated with particle-tracking algorithms. When using particle-tracking algorithms, the velocity vector is determined with only one particle, and hence the reliability and accuracy are of the technique are limited. In addition, interpolation procedures are usually necessary to obtain velocity vectors on the desired regular grid points from the random distributed particle-tracking results (e.g. Fig. 2.4a), and therefore, additional uncertainties are added to the final results. Fortunately, special processing methods can be used to evaluate the μPIV recordings, so that the errors resulting from the low image density can be avoided. In this section two methods are introduced to improve measurement accuracy of μPIV by using a digital image processing technique and by improving the evaluation algorithm, respectively.

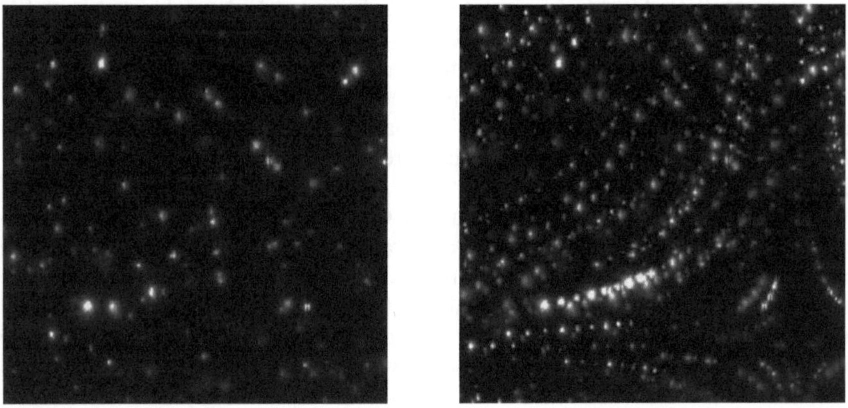

(a) (b)

Fig. 2.3. Example of image overlapping: (a) one of the LID-PIV recordings; (b) result of overlapping 9 LID-PIV recordings. Image size: 256×256 pixels (Wereley, et al., 2001).

2.5.2 Overlapping of LID-PIV Recordings

In early days of PIV, multiple exposure imaging techniques were used to increase the particle image numbers in PIV recordings. Similar to multiply exposing a single frame, high-image-density (HID) PIV recordings can be generated by computationally overlapping a number of LID-PIV recordings with

$$g_o(x,y) = \max\{g_k(x,y), k = 1,2,3,\cdots,N\}, \qquad (2.25)$$

wherein $g_k(x,y)$ is the gray value distributions of the LID-PIV recordings with a total number N, and $g_o(x,y)$ is the overlapped recording. Note that in Equation (2.25) - the particle images are positive, i.e. with bright particles and dark background; otherwise the images should be inverted or the minimum function used. An example of the image overlapping can be seen in Fig. 2.3b for overlapping 9 LID-PIV recordings. The size of the PIV recordings in Fug. 2.3, is 256×256 pixels, and the corresponding measurement area is 2.5×2.5 mm^2. The effect of the image overlapping on the velocity measurement is shown in Fig. 2.4. Figure 2.4a shows the evaluation results for one of the LID-PIV recording pairs with a particle-tracking algorithm (Gui, et al., 1997), and Fig. 2.4b shows the results for the overlapped PIV recording pair (out of 9 LID-PIV recording pairs) with a correlation-based algorithm. The results in Fig. 2.4b are more reliable, more dense, and more regularly spaced than those in Fig. 2.4a.

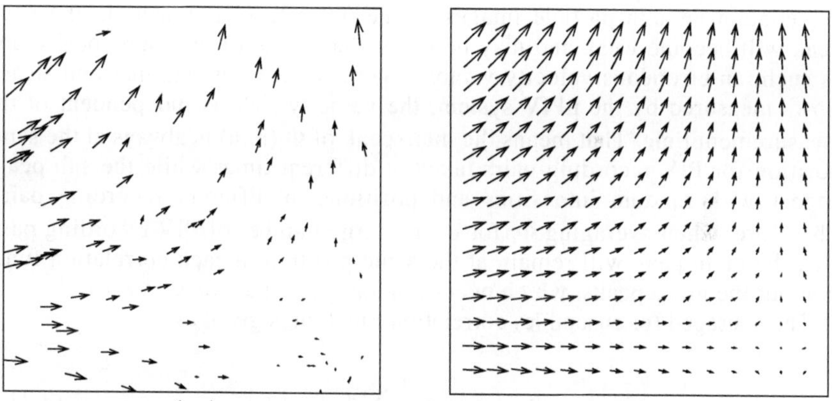

Fig. 2.4. Effect of image overlapping: (a) results for a single LID-PIV recording pair with a particle-tracking algorithm; (b) results for the overlapped PIV recording pair with a correlation-based algorithm (Wereley, et al., 2001).

The image overlapping method is based on the fact that flows in microdomains typically have very low Reynolds numbers, so that the flow can be considered as laminar and steady in the data acquisition period. Note that this method cannot be extended to measurements of turbulent or unsteady flows, and it may not work very well when overlapping HID-PIV recordings or too many LID-PIV recordings because with large numbers of particle images, interference between particle images will occur (Meinhart, et al., 2000). Further study of this technique will be necessary to quantify these limitations but the promise of the technique is obvious.

2.5.3 Correlation Averaging Method

For correlation-based PIV evaluation algorithms the correlation function at a certain interrogation spot is usually represented as

$$\Phi_k(m,n) = \sum_{j=1}^{q} \sum_{i=1}^{p} f_k(i,j) \cdot g_k(i+m, j+n) \tag{2.26}$$

where $f_k(i,j)$ and $g_k(i,j)$ are the gray value distributions of the first and second exposure, respectively, in the kth PIV recording pair at a certain interrogation spot of size of p × q pixels. The correlation function for a singly-exposed PIV image pair has a peak at the position of the particle image displacement in the interrogation spot (or window), which should be the highest among all the peaks of Φ_k. The sub peaks, which result from noise or mismatch of particle images, are usually obviously lower than the main peak, i.e. the peak of the particle image displacement. However, when the interrogation window does not contain enough particle images or the noise level is too high, the main peak will become weak and may be lower than some of the "sub" peaks, and as such, an erroneous velocity vector is generated. In the laminar and steady flows measured by the µPIV system, the velocity field is independent of the measurement time. That means the main peak of $\Phi_k(m,n)$ is always at the same position for PIV recording pairs taken at different times while the sub peaks appear with random intensities and positions in different recording pairs. Therefore, when averaging Φ_k for over a large number of PIV recording pairs (N), the main peak will remain at the same position in each correlation function but the noise peaks, which occur randomly, will average to zero.

The averaged (or ensemble) correlation function is given as

$$\Phi_{ens}(m,n) = \frac{1}{N}\sum_{k=1}^{N} \Phi_k(m,n) \tag{2.27}$$

Just as with the image overlapping method detailed above, the ensemble correlation requires a steady flow. However, in contrast with the image overlapping method, the technique is not limited to LID recordings or to a small number of recordings. The concept of averaging correlation functions can also be applied to other evaluation algorithms such as correlation tracking and the MQD method. This method was first proposed and demonstrated by Meinhart, et al. (2000).

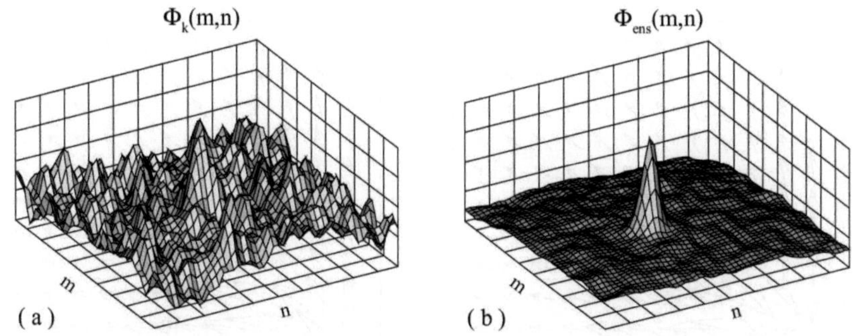

Fig. 2.5. Effect of ensemble correlation: (a) results with conventional correlation for one of the PIV recording pairs; (b) results with ensemble correlation for 101 PIV recording pairs (Wereley, et al., 2001).

The ensemble correlation function technique is demonstrated for 101 LID-PIV recording pairs (Φ_{ens}) in Fig. 2.5 in comparison to the correlation function for one of the single recording pair (Φ_k). These PIV recording pairs are chosen from the flow measurement in a microfluidic biochip for impedance spectroscopy of biological species (Gomez, et al., 2001). With the conventional evaluation function in Fig. 2.5a, the main peak cannot easily be identified among the sub peaks, so that the evaluation result is neither reliable nor accurate. However, the ensemble correlation function in Fig. 2.5b shows a very clear peak at the particle image displacement, and the sub peaks can hardly be recognized.

The effect of the ensemble correlation technique on the resulting velocity field is demonstrated in Fig. 2.6 with the PIV measurement of flow in the microfluidic biochip. All the obvious evaluation errors resulting from the low image density and strong background noise (see Fig. 2.6a) are avoided by using the ensemble correlation method based on 101 PIV recording pairs (Fig. 2.6b). One important note here is that since the bad vectors in Fig. 2.6a all occur at the lower left corner of the flow domain, removal of these bad vectors and subsequent replacement by interpolated vectors will only coincidentally generate results that bear any resemblance to the true velocity field in the device. In addition, if the problem leading to low signal levels in the lower left hand corner of the images is systematic, i.e. larger background noise, etc., even a large collection of images will not generate better results because they will all have bad vectors at the same location.

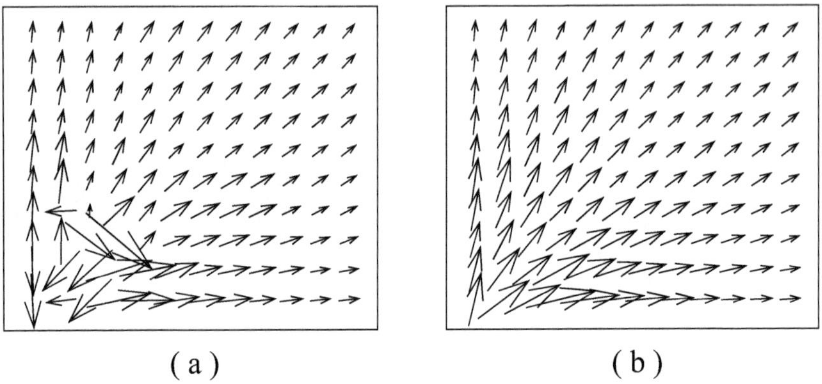

Fig. 2.6. Comparison of the evaluation function of (a) a single PIV recording pair with (b) the average of 101 evaluation functions (Wereley, et al., 2001).

Background Removal

For using the recording overlapping or ensemble correlation techniques, a great number of µPIV recording pairs are usually obtained, enabling removal of the background noise from the µPIV recording pairs. One of the possibilities for obtaining an image of the background from plenty of PIV recordings is averaging these recordings. Because the particles are randomly distributed and quickly move through the camera view area, their images will disappear in the averaged recording. However, the image of the background (including boundary, contaminants on the glass cover, particles adhered to the wall, etc.) maintains the same brightness distribution in the averaged recording, because it does not move or change. Another method is building at each pixel location a minimum of the ensemble of PIV recordings, because the minimal gray value at certain pixel may reflect the background brightness in the successively recorded images (Cowen and Monismith, 1997). The background noise may be successfully removed by subtracting the background image from the PIV recordings.

A data set from a flow in a micro channel is used to demonstrate this point. The size of the interrogation regions are 64×64 pixels and the total sample number is 100 pairs. The mean particle image displacement is about 12.5 pixels from left to right. In one particular interrogation region in the images, the particle images in a region at left side of the interrogation region look darker than those outside this region. This may result from an asperity on the glass cover of the micro-channel. The ensemble correlation function for the 100 image sample pairs without background removal is given in Fig. 2.7a, which shows a dominant peak near zero displacement because the fleck does not move. When the background image is built with the minimum gray value method and subtracted from the image sample pairs, the influence of the asperity is reduced so that the peak of the particle image displacement appears clearly in the evaluation function in Fig. 2.7b.

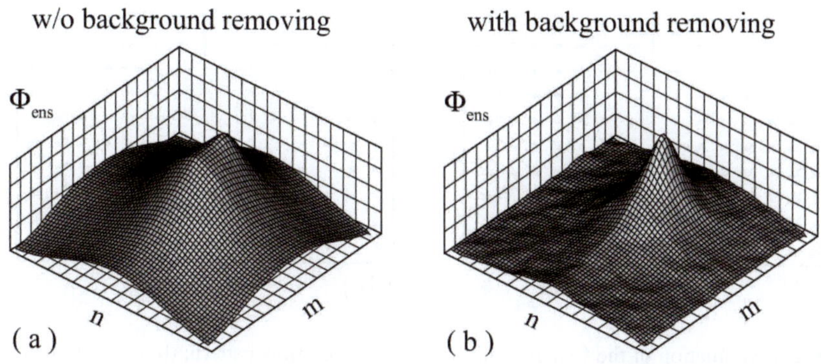

Fig. 2.7. Ensemble correlation function for 100 image sample pairs without (a) and with (b) background removal.

2.5.4 Processing Methods Suitable for Both Micro/Macro PIV

For further improving the reliability and accuracy of μPIV measurements a number of evaluation techniques, which also work well for standard PIV systems, are applied. It is known that the measurement uncertainty of PIV data includes both bias error and precision error. One of the most effective methods for reducing the bias error of PIV measurements in complex flows is the Central Difference Interrogation (CDI) method. For reducing the precision (or random) error, image correction methods are suggested. The CDI method and one of the image correction methods are introduced below.

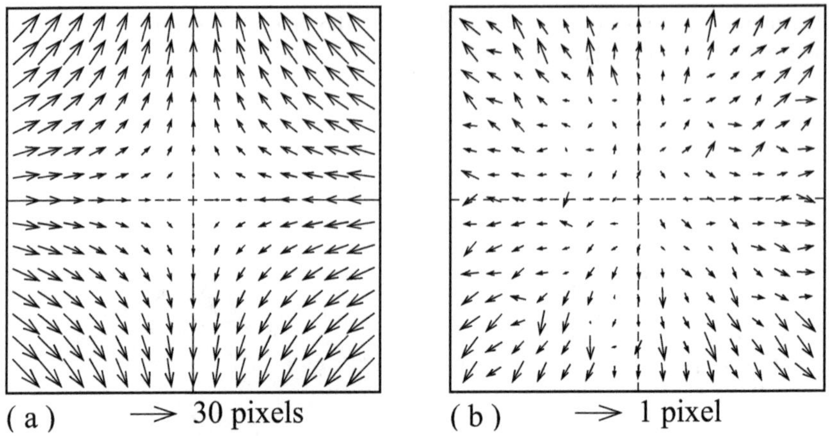

Fig. 2.8. Simulation of the four-roll-mill test: (a) desired flow pattern; (b) evaluation errors with FDI (Wereley, et al., 2001).

2.5.5 Central Difference Interrogation

Currently, adaptive window offsetting is widely used with the FFT-based correlation algorithm for reducing the evaluation error and with the image pattern tracking algorithms for increasing the spatial resolution. The adaptive window offset method, as typically implemented, can be referred to as Forward Difference Interrogation (FDI), because the second interrogation window is shifted in the forward direction of the flow an amount equal to the mean displacement of the particle images initially in the first window. Although the FDI method leads to significant improvements in the evaluation quality of PIV recordings in many cases, there are still some potentially detrimental bias errors that cannot be avoided when using an FDI method. The Central Difference Interrogation (CDI) method was initially introduced by Wereley, et al. (1998), and further developed and explored by Wereley and Meinhart (2001), to avoid the shortcoming of FDI and increase the accuracy of the PIV measurement. The comparison between the CDI and FDI methods is analogous to the comparison between central difference and forward difference discretizations of derivatives wherein the central difference method is accurate to order Δt^2 while the forward difference method is only accurate to order Δt. When using CDI, the first and second interrogation windows are shifted backwards and forwards, respectively, each by half of the expected particle image displacement (see Figure 3; Wereley and Meinhart, 2001). As with many adaptive window shifting techniques, this technique requires iteration to achieve optimum results.

In order to demonstrate the advantage of CDI over the FDI, a typical curvature flow, i.e. the flow in a four-roll-mill, is used here as an example. Based on actual experimental parameters, such as particle image size, concentration, and intensity, PIV recording pairs are simulated with the desired flow field shown in Fig. 2.9a.

The maximal particle image displacement in the PIV recording pair of size of 1024×1024 pixels is about 30 pixels. The corresponding measurement area and the maximal velocity are 10×10 mm^2 and 0.04 mm/s, respectively. When combining the FFT-based correlation algorithm with FDI, evaluation errors of a pair of the simulated recordings are determined by subtracting the desired flow field from the evaluation results and given in Fig. 2.8b. The evaluation errors in Fig. 2.8b are obviously dominated by bias errors that depend on the radial position, i.e. the distance between the vector location and the flow field center.

In this test the bias errors are determined by averaging 500 individual error maps as shown in Fig. 2.9b, and a distribution of RMS values of the random errors is further computed. Dependences of the bias and random errors on the radial position are determined and shown in Fig. 2.9a and Fig. 2.9b for the FDI and CDI, respectively. The total error is defined as the root-sum-square (RSS) of the bias and random error. It is shown in Fig. 2.9 that the evaluation error of FDI is dominated by the bias error, at radial positions greater than 200 pixels.

When CDI is used, the bias error is so small that it can be neglected in comparison to the random error that does not depend on the location.

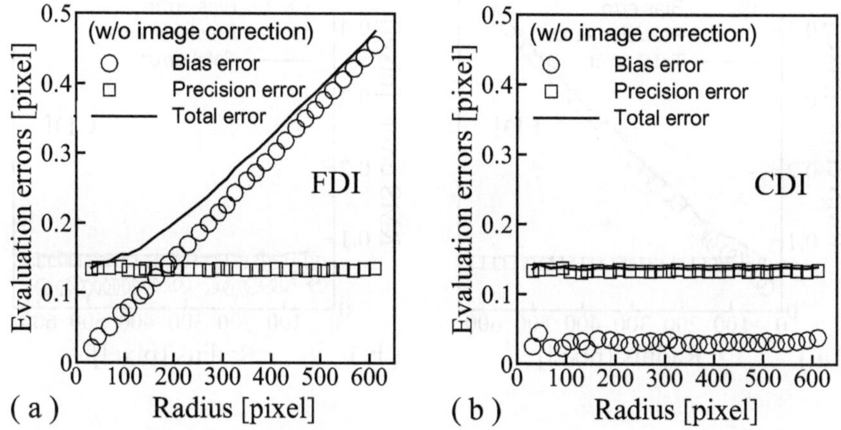

Fig. 2.9. Dependences of evaluation errors on the location (radius) of the evaluation with FDI (a) and CDI (b) for the four-roll-mill test (Wereley, et al., 2001).

2.5.6 Image Correction Technique

In the above example, the bias error of the four-roll-mill test is minimized by using the CDI method. In order to further reduce the measurement uncertainty, i.e. the total error, the random errors must also be reduced. In the four-roll-mill test case, even when the flow is ideally seeded and the PIV recordings are made without any noise, evaluation errors may result from the deformation of the measured flow. To account for the deformation of the PIV image pattern, image correction techniques have been developed. The idea of image correction was presented by

Huang, et al. (1993), and similar ideas were also applied by others. However, since the image correction was a complex and time-consuming procedure, it has not been widely used. In order to accelerate the evaluation, the authors modified the image correction method as follows: Based on previous iterations, the particle image displacements at the four corners of each interrogation window are calculated and used to deform the image patterns in the interrogation area for both exposures of the PIV recording pair using a simple bilinear interpolation, so that the image patterns have a good match despite spatial velocity gradients at the particle image displacement (see Figure 1 in Wereley and Gui, 2001). Combining the modified image correction technique with the FFT-based correlation algorithm, the evaluation can be run at a very high speed. The effect of the image correction is presented in Fig. 2.10. By comparing Fig. 2.9 with Fig. 2.10, the effect of the image correction can be seen to reduce the total error of the measurement scheme by about half.

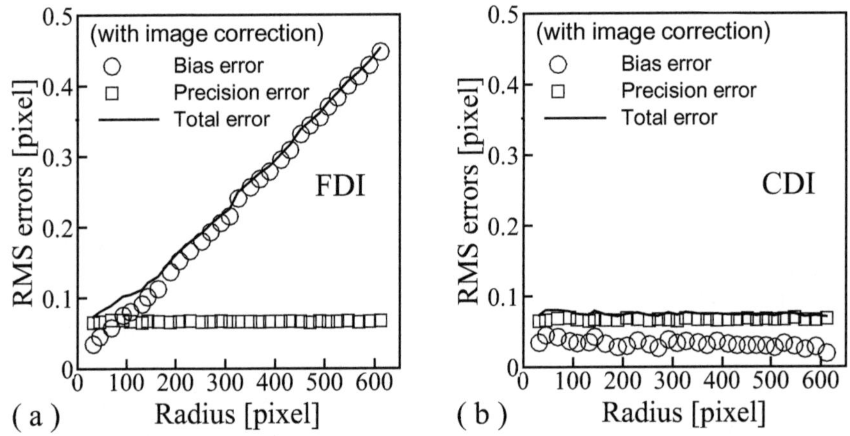

Fig. 2.10. Dependences of evaluation errors on the location of the evaluation with FDI (a) and CDI (b) by using image correction (Wereley, et al., 2001).

2.6 Application Examples of μPIV

2.6.1 Flow in a Microchannel

No flow is more fundamental in fluid mechanics than the pressure driven flow in a straight channel of constant cross section. Since analytical solutions are known for such flows, they prove invaluable for gauging the accuracy of μPIV.

Analytical Solution to Channel Flow

Although the solution to flow through a round capillary is the well-known parabolic profile, the analytical solution to flow through a capillary of rectangular cross section is less well-known. Since one of the goals of this section is to illustrate the accuracy of μPIV by comparing to a known solution, it would be useful here to sketch out the analytical solution. The velocity field of flow through a rectangular duct can be calculated by solving the Stokes equation (the low Reynolds number version of the Navier-Stokes equation), with no-slip velocity boundary conditions at the wall (Meinhart, et al., 1999b). Given dimensions of a rectangular duct of $2H$ for height and $2W$ for width, assuming that $W \gg H$, the coordinates in the vertical and the wall-normal directions can be made nondimensional by the channel half height H (see Fig. 2.9), such that

$$Y = \frac{y}{H} \text{ and } Z = \frac{z}{H}. \tag{2.28}$$

The velocity in the x (or streamwise) direction, scaled by the bulk velocity in the channel is given as

$$\Theta = \frac{v_x}{U} = \frac{3\mu v_x}{H^2(-dP/dx)}. \tag{2.29}$$

The analytical solution to the flow field near the wall for high aspect channels (i.e. $W \gg H$) can be expressed as

$$\Theta = \frac{3}{2}\left(1 - Y^2\right) - 6\sum_{n=0}^{\infty} \frac{(-1)^n}{\lambda_n^3} e^{-\lambda_n Z} \cos \lambda_n Y, \tag{2.30}$$

where $\lambda_n = (n + \frac{1}{2})\pi h$. Sufficiently far from the wall (i.e. Z » 1) the analytical solution in the Y direction (for constant Z), converges to the well known parabolic profile for flow between infinite parallel plates. In the Z direction (for constant Y) however, the flow profile is unusual in that it has a very steep velocity gradient near the wall ($Z < 1$) which reaches a constant value away from the wall ($Z \gg 1$).

Experimental Measurements

A 30 μm × 300 μm × 25 mm glass rectangular microchannel, fabricated by *Wilmad Industries,* was mounted flush to a 170 μm thick glass coverslip and a microscope slide. By carefully rotating the glass coverslip and the CCD camera, the channel was oriented to the optical plane of the microscope within 0.2°, in all three angles. The orientation was confirmed optically by focusing the CCD camera on the microchannel walls. The microchannel was horizontally positioned using a high-precision *x-y* stage, and verified optically to within ~400 nm using epi-fluorescent imaging and image enhancement.

The flow in the glass microchannel was imaged through an inverted epi-fluorescent microscope and a *Nikon Plan Apochromat* oil-immersion objective lens with a magnification $M = 60$ and a numerical aperture $NA = 1.4$. The object plane was placed at approximately 7.5 ± 1 μm from the bottom of the 30 μm thick microchannel. The Plan Apochromat lens was chosen for the experiment, because it is a high quality microscope objective designed with low curvature of field, low distortion, and corrected for spherical and chromatic aberrations.

Since deionized water (refractive index n_w=1.33) was used as the working fluid but the lens immersion fluid was oil (refractive index n_i=1.515), the effective numerical aperture of the objective lens was limited to $NA \approx n_w/n_i = 1.23$ (Inoué & Spring, 1997). A filtered continuous white light source was used to align the test section with the CCD camera and to test for proper particle concentration. During the experiment, the continuous light source was replaced by the pulsed Nd:YAG laser. A *Harvard Apparatus* syringe pump was used to produce a 200 μl hr^{-1} flow through the microchannel.

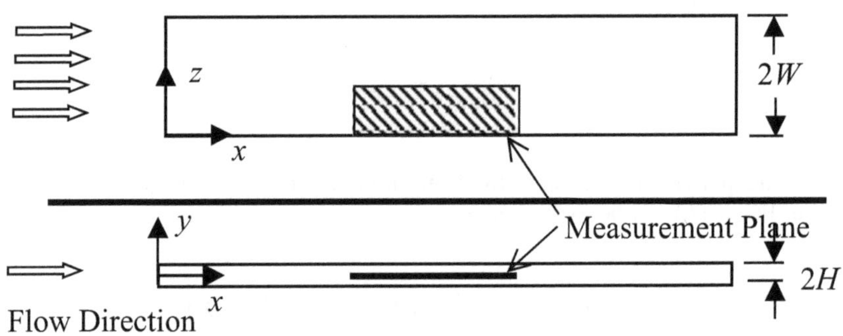

Fig. 2.11. Geometry of the microchannel. The microchannel is $2H$ high and $2W$ wide, and is assumed infinitely long in the axial direction. The measurement plane of interest is orientated in the x-z plane and includes the microchannel wall at $z = 0$. The centerline of the channel is at $y = 0$. The microscope objective images the test section from below, in the lower figure (Stone, et al., 2002).

The particle images were analyzed using a custom-written μPIV interrogation package described in Wereley and Meinhart (1998). Specifically, the images were analyzed using

- correlation averaging,
- background removal based on the minimum function, and
- central difference interrogation (CDI).

For the current experiment, twenty realizations were used because that was more than a sufficient number of realizations to give excellent signal, even with a first interrogation window measuring only 120 × 8 pixels. The high aspect ratio interrogation region was chosen to provide maximal spatial resolution in the wall normal or spanwise direction while sacrificing spatial resolution in the streamwise direction in where there are no velocity gradients at all. The signal-to-noise ratio resulting from these interrogation techniques was high enough that there were no erroneous velocity measurements. Consequently, no measurement validation post-processing was performed on the data after interrogation. The velocity field was smoothed using a 3 × 3 Gaussian kernel with a standard deviation of 1 grid spacing in both directions.

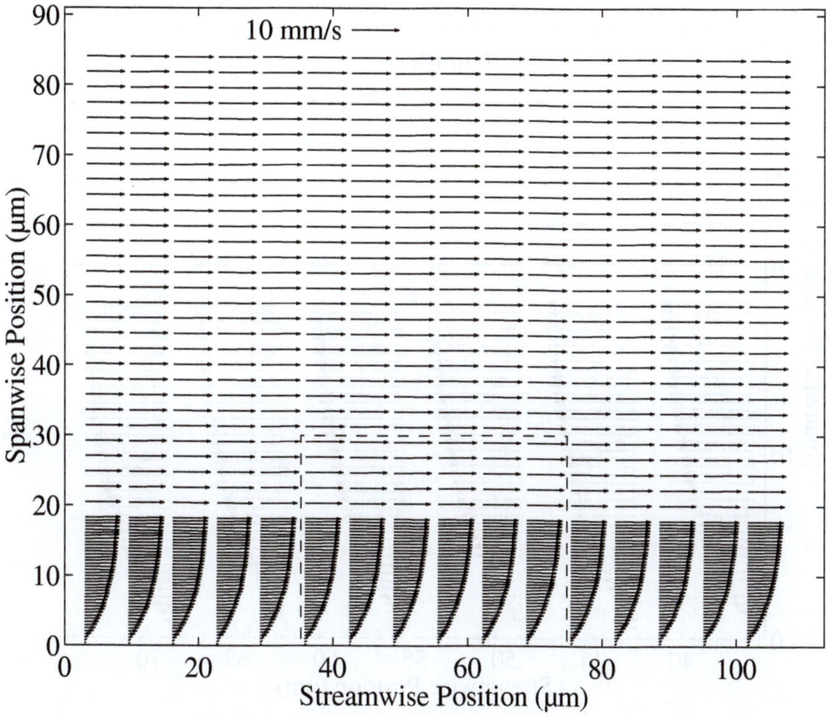

Fig. 2.12a. Large area view of ensemble-averaged velocity-vector field measured in a 30 μm deep × 300 μm wide × 25 mm channel. The spatial resolution, defined by the interrogation spot size of the first interrogation window, is 13.6 μm × 4.4 μm away from the wall, and 13.6 μm × 0.9 μm near the wall (Meinhart, et al., 1999b).

Figure 2.12a shows an ensemble-averaged velocity-vector field of the microchannel. The images were analyzed using a low spatial resolution away from the wall, where the velocity gradient is low, and using a high spatial resolution near the wall, where the wall-normal velocity gradient is largest. The interrogation spots were chosen to be longer in the streamwise direction than in the wall-normal direction. This allowed for a sufficient number of particle images to be captured in an interrogation spot, while providing the maximum possible spatial resolution in the wall-normal direction. The spatial resolution, defined by the size of the first interrogation window was 120 × 40 pixels in the region far from the wall, and 120 × 8 pixels near the wall. This corresponds to a spatial resolution of 13.6 μm × 4.4 μm and 13.6 μm × 0.9 μm, respectively. The interrogation spots were overlapped by 50% to extract the maximum possible amount of information for the chosen interrogation region size according to the Nyquist sampling criterion. Consequently, the velocity vector spacing in the wall-normal direction was 450 nm near the wall. The streamwise velocity profile was estimated by line-averaging the measured velocity data in the streamwise direction.

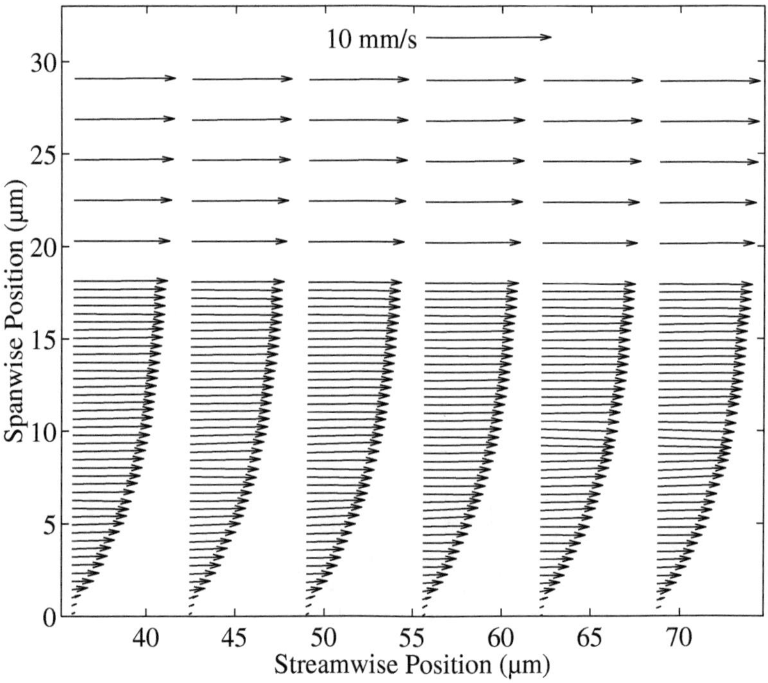

Fig. 2.12b. Near wall view of boxed region from Fig 2.12a (Meinhart, et al., 1999).

Figure 2.13 compares the streamwise velocity profile estimated from the PIV measurements (shown as symbols) to the analytical solution for laminar flow of a Newtonian fluid in a rectangular channel (shown as a solid curve). The agreement is within 2% of full-scale resolution. Hence, the accuracy of μPIV is at worst 2% of full-scale for these experimental conditions. The bulk flow rate of the analytical curve was determined by matching the free-stream velocity data away from the wall. The wall position of the analytical curve was determined by extrapolating the velocity profile to zero near the wall.

Since the microchannel flow was fully developed, the wall-normal component of the velocity vectors is expected to be close to zero. The average angle of inclination of the velocity field was found to be small, 0.0046 radians, suggesting that test section was slightly rotated in the plane of the CCD array relative to a row of pixels on the array. This rotation was corrected mathematically by rotating the coordinate system of the velocity field by 0.0046 radians. The position of the wall can be determined to within about 400 nm by direct observation of the image because of diffraction as well as the blurring of the out of focus parts of the wall.

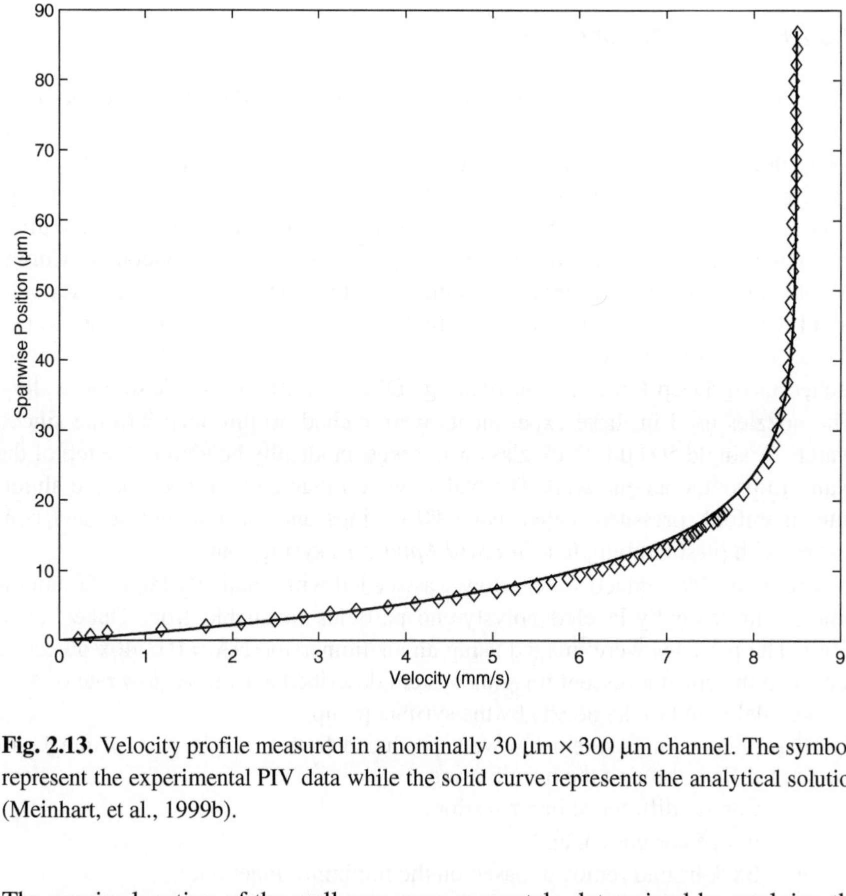

Fig. 2.13. Velocity profile measured in a nominally 30 μm × 300 μm channel. The symbols represent the experimental PIV data while the solid curve represents the analytical solution (Meinhart, et al., 1999b).

The precise location of the wall was more accurately determined by applying the no-slip boundary condition, which is expected to hold at these length scales for the combination of water flowing through glass, and extrapolating the velocity profile to zero at 16 different streamwise positions (see Fig. 2.12a). The location of the wall at every streamwise position agreed to within 8 nm of each other, suggesting that the wall is extremely flat, the optical system has little distortion, and the PIV measurements are very accurate. This technique is the precursor for the microfluidic nanoscope technique which will be explored in greater detail in Section 7.

Most PIV experiments have difficulty measuring velocity vectors very close to the wall. In many situations, hydrodynamic interactions between the particles and the wall prevent the particles from traveling close to the wall, or background reflections from the wall overshadow particle images. By using 200 nm diameter particles and epi-fluorescence to remove background reflections, we have been able to make accurate velocity measurements to within about 450 nm of the wall, see Fig. 2.11.

2.6.2 Flow in a Micronozzle

The flow in a 2-dimensional micronozzle provides a good challenge to the μPIV technique because of the presence of spatial velocity gradients as well as a relatively deep flow. These micronozzles were designed to be operated with supersonic gas flows. In the initial stages of this investigation however, they were operated with a liquid in order to assess the spatial resolution capabilities of the μPIV technique without having to push the temporal envelop simultaneously. Consequently the converging-diverging geometry of the micronozzle served as a very small venturi. The micronozzles were fabricated by Robert Bayt and Kenny Breuer (now at Brown University) at MIT in 1998. The 2-D nozzle contours were etched using Deep Reactive Ion Etching (DRIE) in 300 μm thick silicon wafers. The nozzles used in these experiments were etched 50 μm deep into the silicon wafer. A single 500 μm thick glass wafer was anodically bonded to the top of the wafer to provide an end wall. The wafers were mounted to a macroscopic aluminum manifold, pressure sealed using #0 O-rings and vacuum grease, and connected with plastic tubing to a *Harvard Apparatus* syringe pump.

The liquid (de-ionized water) flow was seeded with relatively large 700 nm diameter fluorescently-labeled polystyrene particles (available from Duke Scientific). The particles were imaged using an air-immersion NA = 0.6, 40x objective lens, and the epi-fluorescent imaging system described above. A flow rate of 4 ml hr^{-1} was delivered to the nozzle by the syringe pump.

These velocity measurements were produced from a single pair of images of the seeded flow through the nozzle using

- Central difference interrogation,
- Image correction, and
- Background removal, based on the minimum function.

Figure 2.14 is the velocity field inside a nozzle with a 15° half angle and a 28 μm throat. The velocity field was calculated using the central difference interrogation (CDI) technique with image overlapping (10 image pairs) and image correction, as explained above. The interrogation windows measured 64 × 32 pixels in the *x* and *y* directions, respectively. When projecting into the fluid, the correlation windows were 10.9 × 5.4 μm in the *x* and *y* directions, respectively. The interrogation spots were overlapped by 50% in accordance with the Nyquist criterion, yielding a velocity-vector spacing of 5.4 μm in the streamwise direction and 2.7 μm in the spanwise direction. The Reynolds number, based upon bulk velocity and throat width, is Re = 22.

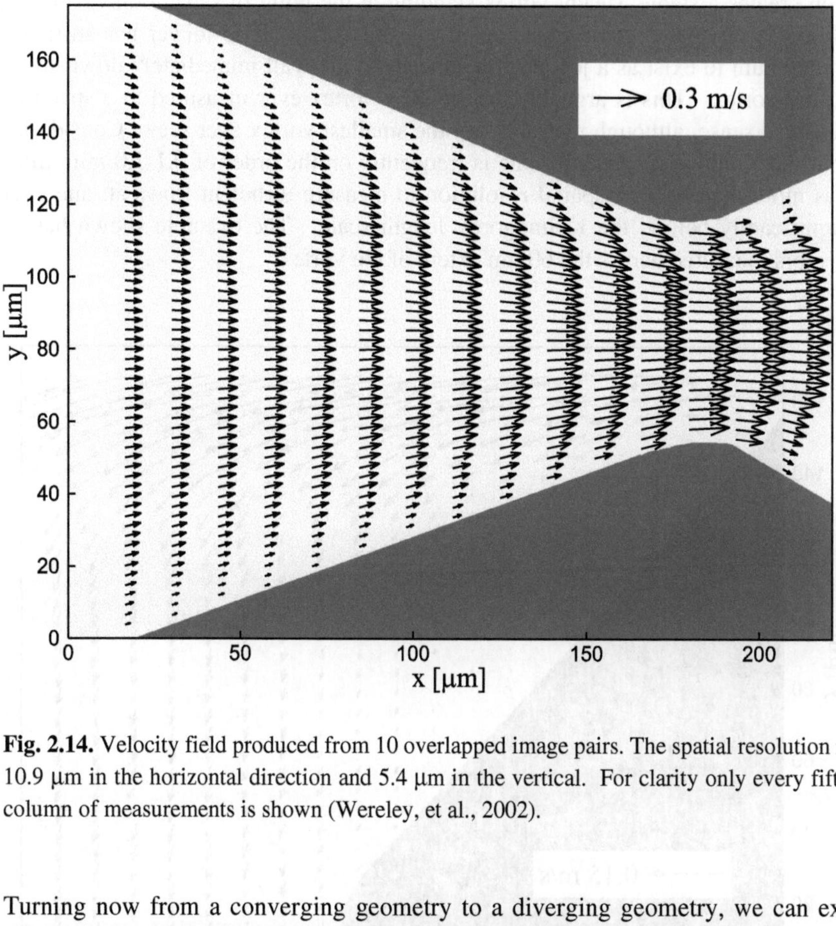

Fig. 2.14. Velocity field produced from 10 overlapped image pairs. The spatial resolution is 10.9 μm in the horizontal direction and 5.4 μm in the vertical. For clarity only every fifth column of measurements is shown (Wereley, et al., 2002).

Turning now from a converging geometry to a diverging geometry, we can explore whether instabilities well predicted by the Reynolds number at macroscopic length scales are indeed as well predicted by the Reynolds number at small length scales. The diffuser has a throat width of 28 μm and a thickness of 50 μm. The divergence half angle is quite large—40°. The expected behavior for this geometry would be that at low Reynolds number the flow would be entirely Stokes flow, i.e. no separation, but at larger Reynolds numbers where inertial effects become important, separation should appear. Indeed this is just what happens. At a Reynolds number of 22, the in the diverging section of the nozzle remains attached to the wall (not shown) while at a Reynolds number of 83, the flow separates as shown in Fig. 2.15a and Fig. 2.15b. These figures are based on a single pair of images and as such represent an instantaneous snapshot of the flow. Figure 2.15b is a close up view of the vortical region of the flow produced from the same velocity data used to produce Figure 2.15a. The interrogation region size measured 32×32 $pixels^2$ or 5.4×5.4 μm^2. A close inspection of Figure 2.15 reveals that the separation creates a stable, steady vortex standing at the point of separation. After the flow has dissipated some of its energy in the vortex, it no longer has sufficient momentum to exist as a jet and it reattaches to the wall immediately downstream of the vortex. This is arguably the smallest vortex ever measured in a spatially-resolved sense, although probably not the smallest vortex ever seen. Considering that the Kolmogorov length scale is frequently on the order of 0.1-1.0 mm, μPIV has more than enough spatial resolution to measure turbulent flows at, and even significantly below, the Kolmogorov length scale. The example shown has 25 vectors measured across the 60 μm extent of the vortex.

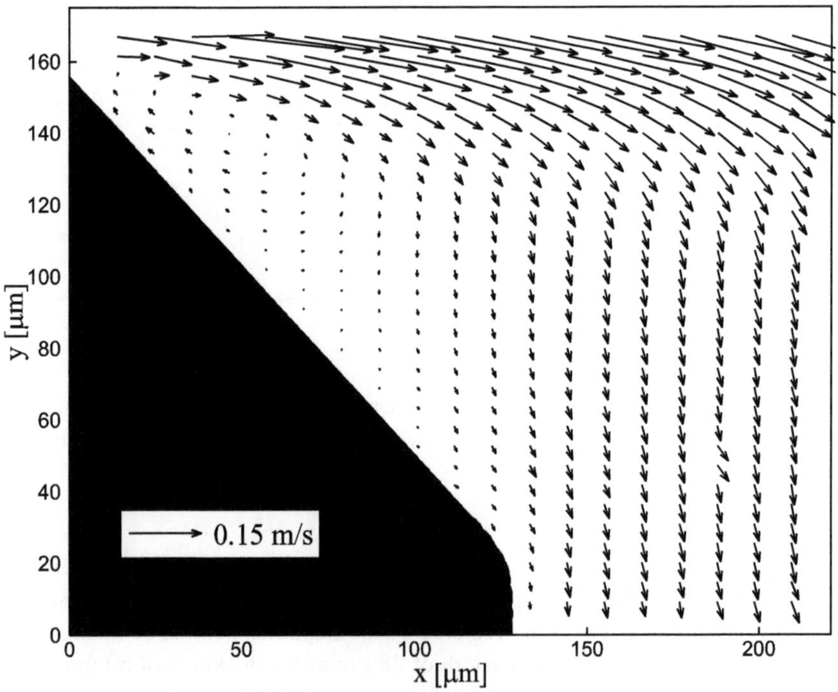

Fig. 2.15a. Recirculation regions in a microdiffuser with spatial resolution of 5.4×5.4 mm^2—only every fourth column and every second row shown for clarity (Wereley, et al., 2001).

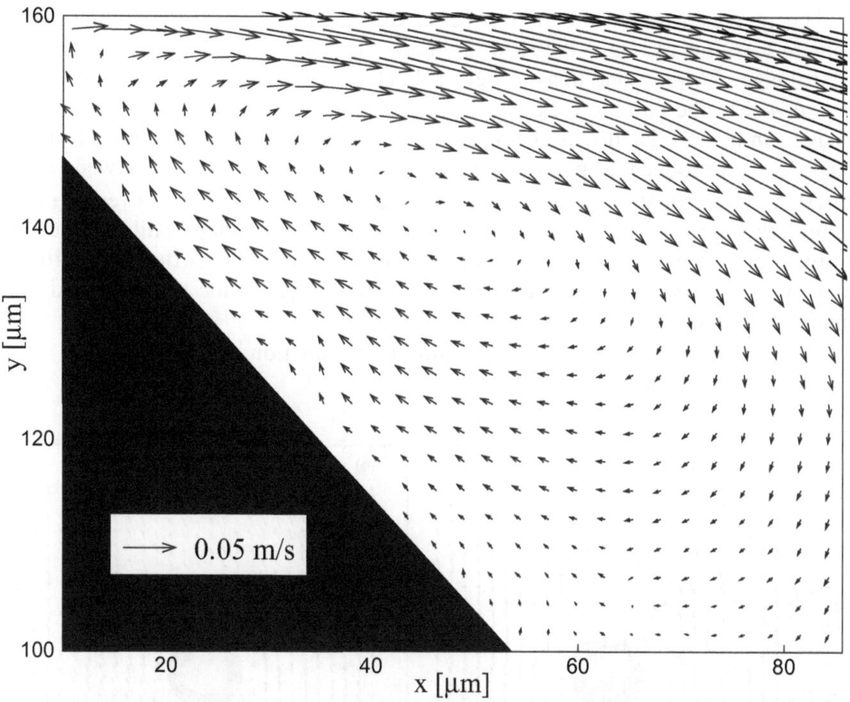

Fig. 2.15b. Recirculation regions in a microdiffuser with spatial resolution of 5.4 × 5.4 μm²—close up view of vortex region with all rows and columns of data shown (Wereley, et al., 2001).

2.6.3 Flow Around Blood Cell

A surface tension driven Hele-Shaw flow with a Reynolds number of 3 x 10^{-4} was developed by placing de-ionized water seeded with 300 *nm* diameter polystyrene particles between a 500 *μm* thick microscope slide and a 170 *μm* coverslip. Human red blood cells, obtained by auto-phlebotomy, were smeared onto a glass slide. The height of the liquid layer between the microscope slide and the coverslip was measured as approximately 4 μm by translating the microscope objective to focus on the glass surfaces immediately above and below the liquid layer. The translation stage of the microscope was adjusted until a single red blood cell was visible (using white light) in the center of the field of view. This type of flow was chosen because of its excellent optical access, ease of setup, and its 4 μm thickness, which minimized the contribution of out of focus seed particles to the background noise. Also, since red blood cells have a maximal tolerable shear stress, above which hemolysis occurs, this flow is potentially interesting to the biomedical community.

The images were recorded in a serial manner by opening the shutter of the camera for 2 ms to image the flow and then waiting 68.5 ms before acquiring the next image. Twenty-one images were collected in this manner. Since the camera is exposed to the particle reflections at the beginning of every video frame, each image can be correlated with the image following it. Consequently, the 21 images recorded can produce 20 pairs of images, each with the same time between exposures, Δt. Interrogation regions, sized 28×28 pixels, were spaced every 7 pixels in both the horizontal and vertical directions for a 75% overlap. Although technically, overlaps greater than 50% over sample the images, they effectively provide more velocity vectors to provide a better understanding of the velocity field. The images were interrogated using:

- Background removal with the minimum function and
- Correlation averaging

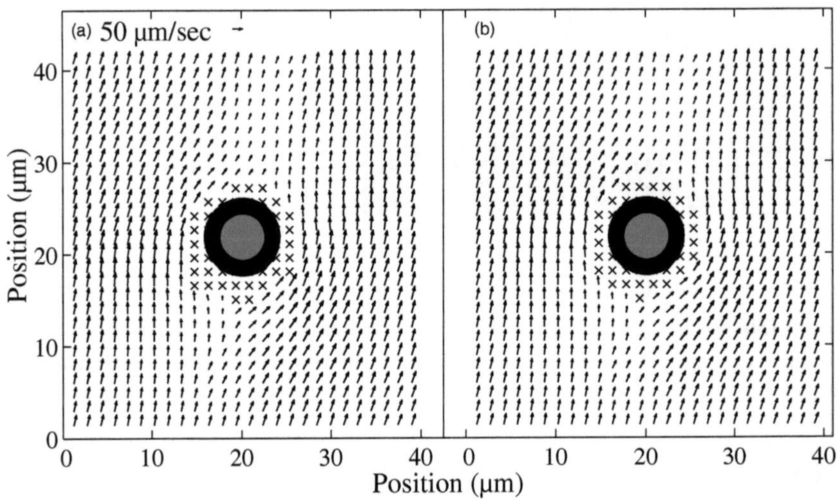

Fig. 2.16. Flow around a single human red blood cell. (a) forward difference adaptive window offset analysis; (b) central difference adaptive window offset analysis. Cross symbols (×) indicate points that cannot be interrogated because they are too close to the cell (Wereley and Meinhart, 2001).

Two velocity fields are shown in Fig. 2.16—the left figure (a) is the result of a forward difference interrogation and the right figure (b) is the result of a central difference interrogation. The differences between these two figures will be discussed below while the commonalities will be considered now. The flow exhibits the features that we expect from a Hele-Shaw flow. Because of the disparate length scales in a Hele-Shaw flow, with the thickness much smaller than the characteristic length and width of the flow, an ideal Hele-Shaw flow will closely resemble a 2-D potential flow (Batchelor, 1987). However, because a typical red blood cell is about 2 μm while the total height of the liquid layer between the slides is 4 μm, there is a possibility that some of the flow will go over the top of the cell instead of around it in a Hele-Shaw configuration. Since the velocity field in Fig. 2.16 closely resembles that of a potential flow around a right circular cylinder, we can conclude that the flow is primarily a Hele-Shaw flow. Far from the cylinder, the velocity field is uniformly directed upward and to the right at about a 75° angle from horizontal. On either side of the red blood cell, there are stagnation points where the velocity goes to zero. The velocity field is symmetric with respect to reflection in a plane normal to the page and passing through the stagnation points. The velocity field differs from potential flow in that near the red blood cell there is evidence of the no-slip velocity condition. These observations agree well with the theory of Hele-Shaw.

For both algorithms, measurement regions that resulted in more than 20% of the combined area of the first and second interrogation windows inside of the blood cell are eliminated and replaced with an 'x' symbol because they will tend to produce velocity measurements with serious errors. The CDI scheme is able to accurately measure velocities closer to the surface of the cell than is the FDI scheme. The CDI scheme has a total of 55 invalid measurement points, equivalent to 59.4 μm^2 of image area that cannot be interrogated, while the forward difference has 57 invalid measurement points or 61.6 μm^2. Although this difference of two measurement points may not seem significant, it amounts to the area that the FDI algorithm cannot interrogate being 3.7% larger than the area the CDI algorithm cannot interrogate. Furthermore, the distribution of the invalid points is significant. By carefully comparing Fig. 2.16a with Fig. 2.16b, it is apparent that the FDI has three more invalid measurement points upstream of the blood cell than does the CDI scheme while the CDI scheme has one more invalid point downstream of the blood cell. This difference in distribution of invalid points translates into the centroid of the invalid area being nearly twice as far from the center of the blood cell in the FDI case (0.66 μm or 7.85% of the cell diameter) versus the CDI case (0.34 μm or 4.05% of the cell diameter). This difference means that the FDI measurements are less symmetrically distributed around the blood cell than the CDI measurements are. In fact, they are biased toward the time the first image was recorded. Computing the average distance between the invalid measurement points and the surface of the blood cell indicates how closely to the blood cell surface each algorithm will allow the images to be accurately interrogated. On average the invalid measurement points bordering the red blood cell generated using the FDI scheme are 12% farther from the cell than the invalid measurement points generated with the CDI scheme. Consequently, the adaptive CDI algorithm is more symmetric than the adaptive FDI algorithm and also allows measuring the velocity field nearer the cell surface.

2.6.4 Flow in Microfluidic Biochip

Microfluidic biochips are microfabricated devices that are used for delivery, processing and analysis of biological species (molecules, cells, etc.). Gomez et al. (2001) successfully used μPIV to measure the flow in a microfluidic biochip for impedance spectroscopy of biological species. The biochip used for the PIV experiment is fabricated in a silicon wafer with a thickness of 450 μm. It has a series of rectangular cavities connected by channels with a depth of 12μm. The surface of the chip is covered with a piece of glass of about 0.2 mm thick, so that the images of seeded flows can be taken from the top. During the experiment, water-based suspensions of fluorescein-labeled latex beads with a mean diameter of 1.88 μm were injected into the biochip. The flow is illuminated with a constant intensity mercury lamp. Images are captured with a CCD camera through an epi-fluorescence microscope and recorded at a video rate (30Hz).

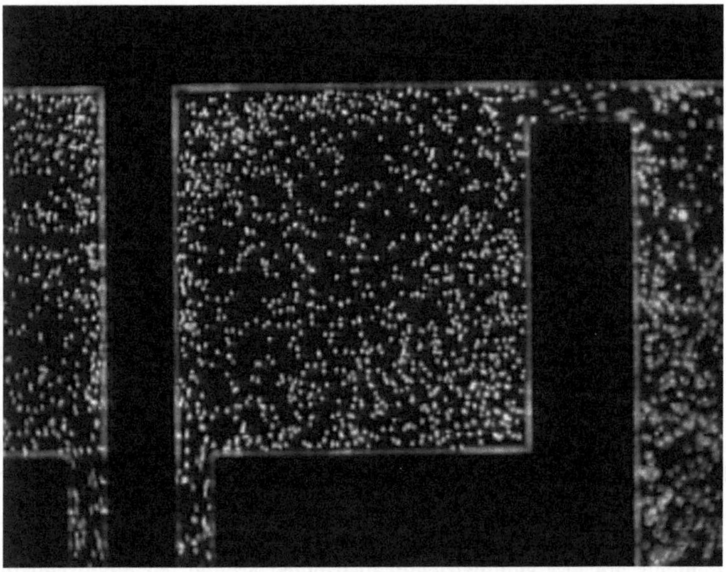

Fig. 2.17. Digital image of the seeded flow in the cavities and channels of the biochip (360×270 pixels, 542×406 μm^2)

One of the PIV images covering an area of 542×406 μm^2 on the chip with a digital resolution of 360×270 pixels is shown in Fig. 2.17. The flow in a rectangular cavity of the biochip is determined by evaluating more than 100 μPIV recording pairs with the ensemble correlation method, CDI and the image correction technique, and the results are given in Fig. 2.18. An interrogation window of 8×8 pixels is chosen for the PIV image evaluation, so that the corresponding spatial resolution is about 12×12 μm^2. The measured velocities in the cavity range from about 100 μm/s to 1600 μm/s.

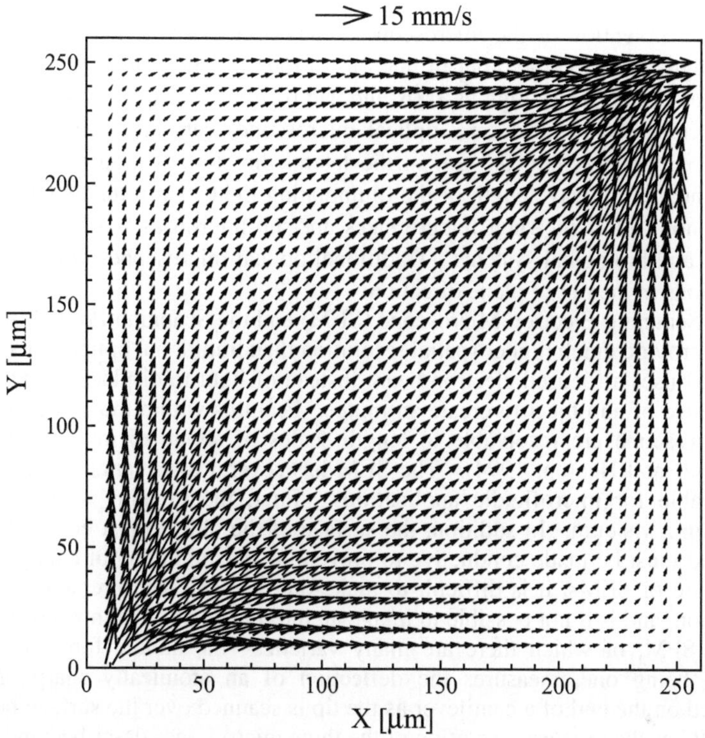

Fig. 2.18. PIV measurement results in a rectangular cavity of the biochip with a spatial resolution of 12×12 μm².

2.7 Extensions of the μPIV Technique

The μPIV technique is very versatile and can be extended in several meaningful ways to make different but related measurements of use in characterizing microflows. One extension involves turning the μPIV system into a high-resolution microscope, called a *microfluidic nanoscope* (Stone, et al., 2002), for probing the location of flow boundaries. Another extension, called micro-particle image thermometry, involves using the μPIV to measure fluid temperature in the same high spatial resolution sense as the velocity is measured. A third extension involves using a similar measurement technique but wavelengths longer than visual, the near infra-red, to measure flows completely encased in silicon—a real benefit in the MEMS field. These extensions will be discussed below.

2.7.1 Microfluidic Nanoscope

Since the invention of the microscope, it has been possible to visualize objects with length scales on the order of microns. Modern optical microscope objectives have magnifications as high as 100x and can be used where there is sufficient optical access. With some care, optical microscopes can have diffraction-limited resolutions approaching 0.5 μm in the lateral directions (Strausser and Heaton, 1994), nearly the wavelength of the illuminating light. Unfortunately this resolution is not sufficient when feature sizes are sub-micron as is the case in many MEMS and biological systems. Traditional optical microscopes have even lower resolutions in the out of plane direction.

The Scanning Electron Microscope (SEM) and the Scanning Probe Microscope (SPM) provide much higher spatial resolution than traditional optical microscopes. An SEM uses a focused electron beam instead of light to displace electrons from the surface of an object to create an image. Features within the plane of view of the microscope are resolvable to length scales of about ±5 nm with the SEM (Strausser and Heaton, 1994). The SEM has several disadvantages that make it undesirable for microfluidic applications. First, the imaging sample must be placed in a vacuum. In addition, the surface of the object must be highly reflective, and must be made conductive to prevent an accumulation of charge. Due to the nature of SEMs, it is difficult to make out-of-plane measurements with high resolution, and is it not possible to image an internal cavity within a device.

The SPM, of which there are many varieties—the atomic force microscope (AFM) being one, measures the deflection of an atomically sharp probe tip mounted on the end of a cantilever as the tip is scanned over the surface being imaged. It has the greatest resolution of the three microscopes described and also the slowest speed. Its resolution is typically ±0.1 to 1.0 nm in the x, y (in-plane) directions and ±0.01 nm in the z (out of plane) direction (Strausser and Heaton, 1994; Revenco and Proksch, 2000). The SPM is the only microscopy technique able to measure with nanometer accuracy in the z direction. The SPM and its derivatives suffer from two primary drawbacks: they have a small depth of focus and the surface must be exposed and accessible to the probe in order to be imaged.

The microfluidic nanoscope is a recent development (Stone, et al., 2002) for measuring the shape of internal cavities and flow channels with a spatial resolution of tens of nanometers. This new technique uses μPIV to measure the motion of fluid near a cavity wall. This information, combined with a model for the fluid's boundary condition, typically the no-slip boundary condition, can be used to determine the wall's location and topology.

The excellent spatial resolution of microfluidic nanoscope technique can be demonstrated by considering again the microchannel flow discussed in Section 2.6.5. By overlapping interrogation regions by 50%, the vector spacing in the spanwise and streamwise directions was 450 nm and 6.8 μm, respectively. In this manner, over 5000 time-averaged velocity measurements were obtained simultaneously, each representing a volume of fluid with dimensions of 0.9 × 13.6 × 1.8 μm. Figure 2.12b shows the velocity data nearest the wall for a 35 μm streamwise section of the microchannel. Careful inspection of the velocity vectors within 2 –

5 particle diameters (i.e. 400 – 1000 nm) of the wall reveals that they seem to be inclined away from the wall. These points must be treated as suspect because of the potential hydrodynamic interactions between the flow-tracing particles and the wall. These points are ignored in the following analysis.

Estimation of the Wall Position

The goal of this technique is to estimate the wall location as accurately as possible using the fluid velocity field. Since at these length scales we expect the fluid to behave as a continuum, it is reasonable to assume that the velocity field will vary continuously. As a further refinement on that assumption, it is also reasonable to assume that the fluid will behave according to the Stokes equation because of the low Reynolds number of this flow. Consequently, we will try to estimate the wall location using two different curve fits, one derived from the analytical solution for laminar flow in a rectangular cross section capillary (Section 2.6.1) and one that is based on a simple polynomial.

Analytical Fit

A velocity profile from the analytical solution of the channel flow was overlaid with steamwise-averaged μPIV velocity measurements (Fig. 2.13). The measured velocity vectors agree with the analytical solution to within 2%. Initial wall positions were estimated as the edge of the particle-image field. By visual inspection of the recorded images, these positions were well inside the channel wall, but were still used as a starting point for the following calculations. A discrete velocity profile was created from the analytical solution given in Equation (2.29) with velocity vectors spaced every nanometer in the spanwise direction. The experimentally measured velocity vectors were grouped into 16 spanwise profiles for the purpose of the fitting process. Each analytical profile was normalized by the average of the far field velocity of the measured profile. Since the wall estimation algorithm essentially matches variations in the measured data versus the variations in the analytical solution, only the region where the velocity profile varies rapidly (close to the wall) is examined. As a result, the mean square error between the analytical and the measured velocity vectors was estimated by averaging over each measurement location only within the nearest 16 μm of the wall for each velocity profile. The zero velocity position of the analytical solution was incremented relative to the experimental data by the resolution of the analytical data (in this case 1 nm) and a new mean square error was estimated. This process was repeated to determine the zero position that minimizes the mean square error, corresponding to the best agreement between the analytical solution and the measured velocity profile. Extrapolating to the location where the analytical solution goes to zero (assuming the no-slip condition) is an estimation of the location of the wall, averaged over the streamwise and out-of-plane resolution of the velocity measurements (13.6 x 1.8 μm in our case). In essence, the wall imparts information into the fluid velocity field in varying locations and wavenumbers via the momentum deficit near the wall.

The location and dynamics of the momentum deficit are directly related to the location of the no-slip boundary. Using this method the location of the microchannel wall was determined with an RMS error of 62 nm.

Second Order Polynomial Fit

Even though an analytical solution matches the streamwise-averaged data profile within 2% error, qualitatively the analytical solution fails to capture the trends of the measured profile very near the wall (Fig. 2.19a). In order to fit a more representative curve, a second order polynomial was fit to the experimental data at each location in the streamwise direction. The polynomial had the following form:

$$x = C_1 U^2 + C_2 U + C_3 \tag{2.31}$$

where x is the distance in the streamwise direction and C_1, C_2 and C_3 are constants. The velocity vectors ranging from 5 – 15 µm from the wall were used to fit the data at each streamwise location. The root of the 2nd order polynomial (where velocity is zero) was assumed to be the location of the wall. Qualitatively, the shape of the 2nd order polynomial corresponded more closely to the shape of the measured profile (Fig. 2.19b) than did the shape of the analytical solution (Fig. 2.19a). Figure 2.5 shows the sixteen velocity profiles of measured data (symbols) overlaying the 2nd order polynomial fit (solid line). The difference between the 2nd order polynomial and the fitted portion of the measured velocity profile was less than 0.1%. Assuming the wall to be flat, the wall position was measured to be flat with an RMS uncertainty of 62 nm. Figure 2.20 shows the results of the wall estimation algorithm versus position in the streamwise direction. Nearly all of the measurements agree to within ±100nm.

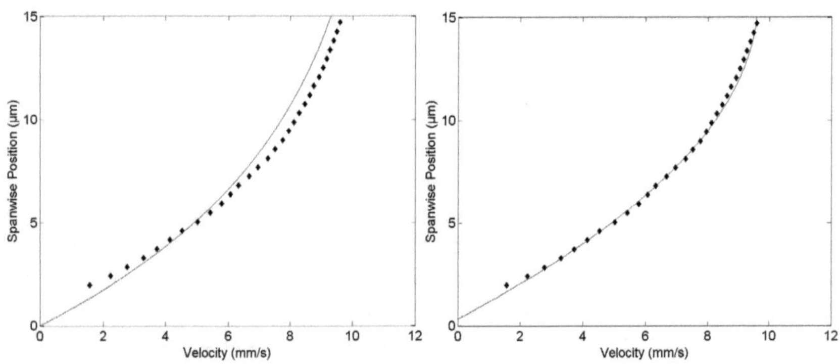

Fig. 2.19. Velocity measurements averaged in the streamwise direction (symbols) compared to (a) the analytical solution (solid curve) and (b) a second order polynomial fit to the velocity measurements (solid curve) (Stone, et al., 2002).

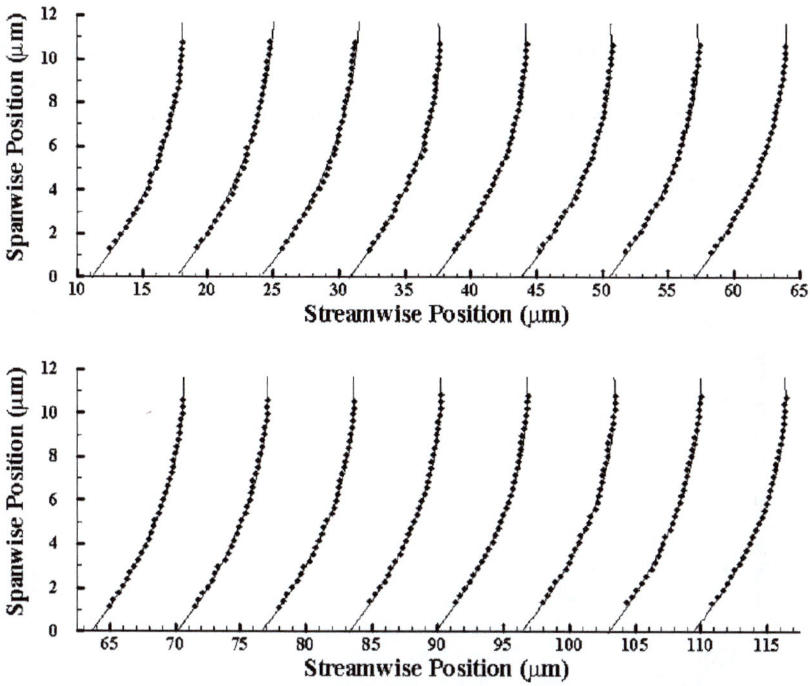

Fig. 2.20. Best-fit curve of the velocity profile (solid line) overlaying measured velocity data (black diamonds). The best-fit curve is a second order polynomial fit to the measured data. Extrapolating the best-fit curve to zero velocity gives an estimate of the location of the channel wall. Zero velocity occurs where the best-fit curve intersects the horizontal axis (Stone, et al., 2002).

Higher order polynomials, beyond 2nd order, were also explored. The higher order polynomials required more data points to be included in the fit, to obtain the same RMS uncertainty, and they often failed to agree qualitatively with the measured data. Near the wall, the higher order polynomials matched the measured velocity profiles quite well. However, in the flatter region away from the wall, the two curves did not agree.

Effect of Noise in Velocity Measurements

Numerical simulations were conducted to determine the effect that noise in the velocity measurements has upon the uncertainty of measuring wall position. A test data set was created by adding unbiased white noise to the analytical channel flow. The magnitude of the random component was a percentage of the magnitude of each velocity vector. The vector spacing was every 450 nm, corresponding to the resolution of the velocity measurements. A randomly prescribed offset was also added to the spanwise position of the test profile. The uncertainty in the wall position was defined as the difference between the actual specified wall position and the wall position determined by the second order polynomial fit. Figure 2.21 is a plot of the RMS uncertainty in estimated wall position versus the percentage error in the velocity measurements. The uncertainty in the wall position scales approximately linearly with the noise in the velocity data. An RMS uncertainty of 62 nm for the wall position of the microchannel corresponds to a noise level of 2.5% in the velocity measurements.

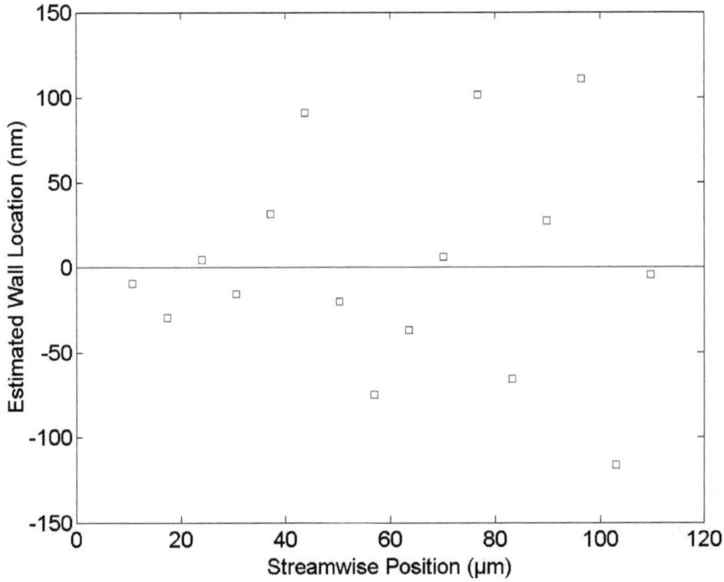

Fig. 2.21. Measurements of wall position by extrapolating the second order polynomial fit to the velocity field to zero. Assuming the wall is approximately flat, the root mean square uncertainty of the measurements is 62 nm (Stone, et al., 2002).

The surface roughness of the test section was assessed by scanning a line on the outside of one of the glass microchannels using a *Sloan* Dektak IIa profilometer. Since the glass microchannel was manufactured by an extrusion process, it was assumed that the inside wall roughness matches the outside wall roughness. The RMS uncertainty of the outside of the glass microchannel was 2.5 nm, which is well below the noise of the nanoscope. Therefore, for all practical purposes the walls are considered to be flat.

The nanoscope is capable of resolving lateral features of ± 62 nm RMS. The close velocity-vector spacing of 450 nm in the spanwise direction (which allows 62 nm resolution) comes at the cost of averaging over a large streamwise distance of 13.6 μm. Streamwise resolution can be improved by either choosing shorter interrogation regions, or by ensemble averaging the correlation function of more image pairs. While the nanoscope presented in this paper is one-dimensional, two-dimensional information can be obtained by varying the *y*-location of the measurement plane.

Hydrogels

There are several scientific and engineering problems that may be examined using the microfluidic-based nanoscope. In principle, the combination of hydrogels and the nanoscope may lead to a new type of chemical sensor. Hydrogels are cross-linked polymers that can undergo volume changes in response to physical and chemical changes in their environment (Kataoka, et al., 1998; Liu, et al., 2000; Osada and Ross-Murphy, 1993). The deformation of the hydrogel can be detected to within tens of nanometers using the μPIV technique. Hydrogel performance is a diffusion-limited process that is rate-limited by surface area. Consequently, macroscale applications of hydrogels have response times of hours to days (Kataoka, et al, 1998). However, the high surface to volume ratios found in microscale applications promote a dramatic decrease in the response time. Lui et al. (2000) reported a hydrogel-based microvalve with a closure time of 39 seconds, while Madou et al. (2000) found that by using micropores, the swelling time of poly (HEMA) hydrogel was approximately 3 minutes.

Olsen, et al., (2000) have reported developing a technique for measuring hydrogel deformation rate related to the microfluidic nanoscope. Since hydrogels are typically made from a liquid prepolymer mixture, fluorescent seed particles can easily be incorporated into this mixture in volume fractions from 0.1% to 1.0%. The prepolymer mixture is then formed into functional structures inside microfluidic channels as described by Beebe, et al. (2000). Since the hydrogel is relatively transparent at visual wavelengths, all the principles of the μPIV technique developed thus far should be applicable to these seed particles despite the fact that they are held fixed with respect to the hydrogel. Figure 2.22 demonstrates how the deformation rate can be measured μPIV. The hydrogel structure is represented by the cylinder in the center of the figure. It is anchored to the top and bottom planes of the figure which represent the top and bottom walls of a microchannel. The sides of the microchannel are not shown. The seed particles are represented as the small black circles distributed randomly throughout the hydrogel. As in the other μPIV apparatus describe here, the entire flow is volume illuminated by a microscope system (not shown) and imaged by the same system. The working distance of the microscope objective lens defines the focal plane of the measurement system which is shown as the gray plane in the vertical center of the microchannel. Deformations of the hydrogel in the focal plane are measured the same way movement of fluid is measured—by acquiring two images and cross correlating them. In the experiments described here, 1 μm seed particles are used in a volume concentration of 1%. The seed particles are illuminated by a Nd:YAG laser and recorded by a CCD camera. The magnification is chosen such that the interrogation regions represent 30 × 30 × 38 μm. The hydrogel, initially at its smallest size of about 400 μm in a solution of pH = 3.0, was immersed in a solution of pH = 12.0 and allowed to expand over the course of ten minutes. Using a relatively long time separation between the images of Δt = 1 second, maximum deformation rates of approximately 10 μm/sec were measured. This technique has the potential to provide important quantitative information about the response of hydrogels to their environment which could be used to optimize hydrogel shape or other properties. The same technique could be used to visualize the deformation of other flexible materials commonly used in microfabrication, such as polydimethylsiloxane (PDMS) and polymethylmethacrylate (PMMA).

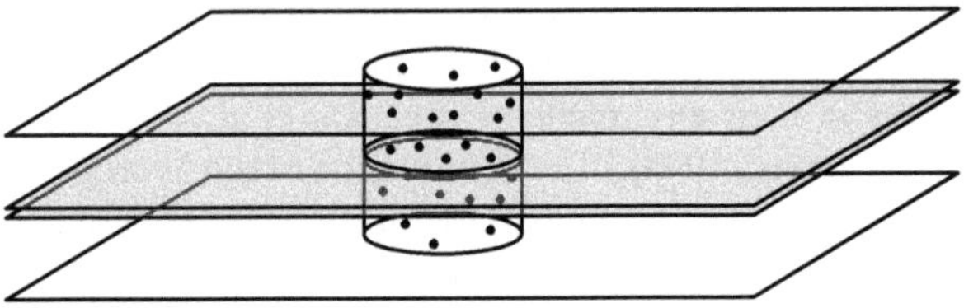

Fig. 2.22. Experimental configuration for measuring hydrogel deformation using µPIV (after Olsen, et al., 2000).

2.7.2 Micro-Particle Image Thermometry

The thermodynamic state of a flowing fluid can be specified by the temperature, pressure, and velocity of the flow, or, in the case of an incompressible fluid, merely the temperature and velocity. Consequently, the ability of a µPIV system to produce high-resolution velocity measurements naturally begins the search for methods that provide temperature measurements with the same high spatial resolution. The small scales of MEMS devices often make invasively probing a flow impractical, as even the smallest probe would likely be on the order of the size of the device itself. This condition puts minimally invasive measurement techniques, such as µPIV, at a premium.

Early literature on µPIV noted that for small seed-particles (<1 µm) and low speed flows (<1 mm/s) Brownian particle motion was measurable and could be significant enough to introduce considerable error into velocity measurements. Because it was viewed as an undesirable effect on velocity data, the effect of Brownian motion on the PIV correlation function—namely a width-wise spreading of the correlation peak which added to the uncertainty of locating the peak center—was often intentionally and substantially reduced through ensemble averaging over multiple images for a given flow field. However, Olsen and Adrian (2001) postulated that such spreading of the correlation peak could be used to deduce fluid temperature since Brownian motion has a direct, explicit temperature dependence (Hohreiter, et al., 2001). Furthermore, since peak location (which yields velocity information) and peak width are independent parameters it is conceivable that PIV may be used to simultaneously measure both temperature and velocity.

The following sections detail an experimental measurement of the temperature in a stagnant fluid and relate the variations in correlation peak broadening to variations in temperature. This technique is sensitive to both velocity and temperature at the same time—particle image velocimetry and thermometry (PIVT and µPIVT).

Theory of PIV-Based Thermometry

The theoretical basis for the hypothesis of the current work—that temperature measurements can be deduced from the images of individual particles in a flow—rests in the theory of particle diffusion due to Brownian motion. Constant random bombardment by fluid molecules results in a random displacement in the seed-particles. This random particle displacement will be superimposed on any particle displacement due to the fluid velocity. This phenomenon, previously discussed in Section 3, is described by

$$D = \frac{\kappa T}{3\pi\mu \mathrm{d}_{\mathrm{p}}} \tag{2.32}$$

where the diffusivity D of particles of diameter d_p immersed in a liquid of temperature T and dynamic viscosity μ. K is Boltzmann's constant. Noting the dimension of D is [length^2/time], the square of the expected distance traveled by a particle with diffusivity D in some time window Δt is given by

$$< s^2 > = 2D\Delta t \tag{2.33}$$

Combining Equations (2.32) and (2.33), it can be observed that an increase in fluid temperature, with all other factors held constant, will result in a greater expected particle displacement, $\sqrt{< s^2 >}$. However, dynamic viscosity, μ, is a strong function of temperature and $< s^2 > \propto T/\mu$. The effect of this relationship depends on the phase of the fluid. For a liquid, increasing temperature decreases absolute viscosity—so the overall effect on the ratio T/μ follows the change in T. For a gas, however, increasing temperature increases absolute viscosity meaning that the effect on T/μ, and hence $< s^2 >$, would need to be determined from fluid specific properties.

Relating changes in fluid temperature to changes in the magnitude of random seed-particle motion due to Brownian motion is the key to measuring temperature using PIV. To demonstrate the feasibility of using PIV for temperature measurement, an analytical model of how the peak width of the spatial cross-correlation varies with relative Brownian motion levels must be developed.

In a typical PIV experiment, two images are taken of the flow field at times t_1 and $t_2 = t_1 + \Delta t$. If these two images are denoted by $I_1(X)$ and $I_2(X)$, then the spatial cross-correlation can be estimated by the convolution integral (following Keane and Adrian, 1992)

$$R(\mathrm{s}) = \int I_1(\mathrm{X}) I_2(\mathrm{X} + \mathrm{s}) d\mathrm{X} \tag{2.34}$$

R(s) can be decomposed into three components, such that

$$\mathrm{R}(\mathbf{s}) = \mathrm{R_C}(\mathbf{s}) + \mathrm{R_F}(\mathbf{s}) + \mathrm{R_D}(\mathbf{s}) \tag{2.35}$$

where $R_C(\mathbf{s})$ is the convolution of the mean intensities of the two images and is a broad function of s with a diameter of the order of the interrogation spot diameter, $R_F(\mathbf{s})$ is the fluctuating noise component, and $R_D(\mathbf{s})$ is the displacement component of the correlation function, and as such gives the particle displacement from time t_1 to t_2. Thus $R_D(\mathbf{s})$ contains the information necessary to calculate the velocity vector, i.e., it is the PIV signal peak.

The displacement and width of the signal peak are dependent on the probability function $f(\mathbf{x}',t_2;\mathbf{x},t_1 \mid \mathbf{u}(\mathbf{x}),T)$ where f is the probability that a particle initially at $(\mathbf{x},t_1)$ moves into the volume $(\mathbf{x}',\mathbf{x}'+d\mathbf{x})$ at t_2 for a given velocity field $\mathbf{u}(\mathbf{x})$ and temperature T. Letting $\Delta\mathbf{x} = \mathbf{u}(\mathbf{x},t)\Delta t$ be the displacement undergone by a particle that was initially at $(\mathbf{x},t_1)$, in the absence of Brownian motion f is simply described by a delta function, i.e.,

$$f(\mathbf{x}',t_2;\mathbf{x},t_1 \mid \mathbf{u}(\mathbf{x}),T) = \delta(\mathbf{x}' - \mathbf{x} - \Delta\mathbf{x}) \tag{2.36}$$

because for a given velocity field, there is only one possible end location for the particle.

When Brownian motion is present, however, *any* displacement $\Delta\mathbf{x}$ is possible, and f will no longer be a delta function. Instead, f will have a probability distribution centered at $\mathbf{x}' = \mathbf{x} + \Delta\mathbf{x}$ with a shape defined by the space-time correlation for Brownian motion derived by Chandrasekhar (1941) (cf. Edwards et al., 1971)

$$f(\mathbf{x}',t_2;\mathbf{x},t_1 \mid \mathbf{u}(\mathbf{x}),T) = (4\pi D\Delta t)^{-3/2} \times exp\left(\frac{-(\mathbf{x}' - \mathbf{x} - \Delta\mathbf{x})^2}{4D\Delta t}\right) \tag{2.37}$$

This change in f due to Brownian motion has two effects on the signal peak: it broadens it and reduces its height. It is the broadening of the signal peak in the cross-correlation function that is the key to measuring temperature using PIV. This effect is demonstrated in Fig. 2.23 for a pair of experimental PIV images.

Olsen and Adrian (2001) derived analytical equations describing the shape and height of the cross-correlation function in the presence of Brownian motion for both light-sheet illumination and volume illumination (as is used in μPIV). In both cases the signal peak in the cross-correlation has a Gaussian shape with the peak located at the mean particle displacement.

One of the key differences between light-sheet PIV and μPIV (volume illumination PIV) lies in the images formed by the seed particles. In light-sheet PIV, if the depth of focus of the camera is set to be greater than the thickness of the laser sheet, then all of the particle images will (theoretically) have the same diameter and intensity. The relationship between a particle's actual cross-sectional area and that of its image will be governed by the characteristics of the imaging optics (Adrian, 1991). The image of a particle will be the convolution of two quantities: the geometric image of the particle and, given a diffraction-limited lens, the point response function of the imaging system. The point response function is an Airy function with diameter given by

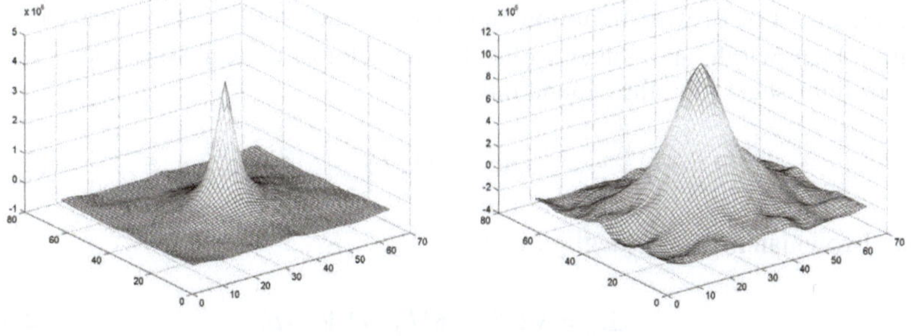

Fig. 2.23. A pair of correlation functions demonstrates possible variations in peak width. Note also that the height of the correlation peak reduces from 5×10⁶ to 1.2×10⁶ (Hohreiter, et al., 2001).

$$d_s = 2.44(1 + M)\, f^{\#} \lambda \quad (2.38)$$

where M is the magnification of the lens, $f^{\#}$ is the f-number of the lens, and λ is the wavelength of light reflected, scattered, or fluoresced by the particle. Adrian and Yao (1985) found that the Airy function can be approximated accurately by a Gaussian function. If both the geometric image and the point response function are approximated by Gaussian functions, the following approximate formula for particle image diameter is obtained

$$d_e = (M^2 d_p^{\,2} + d_s^2)^{1/2} \quad (2.39)$$

where d_p is the actual particle diameter and M is the magnification of the lens.

In μPIV, the particle images are a bit more complex. Because the entire volume of fluid is illuminated in μPIV, all of the particles throughout the depth of the flow field will contribute to the resulting PIV image. Those particles close to the focal plane will form sharp, bright images, while particles farther from the focal plane will form blurry, dim images. Olsen and Adrian (2001) found that the image formed by a particle in μPIV can be approximated by

$$d_e = (M^2 d_p^{\,2} + d_s^2 + d_z^2)^{1/2} \quad (2.40)$$

where

$$d_z = MzD_a \,/\, (x_o + z) \quad (2.41)$$

and z is the distance of the particle from the object plane, D_a is the aperture diameter of the microscope objective, and x_o is the object distance (typically, $x_o \gg z$, and the image diameter as a function of distance from the focal plane is a hyperbola).

From their analysis of cross-correlation PIV, Olsen and Adrian (2001) found that one effect of Brownian motion on cross-correlation PIV is to increase the correlation peak width, Δs_0—taken as the $1/e$ diameter of the Gaussian peak. For the case of light-sheet PIV, they found that

$$\Delta s_{0,a} = \sqrt{2} d_e / \beta \tag{2.42}$$

when Brownian motion is negligible, to

$$\Delta s_{0,c} = \sqrt{2}(d_e^{\,2} + 8M^2\beta^2 D\Delta t)^{1/2}/\beta. \tag{2.43}$$

when Brownian motion is a significant (note that in any experiment, even one with significant Brownian motion, $\Delta s_{0,a}$ can be determined by computing the autocorrelation of one of the PIV image pairs). It can be seen that Equation (2.43) reduces to Equation (2.42) in cases where Brownian motion is a negligible contributor to the measurement (i.e., when $D\Delta t \to 0$). The constant β is a parameter arising from the approximation of the Airy point-response function as a Gaussian function. Adrian and Yao (1985) found a best fit to occur for β^2=3.67.

For the case of volume illumination PIV, the equations for Δs_0 are a bit more complex. The equations have the same form, but because of the variation of d_e with distance from the focal plane, instead of being constants, the d_e terms in Equations (2.42) and (2.43) are replaced with integrals over the depth of the device.

The difficulty in calculating the integral term for d_e for volume illumination PIV can be avoided by strategic manipulation of Equations (2.42) and (2.43). Squaring both equations respectively, taking their difference, and multiplying by the quantity $\pi/4$ converts the individual peak width (peak diameter for a 3-D peak) expressions to the difference of two correlation peak areas—namely the difference in area between the auto- and cross-correlation peaks. Performing this operation and substituting Equation (2.32) in for D yields

$$\Delta A = \pi/4\ (\Delta s_{0,c}^{\ 2} - \Delta s_{0,a}^{\ 2}) = C_0\ (T/\mu)\ \Delta t \tag{2.44}$$

where C_0 is the parameter $2M^2K/3d_p$. The expected particle displacement, $\sqrt{<s^2>}$, of classical diffusion theory can now be tied to the peak width of the correlation function, Δs_0, or the change in peak area, ΔA, through the diffusivity, D.

Modeling

Before any measurements were made using the µPIV system, an experimental model and feasibility analysis were designed using simulated particle images and the cross-correlation PIV algorithm. The initial analysis allowed for the characterization of the algorithm's sensitivity to particle displacement and anticipate the likelihood that good experimental images would result in measurable trends.

The particle image simulation code starts with an n x n pixel black image (n indicating a user prescribed image size) and creates a number of white particles analogous in size and number density (particles / pixel area) to an expected experimental particle image. Particle placement within the image frame is set by uniformly distributed random-numbers assigned to x and y coordinates. This is done to simulate the actual random distribution of particle locations within an experimental image. The light intensity of the simulated particles is given a Gaussian distribution because a spherical particle image is a convolution of an Airy point-spread function and a geometric particle image–both of which are well-modeled as Gaussian functions.

After an initial particle image was generated, a random number generator (mean-zero, normal distribution) was used to impart a random shift to the x and y position of each particle. The particle shift routine was repeated several times, each time imparting a random shift from the previous particle positions, in order to produce an image set. These successive shifts approximated the spatial shifts that the experimental particles undergo between successive frames of video.

The simulated particle images were then cross-correlated and the trends in peak broadening and peak location observed. Assuming truly random shifts, it was expected that the average correlation would indicate a net-zero velocity. Furthermore, because the shifts were done in an additive fashion, a simulated sequence of images, 1-2-3, should yield an increase in peak-width from a correlation of 1-2 to a correlation of 1-3, and so on.

The major difference between the simulated images and experimental μPIV images is that the effects of out-of-focus particles are not present—out-of-focus particles negatively contribute to the image by varying the particle image size and luminous intensity, raising the signal-to-noise ratio, and ultimately affecting the correlation (Meinhart, et al., 1999a). However, Equation (2.44) demonstrates that these effects, which are present in both the auto-correlation and cross-correlation peak morphology, are removed from consideration by using the difference of the cross-correlation and auto-correlation peak widths to infer temperature. Therefore, even though the simulated images more closely approximate PIV images under light-sheet illumination than volume illumination, they should provide considerable insight into the volume-illumination case.

Experimental Technique

An Olympus BX50 system microscope with BX-FLA fluorescence light attachment (housing the dichroic mirror/prism and optical filter cube) was used to image the particle-laden solution. All experiments were carried out with a 50X objective (NA=0.8). A Cohu (model 4915-3000) 8-bit CCD video camera was used—the CCD array consisted of 768 (horizontal) × 494 (vertical) pixels and a total image area of 6.4 × 4.8 mm. The particles—700nm diameter polystyrene latex microspheres (Duke Scientific, Palo Alto, CA)—had a peak excitation wavelength at 542nm and peak emission at 612nm. A variable intensity halogen lamp was used for illumination—optical filters were used to isolate the wavelength bands most applicable to the particles—520-550nm for the incident illumination, and >580nm for the particle fluorescence.

In the experiments voltage supplied to a patch heater (see Fig. 2.24) was adjusted incrementally and several successive image of the random particle motion was captured at each of several temperature steps. At each temperature, the system was allowed 5 minutes to come to a steady temperature as recorded by a thermocouple. The gating between frames was fixed by the camera frame rate of 30 frames per second. In order to get numerical data, the individual frames were cross-correlated using a custom-written PIV interrogation code capable of out putting the correlation function. The first frame in each sequence was correlated with itself (i.e. autocorrelated) to provide a reference value of correlation peak width. Then the first frame was cross-correlated with the second frame, and then with the third, and the fourth, and so on—time between cross-correlated frames linearly increased. Each individual cross-correlation of such successive pairs of images produced one correlation peak (the average over each interrogation region peak). The width of each peak was recorded and trends, both temporal and thermal dependence, in the measurements of peak widths were observed. Temperatures from 20°C to 50°C were measured in this way.

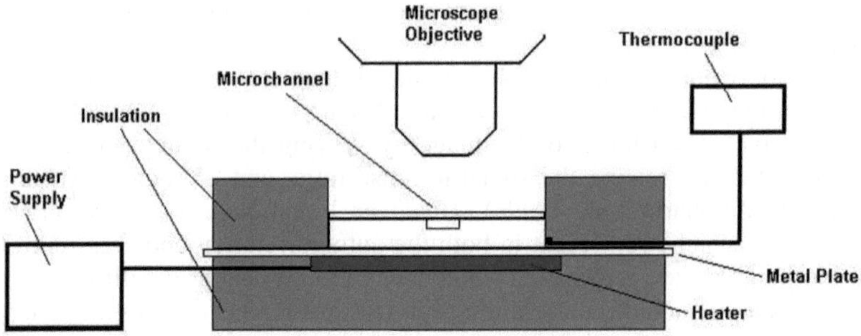

Fig. 2.24. Microchannel, heater, and thermocouple arrangement used for experimentation (Hohreiter, et al., 2001).

Results

The results of the simulated particle images are shown in Fig. 2.25 (left) while the experimental results are shown in Fig. 2.25 (right) for a certain fixed temperature. In both figures, the PIV-determined peak area data are plotted as the rhomboid symbols while the line is a best-fit linear profile. The salient feature of these two plots is that the area increase is very nearly proportional to time, as predicted by Equation (2.44). From a set of such figures, it is possible to extract a calibration constant representing the particle diameter, Boltzmann's constant, pi, etc. The quality of the linear fit gives an estimate of the uncertainty of the technique. The root-mean-squared (RMS) difference between experimental and theoretical values of peak area increase (at each data point) was taken for many such curves. This RMS difference in square-pixels was converted to an equivalent temperature difference, which is the nominal value of temperature resolution given above. The average error over all the test cases is about ± 3°C. By combining many such data sets, the temperature at many different values can be assessed and compared to the thermocouple measurements, as in Fig. 2.26.

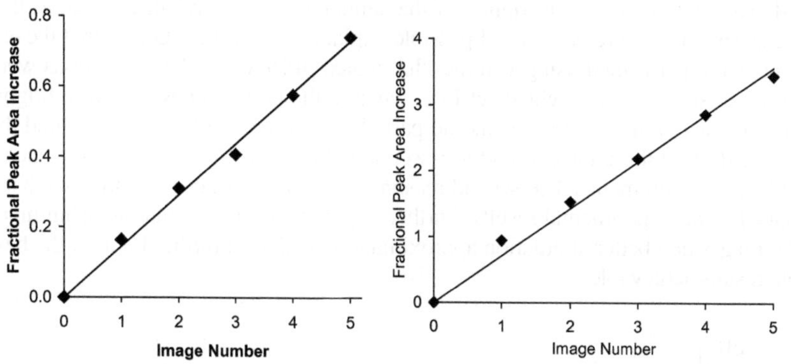

Fig. 2.25. Measured versus theoretical peak broadening trend for particle diffusion in simulated images (left) and actual experimental images (right) (After Hohreiter, et al., 2001).

Experimental Uncertainty

To examine the uncertainty of the temperature measurement technique, the root-mean-squared (RMS) difference between experimental and theoretical values of peak area increase (at each data point) was computed for a wide range of operating conditions. This RMS difference in square-pixels was converted to an equivalent temperature difference, which is the nominal value of temperature resolution given above. The average error over all the test cases is about ± 3°C.

To explore further the uncertainty of the measurements, Equation (2.44) will be used in a standard uncertainty analysis to find

$$\delta T = \pm T \cdot \left[1 - \frac{T}{\mu}\frac{d\mu}{dT}\right]^{-1} \cdot \sqrt{\left(\frac{\delta(\Delta A)}{\Delta A}\right)^2 + \left(2\frac{\delta M}{M}\right)^2 + \left(\frac{\delta(\Delta t)}{\Delta t}\right)^2 + \left(\frac{\delta d_p}{d_p}\right)^2} \qquad (2.45)$$

The one unusual result in this uncertainty calculation is the term raised to the negative one power that comes from the temperature dependence of the viscosity combined with the assumption that the viscosity is a known property of the fluid dependent only on the temperature. The values of the parameters in Equation (2.44) used in the current work can by substituted into Equation (2.44) to find the expected accuracy of the technique. At this stage we will assume that the particles are mono-disperse (δd_p=0), that the laser pulse separation is exactly known ($\delta(\Delta t)$=0), and that the magnification of the microscope is exactly known (δM=0). These assumptions are reasonable because the uncertainty in the area difference $\delta(\Delta A)$ dominates the right hand side of Equation (2.44). As an estimate of the uncertainty in area difference $\delta(\Delta A)$, we can use the standard error between the data points and the curve fits in Fig. 2.25. For the simulations, $\delta(\Delta A)$=0.95 pixels^2 and ΔA=42 pixels^2 while for the experiments, $\delta(\Delta A)$=5.0 pixels^2 and ΔA=126 pixels^2. Using these values we can plot in Fig. 2.27 the expected uncertainty of the measurements and simulations over the range for which water is normally a liquid. The measurement uncertainty of the simulations is about half as large as that of the experiments. There are several possible explanations for this. One is that the experiments were performed using volume-illuminated µPIV while the simulations were done more in keeping with light sheet PIV, wherein the particles have uniform brightness and size within the light sheet and no particles are visible in front of or behind the light sheet. Both of these factors tend to lower signal-to-noise ratio and raise the uncertainty of the measurements. The second reason is that the statistics may not have been stationary for the experimental results. Further experiments and simulation using more particle images and better simulation approximations will shed further light on the best possible results achievable.

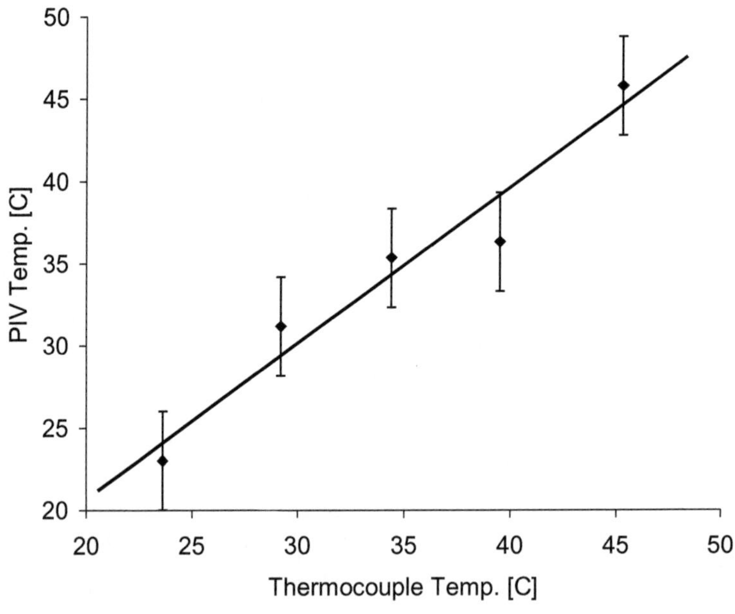

Fig. 2.26. Temperature inferred from PIV measurements plotted versus thermocouple-measured temperature. Error bars indicate the range of average experimental uncertainty, ± 3°C (After Hohreiter, et al., 2001).

Simultaneous Velocity and Temperature Measurement

In the introduction section of this work, the potential for the simultaneous measurement of both velocity and temperature was noted. While it is true that all experimental measurements reported in the current work were made using fluids with a net-zero velocity, it is also true that the correlation peak location (from which the velocity measurement is derived) and the correlation peak width (which yields the temperature measurement) are independent measurements whose convolution results in the correlation function. Therefore, it is not mere speculation to say that the two may be simultaneously measured. The key is finding the range of flow parameters over which both may be measured. The following analysis, based on the results of this work, establishes a range over which both velocity and temperature may be measured using PIV.

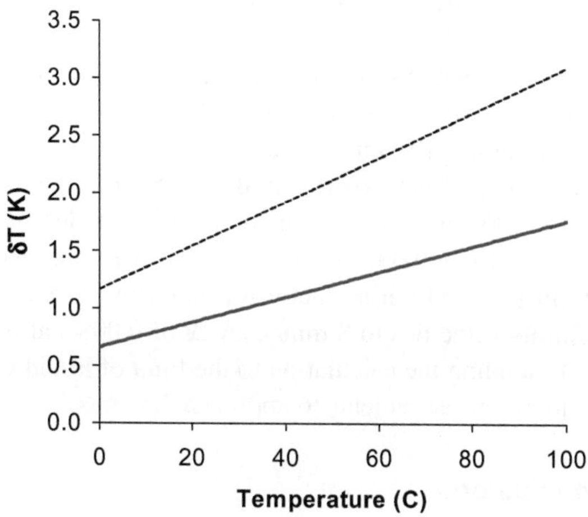

Fig. 2.27. Measurement uncertainty over the range of temperatures for which water is a liquid (After Hohreiter, et al., 2001).

For a control surface, take a standard *n x n* pixel interrogation region (IR) in a larger image of a particle-seeded fluid at some temperature *T* and some steady, bulk velocity *V*. A set of images is recorded—with some time delay between each image—for the purposes of measuring *T* and *V*. The time delay, Δt, must satisfy two criteria: (a) it needs to be sufficiently long to allow measurable particle motion to take place, yet (b) short enough that a significant fraction of the particles in the first image also be present in the second. The former criterion is imposed by Brownian particle motion, the latter by bulk fluid motion.

The first criterion establishes a minimum Δt and requires that particles move beyond a measurable threshold—a property of the optical system—in order to be accurately resolved. With a precision micrometer and stationary fluorescing particles (dried onto a microscope slide) under the experimental (50X) microscope objective, the threshold of the current system was found to be about 100 nm.

The second criterion establishes a maximum Δt and requires that particles not leave the interrogation region between frames. While there are two possible ways a particle can leave an IR—either by convection, following a streamline of the flow or by diffusion, following a Brownian path—for bulk flows with velocities greater than 10 μm/s (using particles on the order of 100 nm), bulk motion will dominate diffusion in violating the second criterion. Furthermore, judicious window shifting can allow particles to move a distance bounded only the size of the CCD array—much farther than the size of an interrogation region, which is the bound that exists without a window shifting scheme.

Combining these two constraints yields

$$\sqrt{< s^2 >} = (KT\Delta t / 3\pi\mu d)^{1/2} \tag{2.46}$$

which gives the average particle displacement due to Brownian motion in terms of experimental parameters. This value is bounded below by the measurement threshold of the system, about 100 nm, and above by the size of the CCD. Constraining the analysis to the current experimental parameters—the minimum Δt required to get a $\sqrt{<s^2>}=100$ nm, for 700 nm diameter particles in liquid water, ranges from 0.016 s for 20°C to 0.008 s for 50°C. Furthermore, using the size of the CCD array (6.4 mm) as the limiting factor for bulk flow, a Δt of 0.016 s under 50X magnification limits velocities to 8 mm/s. A Δt of 0.008 s allows for velocities up to 16 mm/s. Extending the calculation to the limit of liquid water, a 100°C pool would allow velocity measurements to approach 3.5 cm/s.

Thermometry Conclusions

The random component of Brownian particle motion is directly related to the temperature of a fluid through the self-diffusion mechanism. Changes in fluid temperature result in changes in the magnitude of Brownian particle motions. Such fluctuations can be detected by analyzing a spatial cross-correlation of successive particle images.

A cross-correlation PIV algorithm provides a reliable spatial cross-correlation. Where standard PIV looks at correlation peak location to measure velocity, PIV thermometry focuses on changes in correlation peak area—the cross-sectional peak area being a measure of the average magnitude of Brownian motion. Experimentally, temperatures were measured for zero-velocity pools of particle-seeded water over the range 20-50 °C using a cross-correlation PIV system. Results for experimentally measured temperatures, when compared with thermocouple-measured temperatures, agreed within a range of ±3°C.

Experimental error for PIV thermometry is tied closely to the optical resolution of the PIV system being used—the higher the optical resolution the more accurately fluid temperatures can be measured using this technique. Increasing optical resolution also has effects on the potential for PIV to simultaneously measure both velocity and temperature. The results of the current work indicate that, using water as the fluid, measurements of fluid velocity less than or equal to 8 mm/s can be made while simultaneously measuring temperatures greater than 20°C.

2.7.3 Infrared μPIV

Another recent extension of μPIV that has potential to benefit microfluidics research in general and silicon MEMS research in particular is that of IR-PIV (Han, et al., 2004). The main difference between the established technique of μPIV and IR-PIV is the wavelength of the illumination which is increased from visible wavelengths to infrared wavelengths to take advantage of Silicon's relative transparency at IR wavelengths. While this difference may seem trivial, it requires several important changes to the technique while enabling several important new types of measurements to be made.

Differences Between μPIV and IR-PIV

The fluorescent particles that allow the use of epi-flourescent microscopes for μPIV are not available with both absorption and emission bands at infrared wavelengths (Han, et al., 2004). Consequently elastic scattering must be used in which the illuminating light is scattered directly by the seed particles with no change in wavelength. Using this mode of imaging, it is not possible to separate the images of the particles from that of the background using colored barrier filters as in the μPIV case. The intensity of elastic scattering intensity I of a small particle of diameter d varies according to

$$I \propto \frac{d^6}{\lambda^4} \tag{2.47}$$

where λ is the wavelength of the illuminating light. Thus a great price is exacted for imaging small particles with long wavelengths. The main implication of Equation (2.47) is that there is a trade off between using longer wavelengths where Silicon is more transparent and using shorter wavelengths where the elastic scattering is more efficient. Typically infrared cameras are also more efficient at longer wavelengths. Han, et al. (2004) found a good compromise among these competing factors by using 1 μm polystyrene particles and an illumination wavelength of $\lambda = 1200$ nm.

An experimental apparatus suitable for making IR-PIV measurements is described by Han, et al. (2004) and is shown in Fig. 2.28. As with μPIV, a dual-headed Nd:YAG laser is used to illuminate the particles. However in this case, the 532 nm laser light is used to drive an Opto-Parametric Oscillator (OPO)—a nonlinear crystal system that transforms the 532 nm light into any wavelength between 300 nm and 2000 nm. The laser light retains its short pulse duration when passing through the OPO. The output of the OPO is delivered via fiber optics to the microfluidic system being investigated. Han, et al. (2004) use an off-axis beam delivery, as shown in Fig. 2.28, with an angle of 65° between the surface normal of the device and the axis of the beam. Alternatively, dark field illumination could be used. The light scattered by the particles is collected by a Mititoyo near infrared (NIR) microscope objective (50×, *NA*=0.42) mounted on a 200 mm microscope tube and delivered to a Indigo Systems Indium Gallium Arsenide (InGaAs) NIR camera. The camera has a 320×256 pixel array with 30 μm pixels—a relatively small number of relatively large pixels compared to the high resolution cameras typically used for μPIV applications. The NIR is a video rate camera which cannot be triggered, meaning that the PIV technique needs to be modified slightly. Instead of using the computer as the master for the PIV system, the camera is the master, running at its fixed frequency of 60 Hz. The laser pulses are synchronized to the video sync pulses generated by the camera and can by programmed to occur at any point within a video frame. For high speed measurements a process called frame straddling is used in which the first laser pulse is timed to occur at the very end of one frame and the second laser pulse is timed to occur at the very beginning of the next video frame. Using the frame straddling technique the time between images can be reduced to as little as 0.12 ms—suitable for measuring velocities on the order of cm/s. Higher speed flows can be measured by recording the images from both laser pulses on a single video frame. The SNR of the double exposed images is decreased somewhat when compared to the single exposed images but flows on the order of hundreds of meters per second can be measured with the double exposed technique.

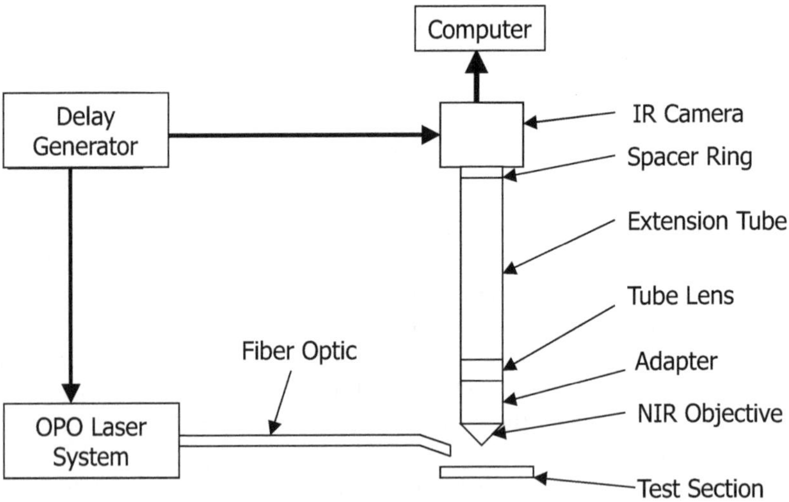

Fig. 2.28. Schematic of the experimental apparatus for IR-PIV (after Han, et al., 2004).

Han, et al. (2004) demonstrated their system on a flow through a silicon micronozzle constructed using deep reactive ion etching (DRIE). The nozzle was 300 μm deep into a 500 μm thick silicon wafer. The nozzle was sealed by fusion bonding a second, planar silicon wafer to the wafer with the nozzle geometry. The nozzle, shown in Fig. 2.29 had a 40 μm throat width. The measurements were made downstream of the throat in an area where the nozzle had expanded to 1000 μm wide. For the initial experiments, Han, et al. (2004) measured a water flow through the nozzle. The flow tracing particles were 1 μm polystyrene particles with a refractive index of 1.56 at 589 nm. These particles, combined with the imaging system, produce images on the CCD array of 181 μm in diameter. This value would be prohibitively large for a visual wavelength CCD imager—which typically have pixels of 6 to 8 μm. Fortunately, pixels in IR imagers tend to be larger—on the order of 30 μm and so the particle images are only 6 pixels across instead of 30 pixels across. Han, et al. (2004) successfully made measurements in two regions of the nozzle—a high speed region with flow on the order of 3 cm/s and a low speed region with flow on the order of 50 μm/s. These regions are labeled 'Hi' and 'Lo' in Fig. 2.29. Although this technique is still being developed, it shows great promise for making measurements inside devices that would otherwise be inaccessible.

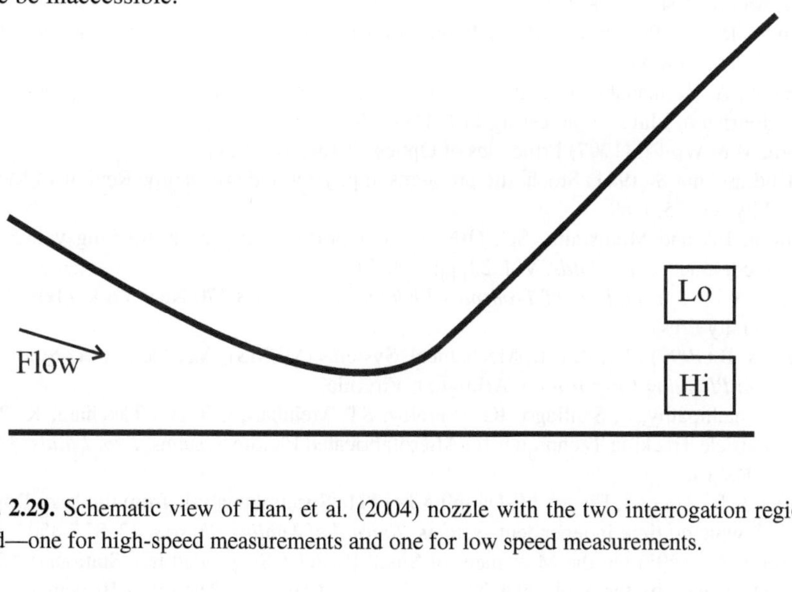

Fig. 2.29. Schematic view of Han, et al. (2004) nozzle with the two interrogation regions used—one for high-speed measurements and one for low speed measurements.

2.8 Conclusions

Currently, μPIV is able to deliver thin 2-D planes of velocity measurements that can be scanned in the 3rd dimension to construct 2-component, 3-dimensional velocity measurements within a volume. By applying the advanced experimental and analytical techniques outlined in this chapter, the maximum spatial resolution of the μPIV technique stands at approximately 1 μm. By using smaller seed particles that fluoresce at shorter wavelengths, this limit could be reduced by a factor of 2 to 4. This lower limit of approximately 250 nm should be regarded as a hard limit for correlation-based PIV using visual wavelength light. Higher spatial resolutions could still be obtained by adding a particle tracking step after the correlation-based PIV. Spatial resolutions an order of magnitude smaller could then reasonably be reached.

References

Adrian RJ (1991) Particle-imaging techniques for experimental fluid mechanics. *Annual Review of Fluid Mechanics*, 23, 261-304

Adrian RJ, Yao CS (1985) Pulsed laser technique application to liquid and gaseous flows and the scattering power of seed materials. *Applied Optics*, 24, 44-52

Batchelor, GK, (1987), An introduction to fluid dynamics, *Cambridge University Press.*

Beebe, DJ, Moore, JS, Bauer, JM, Yu, Q, Liu, RH, Devadoss, C, and Jo, BH (2000) Functional hydrogel structures for autonomous flow control inside microfluidic channels. Nature, 404, 588-590.

Bendat JS and Piersol JG (1986) Random data : analysis and measurement procedures. Wiley, New York

Beskok, A, Karniadakis, GE, and Trimmer, W (1996). "Rarefaction and Compressibility." Journal of Fluids Engineering **118**: 448-456.

Born, M & Wolf E (1997) Principles of Optics. *Pergamon Press.*

Chandrasekhar S (1941) Stochastic problems in physics and astronomy. Review of Modern Physics, 15, 1-89

Cowen, EA and Monismith, SG, (1997), 'A hybrid digital particle tracking velocimetry technique,' *Exp. Fluids*, Vol. 22, pp. 199-211.

Deen, W (1998) *Analysis of Transport Phenomena.* pp. 268-270 New York, Oxford University Press.

Detlefs, B (1999) MicroElectroMechanical Systems (MEMS), An SPC Market Study, *System Planning Corporation*, Arlington, Virginia.

Devasenathipathy, S, Santiago, JG, Wereley, ST, Meinhart, CD, and Takehara, K (2003) Particle Tracking Techniques for Microfabricated Fluidic Systems. *Exp. Fluids*, 34: pp. 504-514.

Edwards R, Angus J, French M, Dunning J (1971) Spectral analysis from the laser Doppler flowmeter: time-independent systems. *Journal of Applied Physics*, 42, 837-850

Einstein A. (1905) On the Movement of Small Particles Suspended in a Stationary Liquid Demanded by the Molecular-Kinetic Theory of Heat. In: Theory of Brownian Movement. Dover Publications, Inc, New York, pp. 1-18

Gad-el-Hak M (1999) The Fluid Mechanics of Microdevices – The Freeman Scholar Lecture, *J. Fluids. Eng.* 121, pp. 5-33.

Gomez, R., Bashir, R., Sarakaya, A., Ladisch, M.R., Sturgis, J., Robinson, J.P., Geng, T., Bhunia, A.K., Apple, H.L., and Wereley, S.T., "Microfluidic Biochip for Impedance Spectroscopy of Biological Species," *Biomedical Microdevices*, Vol. 3, No. 3, 201-209 (2001).

Gui L, Merzkirch W, Shu JZ 1997, Evaluation of low image density PIV recordings with the MQD method and application to the flow in a liquid bridge. *J. Flow Vis. and Image Proc.*, Vol. 4, No. 4, pp. 333-343

Han, GX., Bird, JC, Westin, JK, Cao, ZQ, and Breuer, KS (2004) Infrared Diagnostics for measuring fluid and solid motion inside silicon microdevices. *Microscale Thermophysical Engineering*, 8, p 169-182

Hohreiter, V, Wereley, ST, Olsen, MG, Chung, JN, (2002) Cross-correlation analysis for temperature measurement *Meas. Sci. Technol.* 13, pp. 1072-1078.

Inoué, S & Spring, KR (1997) Video Microscopy, Second Edition, *Plenum Press.*

Kataoka, K., Miyazaki, H., Bunya, M., Okano, T. and Sakurai, Y. (1998) Totally Synthetic Polymer Gels Responding to External Glucose Concentration: Their Preparation and Application to On-Of Regulation of Insulin Release. *J. Am. Chem. Soc.*, **120**: 12694-5.

Keane RD, Adrian RJ (1992) Theory of cross-correlation analysis of PIV images. *Applied Scientific Research*, 49, 1-27

Koutsiaris, AG, Mathioslakis, DS & Tsangaris, S (1999) Microscope PIV for velocity-field measurement of particle suspensions flowing inside class capillaries, *Meas. Sci. Technol.* 10, pp. 1037-1046.

Liu, R, Yu, Q, Bauer, JM, Jo, BH, Moore, JS and Beebe, DJ (2000) In-channel processing to create autonomous hydrogel microvalves. In: *Micro Total Analysis Systems 2000*, (ed. A. van den Berg et al.) pp. 45-48, Netherlands: Kluwer Academic.

Madou, M He, K and Shenderova, A (2000) Fabrication of artificial muscle based valves for controlled drug delivery. In: *Micro Total Analysis Systems 2000*, (ed. A. van den Berg et al.) pp. 147-150, Netherlands: Kluwer Academic.

Meinhart CD & Zhang HS (2000) The flow structure inside a microfabricated inkjet printhead. *Journal of MEMS* Vol. 9, (no.1) IEEE March 2000, pp. 67-75.

Meinhart CD, Gray MHB, Wereley ST (1999a), PIV Measurements of High-speed flows in Silicon-micromachined nozzles, (AIAA/ASME/SAE/ASEE Joint Propulsion Conference and Exhibit, 35th, Los Angeles, CA, June 20-24, 1999) AIAA-99-3756

Meinhart CD, Wereley ST & Santiago JG (1999b) PIV Measurements of a Microchannel Flow. *Exp. in Fluids*, Vol. 27, pp. 414-419.

Meinhart CD, Wereley ST, Santiago JG (2000), A PIV algorithm for estimating time-averaged velocity fields, *Journal of Fluids Engineering*, Vol. 122, 285-289

Melling, A (1986). Seeding Gas Flows for Laser Anemometry**:** 8.1-8.11.

Olsen, MG, Bauer, JM, and Beebe, DJ (2000) Particle imaging technique for measuring the deformation rate of hydrogel microstructures. *Applied Physics Letters*, 76, 3310-3312.

Osada, Y. Ross-Murphy, S. (1993) Intelligent Gels *Scientific American*, **268**: 82-87.

Pong KC, Ho CM, Liu J, & Tai YC (1994). Nonlinear pressure distributin in uniform microchannels. *ASME FED* 197:51-6.

Prasad AK; Adrian RJ; Landreth CC, Offutt PW (1992) Effect of resolution on the speed and accuracy of particle image velocimetry interrogation. *Exp Fluids* 13: 105-116

Probstein RF (1994) Physicochemical Hydrodynamics : an introduction, John Wiley & Sons, New York

Revenco, I and Proksch, R (2000) Magnetic and acoustic tapping mode microscopy of liquid phase phospholipid bilayers and DNA molecules. *J. App. Phys.*, **87**: 526-533

Santiago, JG (2001) Electroosmotic Flows in Microchannels with Finite Inertial and Pressure Forces, *Anal. Chem.* 73, pp. 2353-2365.

Santiago, JG, Wereley, ST, Meinhart, CD, Beebe, DJ & Adrian, RJ (1998) A micro particle image velocimetry system. *Exp. Fluids*, Vol. 25 No.4, pp 316-319.

Stone, SW, Meinhart, CD & Wereley, ST (2002) A Microfluidic-based Nanoscope, *Exp. Fluids*, Vol. 33, 613-619.

Strausser, Y and Heaton, M (1994) An introduction to scanning probe microscopy. *American Laboratory*. **26**: April.

Tretheway D & Meinhart CD (2002) Fluid slip near hydrophobic microchannel walls, *Phys. of Fluids*, 14 (3), L9-L12.

Van Kampen NG (1997) Stochastic Processes in Physics and Chemistry, Elsevier

Wereley, ST, Gui, LC, and Meinhart, CD (2001) "Flow Measurement Techniques for the Microfrontier," Paper 2001-0243, American Institute of Aeronautics and Astronautics Annual Meeting, Reno, NV, Jan. 2001.

Wereley, ST, Gui, LC, and Meinhart, CD (2002) "Advanced algorithms for microscale particle image velocimetry," *J. AIAA*, Vol. 40, No. 6, pp 1047-1055.

Wereley ST, Meinhart CD (2001), Adaptive second-order accurate particle image velocimetry, *Exp. Fluids*, Vol. 31, 258-268

Wereley ST, Santiago JG, Meinhart CD, Adrian RJ 1998, Velocimetry for MEMS Applications. *Proc. of ASME/DSC,* Vol. 66, (*Micro-fluidics Symposium*, Nov. 1998, Anaheim, CA)

3. Electrokinetic Flow Diagnostics

S. Devasenathipathy and J.G. Santiago

The advent of microfabricated chemical analysis systems has led to a growing interest in microfabricated fluidic systems with characteristic scales in the range of one micron to one millimeter. A motivation to integrate components in a manner analogous to modern microelectronics is coupled with a potential for achieving massively parallel functions, and the field is rapidly developing. Most microfluidic systems rely on two modes of fluid transport: pressure-driven and electrokinetically-driven flow.

An important class of microfluidic systems is systems that aim to perform basic chemical assays and other processing steps on a fluidic chip. Fluid motion in these chemical biochip systems is often achieved using electroosmotic flow, which enjoys several advantages over pressure-driven flows. Chiefly, electroosmotic flow produces a nearly uniform "plug" profile, which results in reduced sample species dispersion as compared to the velocity gradients associated with pressure-driven flows. This important contrast between pressure-driven and electroosmotic flows is demonstrated by the visualization data in Figure 3.1. This sequence of images was obtained with a molecular tagging technique (caged fluorescence visualization) described later in this chapter. In electroosmotic flow systems, fluid pumping and valving can be controlled without moving parts and simple devices are capable of wide variety of processes including mixing, molecular separation, and the generation of pressure work. Many of these systems also employ electrophoresis; another electrokinetic phenomena [2] which describes the Coulombic-force-driven motion of suspended molecular or microparticle species in solution. Ease of fabrication (e.g., using standard lithographic masking and wet-etching techniques), allows for the rapid development of system design concepts and a rapid evolution in the functionality of electroosmotic flow systems. As device-design technologies and a basic understanding of the underlying physics improve, electroosmotic microscale flow devices may also find niche applications in areas outside of chemical analysis and processing. For example, electroosmotic flow pumping is being applied to the generation of high pressure (> 2 atm) and high flow rate (> 10 ml/min) in two-phase cooling systems for microelectronics [3,4].

As on-chip electroosmotic and electrophoretic systems grow in complexity and designs are optimized, the need for a detailed understanding of the underlying flow physics of such systems grows ever more critical. Experimental studies of these flows as well as experimentally-validated flow models are needed to facilitate the development of microfabricated electroosmotic systems. This chapter presents a review of flow diagnostics that have been applied to the study of electrokinetic flow systems. An emphasis is placed on flow diagnostics that are applicable to on-chip electroosmosis and electrophoresis devices.

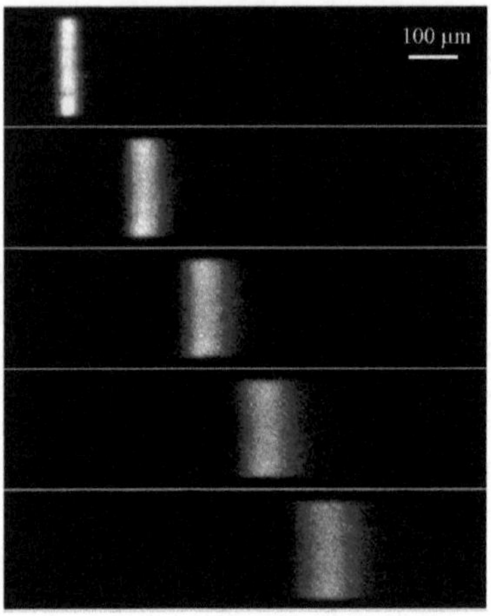

(a)

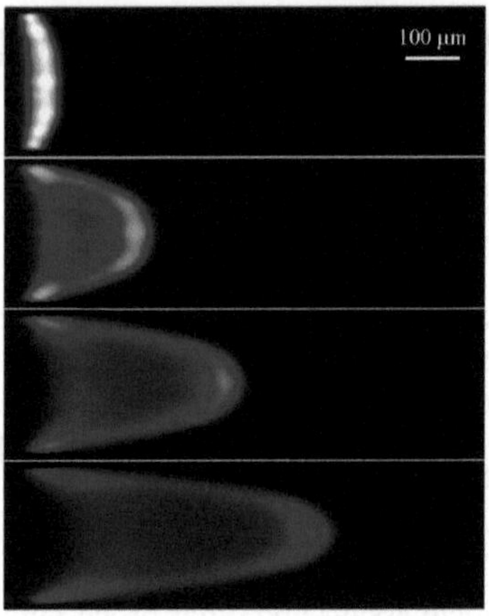

(b)

Fig. 3.1. These images show a fundamental difference in the dynamics of sample dispersion between electroosmotically-driven and pressure-driven flows. This visualization was performed using a molecular tagging technique (caged fluorescence visualization described later on in the chapter) and shows the reduced sample dispersion for (a) electroosmotic flow (in a capillary with a rectangular cross section 200 μm wide and 9 μm deep) as compared to (b) pressure-driven flow (rectangular cross-section 250 μm wide and 70 μm deep). The images are adapted from recent work by Molho [1].

3.1 Theory

A brief introduction to the theory of electrokinetics is presented here in order to facilitate discussions regarding flow diagnostics and identify the major flow parameters of interest. Readers who desire a more detailed explanation of electrokinetic flow physics are referred to Probstein [2] and Hunter [5]. A brief summary of both electrokinetic and pressure-driven flow physics in microchannels is also given by Sharp et al. [6] The phenomenon of electrokinetics may be broadly classified into four types [2]: a) electroosmosis, b) electrophoresis, c) streaming potential, and d) sedimentation potential. These can be qualitatively described as follows:

a) Electrosmosis is the motion of the bulk liquid in response to an applied electric field in a channel with electric double layers on its wetted surfaces.
b) Electrophoresis is the motion (relative to the bulk liquid) of charged colloidal particles or molecules suspended in a solution that results upon the application of an electric field.
c) Streaming potential is the electric potential that develops along a channel with charged walls when a liquid is driven using pressure forces. The electric Joule current associated with this advective charge transport effect is called the streaming current.

d) Sedimentation potential is the electric potential that develops when charged colloidal particles are set in motion with respect to a stationary liquid. The driving force for this effect is typically gravity.

In this chapter, we will not discuss sedimentation potential as it is not typically important in electrokinetic microchannel systems. We will limit our discussion of streaming potential in the context of its application in determining the zeta potential of microchannels (i.e., streaming potential measurements).

3.1.1 Electroosmosis

When an electrolyte is brought in contact with a solid surface, a spontaneous electrochemical reaction typically occurs between the liquid and the surface, resulting in a redistribution of charges. For microfluidic electrokinetic systems fabricated from glass or fused silica, silanol groups on the surface deprotonate when brought in contact with an electrolyte [5]. The extent of deprotonation depends on the local pH and the ion concentration of the solution [7]. Polymer-based microchannels also characteristically acquire a surface charge when in contact with a liquid [8]. In the cases of interest, an electric double layer (EDL) is formed that consists of a charged solid surface and a region near the surface that supports a net excess of counter-ions. In classical theory, these counter-ions are considered to reside in two regions: the Stern and Gouy-Chapman Diffuse Layers [9]. The immobile counterions adsorbed to and immediately adjacent to the wall form the Stern layer, while the Gouy-Chapman Layer comprises the diffuse and mobile counter-ion layer that is set in motion upon the application of an external electric field. The shear plane separates the Stern and Gouy-Chapman layers and, in simple models of the EDL, is the location of the fluid motion's no slip condition. The potential at the shear plane is called the zeta potential, ζ. A sketch of the potential associated with the EDL is shown in Figure 3.2. The magnitude of the potential decays away from the wall and the bulk fluid far from the wall is assumed net neutral. A review of modern EDL theory including recent descriptions and formulations of the basic structure (and component regions) of the EDL is given by Dukhin et al. [10].

The concentration profile in the diffuse ion region of the EDL can be described by the Boltzmann distribution and is a result of the balance between electromigration and diffusive fluxes [11]. For the EDL on a flat plate, the Boltzmann distribution of ions of species i, c_i, is

$$c_i(y) = c_{\infty,i}\ \exp\left(-\frac{z_i e\phi(y)}{kT}\right) \tag{3.1}$$

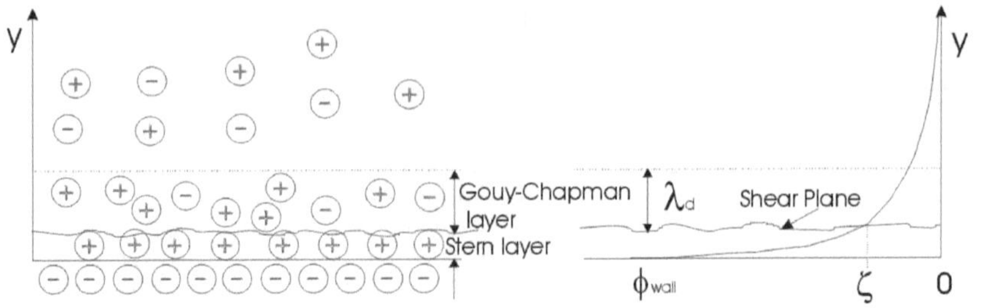

(a) (b)

Fig. 3.2. a) Schematic of a simple EDL model showing the shielding of a negatively charged wall by a stagnant layer of counter-ions (Stern layer) and a layer of mobile ions called the Gouy-Chapman layer. The two layers are separated by the shear plane, and the solution far from the wall is neutral. b) A plot of electric potential versus distance from the wall. The wall potential ϕ_{wall} falls sharply to the zeta potential (ζ) at the shear plane and then decays to zero far from the wall. The Debye length (λ_d) of the solution is shown in the schematic.

where $c_{\infty,i}$ is the concentration of ion i in the liquid far from the wall, $\phi(y)$ is the electrical potential associated with the EDL charges of the Gouy-Chapman layer, z_i is the valence number of ion i, and T is the temperature of the liquid. The wall coordinate y is as shown in Figure 3.2, where $y = 0$ is the shear plane. The net charge density in the EDL, ρ_E, is related to the molar concentrations of N species by

$$\rho_E = F\sum_{i=1}^{N} z_i c_i \tag{3.2}$$

The net charge density can also be related to the local potential in the diffuse EDL by the Poisson equation

$$\nabla^2\phi = \frac{-\rho_E}{\varepsilon} \tag{3.3}$$

Combining the Boltzmann distribution and the relation for the net charge density with the Poisson equation, we obtain

$$\frac{d^2\phi}{dy^2} = \frac{-F}{\varepsilon}\sum_{i=1}^{N} z_i c_{\infty,i} \exp\left(-\frac{ze\phi(y)}{kT}\right) \tag{3.4}$$

For symmetric electrolyte, we can obtain a well-known form of the non-linear Poisson-Boltzmann equation:

$$\frac{d^2\phi}{dy^2} = \frac{2Fzc_\infty}{\varepsilon}\sinh\left(\frac{ze\phi(y)}{kT}\right) \tag{3.5}$$

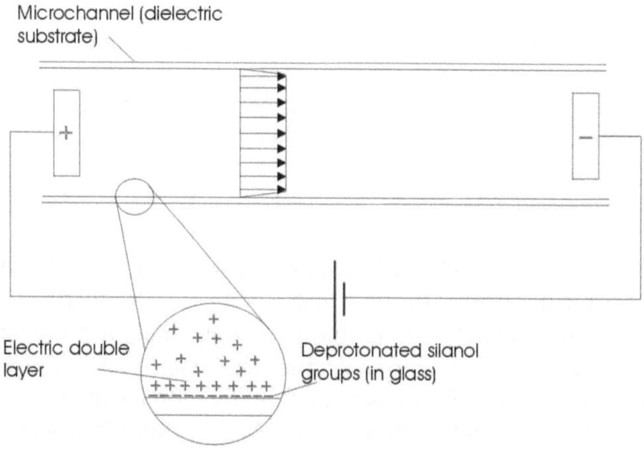

Fig. 3.3. Electroosmotic field schematic with applied electric field and detail of double layer. Electroosmotic flow results in nearly plug-like velocity profile for the case of thin electric double layer. The charges in the double layer are set into motion on the application of an external electric field and drag the bulk fluid through viscous interaction.

The Debye-Huckel limit of the EDL is the case where $ze\phi(y)/kT$ is small enough such that the hyperbolic sine function above can be approximated by its argument and the Poisson-Boltzmann equation above reduces to the following linear form:

$$\frac{d^2\phi}{dy^2} = \frac{\phi(y)}{\lambda_D^2} \tag{3.6}$$

Here λ_D is the Debye length of the electrolyte, defined as $\lambda_D \equiv \left[\varepsilon kT/\left(2z^2F^2c_\infty\right)\right]^{\frac{1}{2}}$. The Debye length describes the characteristic thickness of the EDL and, in the Debye-Huckle limit, λ_D is the length from the shear plane at which the EDL potential has fallen to its e^{-1} value of ζ. Note that this thickness can be thought of as a property of the solution of interest and is a length scale that varies inversely with the square root of ion molar concentration, c_∞.

A relation for the velocity field in an arbitrarily shaped microchannel of uniform cross-section can be derived [6] starting with the equation of motion for a low Reynolds number, incompressible liquid:

$$\nabla p = \mu\nabla^2\bar{\mathbf{u}} + \rho_\varepsilon\bar{\mathbf{E}} \tag{3.7}$$

where $\bar{\mathbf{E}}$ is the applied electric field. As described by Sharp et al. [6] the potential field in the problem can be separated into two components (for applied field and EDL charge field) and substituting Equation 3.3 yields

$$\frac{\nabla p}{\mu} = \nabla^2\left(\bar{\mathbf{u}} - \frac{\varepsilon\bar{\mathbf{E}}\phi}{\mu}\right) \tag{3.8}$$

Equation 3.8 is linear allowing the velocity components due to the electric field, $\bar{\boldsymbol{u}}_{eof}$, and pressure gradient, $\bar{\boldsymbol{u}}_{pres}$, to be considered separately. For a microchannel with a cross-section in the y-z plane which is uniform along the x direction and is subject to a field directed along the x-axis, the expression for the x-component electroosmotic velocity, implicit in terms of the EDL potential, is then:

$$u_{eof}(y,z) = \frac{-\varepsilon E \zeta}{\mu}\left[1 - \frac{\phi(y,z)}{\zeta}\right] \tag{3.9}$$

There are a significant number of solutions for $\bar{\boldsymbol{u}}_{pres}$ available [12] which can be applied to solve for the total velocity $\bar{\boldsymbol{u}} = \bar{\boldsymbol{u}}_{pres} + \bar{\boldsymbol{u}}_{eof}$ which satisfies Equation 3.8. For simple "straight" channels with uniform zeta potential, the problem reduces to finding solutions for the (uncoupled) electric potential distribution, $\phi(y,z)$, in the channel. A schematic of the electroosmotic flow field on the application of an external electric field is shown in Figure 3.3. Expressions for electroosmotic flow in a cylindrical capillary and between two parallel plates are given by Rice and Whitehead [13] and Burgreen and Nakache [14], respectively.

Numerical solutions to predict electroosmotic flows for all relevant length scales in complex geometries with arbitrary cross-sections are difficult for Debye lengths much smaller than the characteristic dimensions of the channels (e.g., the hydraulic diameter) [15]. Indeed, this is the case for typical microfluidic electrokinetic systems which have Debye length-to-channel-diameter ratios of order 10^{-4} or less. For these cases, thin EDL assumptions are often appropriate as an approximation of electroosmotic flow solutions in complex geometries. For the case of thin EDL, the electric potential throughout most of the cross-sectional area of a microchannel is zero and Equation 3.9, for the case of zero pressure gradients, reduces to

$$u = -\frac{\varepsilon \zeta E}{\mu} \tag{3.10}$$

which is the Helmholtz-Smoluchowski relation for electroosmotic flow.

Two important electroosmotic flow parameters relevant to experimental measurements follow from this discussion. The first is the electroosmotic mobility, μ_{eo}, of a microchannel defined as the field-specific velocity of an electroosmotic channel with zero pressure gradient: $\mu_{eo} = u/E$. The mobility is a fairly generally applicable concept as it describes the empirically observed proportionality between electric field and fluid velocity. For cases where Joule heating effects are negligible, the mobility is considered a constant of proportionality for a given wall material and solution chemistry. A second electroosmosis parameter revealed is the zeta potential. The zeta potential is often measured indirectly using velocity or flow rate measurements and its quantification typically incorporates (i.e., assumes) aspects of electric double layer theory. Some techniques, such as streaming potential measurements, attempt to measure zeta potential directly, but even these are subject to assumptions regarding charge layers such as the form of the relations governing so-called surface conductance [16].

3.1.2 Electrophoresis

Electrophoresis is the induced motion of colloidal particles or molecules suspended in ionic solutions that results from the application of an electric field. The electromigration of these species are classified into two regimes, based on the ratio of the size of the particle or molecule to the Debye length of the solution, as depicted in Figure 3.4. First, consider the electrophoresis of ionic molecules and macromolecules whose characteristic diameter are much smaller than the Debye length of the solution of interest. The motion of these molecules can be described as a simple balance between the electrostatic force on the molecule and the viscous drag associated with its resulting motion. As a result, the electrophoretic mobility of molecules is a function of the molecule's effective size (and molecular weight) and directly proportional to their valence number

$$\bar{\mathbf{u}} = \frac{q\bar{\mathbf{E}}}{3\pi\mu d} \tag{3.11}$$

where q is the total charge on the molecule, $\bar{\mathbf{E}}$ is the applied field, and d is the diameter of a Stokes sphere in a continuum flow with a drag coefficient equal to that of the molecule [11]. For molecules, the shielding layer of counter-ions surrounding molecule have a negligible effect on the externally applied electric field.

A second limiting situation arises during electrophoresis of relatively large particles. Examples of large particles relevant to microfluidics include 100–10,000 nm diameter polystyrene spheres and ~10 μm diameter cells or single-celled organisms. In this second limiting case the electrophoretic velocity is a function of the electrostatic forces on the surface charge, the electrostatic forces on their charge double layers, and the viscous drag associated with both the motion of the body as well as the motion of the ionic cloud around the body. For a wide range of cases where the particle diameter-to-Debye length ratio is large so that, locally, the ionic cloud near the particle surface can be approximated by the EDL relations for a flat plate, the velocity of an electrophoretic particle reduces simply to

$$\bar{\mathbf{u}} = \frac{\varepsilon\zeta\bar{\mathbf{E}}}{\mu} \tag{3.12}$$

The 100–1000 nm diameter seed particles described later in this chapter typically fall into this thin EDL particle flow regime. As in the discussion above for electroosmotic flows, Equations (3.11) and (3.12) demonstrate a direct proportionality between velocity and electric field which can be used to formulate an empirical mobility parameter of the form $\mu_{eph} = u/E$. Applying the theoretical models discussed above, the two definitions of mobility are $q/3\pi\mu d$ and $\varepsilon\zeta/\mu$ for particles diameters small and large with respect to Debye length, respectively.

Lastly, note that theory relating the two limits described above has long been a subject of interest as discussed by Russel et al. [17]. As will be discussed later in this chapter, most visualization applications of electrokinetic flows (i.e., using either fluorescent molecular dyes or micron-sized ploymer seed particles) are well approximated by one of these two limits.

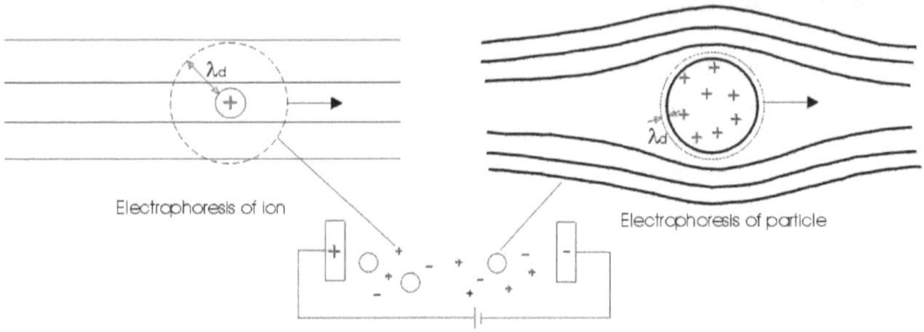

Fig. 3.4. Two limits of the electrophoretic behavior of ions and particles. The schematic on the left depicts the electrophoresis of an ion, where the EDL is much larger than the characteristic size of the ion. The electric field lines are not appreciably distorted by the presence of the ion. To the right is a depiction of the electrophoresis of a micron-sized sphere whose EDL thickness is much smaller than its diameter. The surface/charge layer interaction is therefore similar to that of the flat-wall electroosmotic flow.

3.1.3 Similarity Between Electric Field and Velocity Field for Fluid

One other simplification of electroosmotic flow in microsystems occurs in the case of non-inertial flow of uniform property liquids in channels with uniform zeta potentials and thin EDLs. For this simple case, the velocity field throughout an arbitrarily-shaped flow device with no applied pressure gradients can be expressed as

$$\bar{\mathbf{u}}(x, y, z, t) = \frac{\varepsilon\zeta}{\mu}\bar{\mathbf{E}}(x, y, z, t) \tag{3.13}$$

where $\bar{\mathbf{E}}$ is the electric field in the structure. This simplification is very useful in approximating electroosmotic flow fields as only simple Laplace equation solutions (of the shape of the electric field), together with an estimate of zeta potential, are required. Note that electrophoretic motion in these simple systems is also always similar to the electric field. Overbeek [18] first suggested that the electroosmotic velocity is everywhere parallel to the electric field for simple electroosmotic flows at low Reynolds numbers. A set of sufficient conditions for the velocity field to be similar to the electric field is given by Santiago [19], and the issue is also discussed by Cummings et al. [20].

This result greatly simplifies the modeling of simple electroosmotic flows since Laplace equation solvers can be used to solve for the electric potential and the Helmlholtz-Smoluchowski equation can then be used to solve for the velocity field of the flow outside of the EDL. This approach has been applied to the optimization of microchannel geometries and has been verified experimentally [19–21].

3.2 Diagnostics

3.2.1 Capillary Electrophoresis: Electrokinetic System Background

On-chip applications of electrokinetics are relatively new, most arising in the last decade [22,23] Traditionally, the most important application for electrokinetic systems has been capillary electrophoresis (CE). Electrophoresis as a separation tool was first introduced by A.W.K.Tiselius (1937) for which he was awarded a Nobel Prize in 1948. Over the years, research in this field has evolved from gel-based electrophoresis in the slab-format (which is still in use) to capillary-based electrophoretic separations. Conventional CE systems use pulled, free-standing, fused-silica capillaries with inner diameters of order 10 μm to achieve electrophoretic separation of samples using applied electric fields approximately in the range of 100-1000 V/cm [24,25]. The separation media may be aqueous solutions (e.g., as in capillary zone electrophoresis) or gel matrices (as in capillary gel electrophoresis). Samples include amino acids, proteins, DNA, RNA, and organic molecules. Electroosmosis in systems that apply capillary zone electrophoresis allows for the detection of positive, neutral, and negative ions with a single point-wise detector. The literature of the CE field is extensive and has grown exponentially [26] with several good reviews available [26–31]. We here present a comparison of the detection limits of various point-wise CE detection modalities which is adapted from a book by Landers [26]. This comparison is an effort to characterize and summarize the many point-wise detection methods and serves as a short introduction to the electroosmotic flow diagnostics systems discussed in this chapter. Figure 3.5 shows the detection limits of CE detection systems as a function of their molar sensitivity. Molar sensitivity is plotted on the abscissa, and is formulated here as the number of sample moles loaded onto the capillary column. The ordinate of the graph shows the concentration of the sample of interest. The concentration limit of detection for a given sample amount is then dictated by the detection technique used. Trends are apparent for three detection schemes: electrochemical, fluorescence and ultraviolet (UV) absorbance.

Electrochemical detection includes amperometry, conductivity, and potentiometry. The drawback with this detection scheme is the requirement for integrated electrode structures within the microchannel. In contrast to electrochemical detection, the sensitivity of UV absorbance is weak but is still very popular due to its simplicity of operation and the fact that untagged samples are detectable. A majority of the samples of interest, including peptides and proteins, absorb in UV wavelengths. Despite its popularity in free-standing capillary systems, UV detection is not easily applicable to microchannel systems etched in planar glass substrates due to the short optical path lengths available from the shallow channel depths, and the difficulties associated with transmitted light optics in an etched microchannel. One approach to increase absorbance sensitivity is to fabricate a multi-reflection absorbance cell onto the microfluidic device [32]. The third detection scheme, fluorescence, offers the highest sensitivity. Advances in derivatization chemistry have led to the effective tagging of several thousand analytes [33].

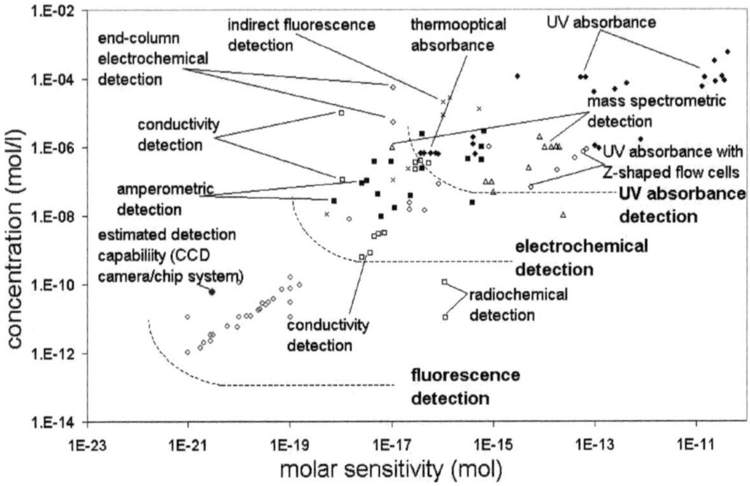

Fig. 3.5. Detection techniques for capillary electrophoresis (adapted from the CRC Handbook of Capillary Electrophoresis [26], with permission). Molar sensitivity (here defined as the number of moles which are detected) and concentration are plotted on the abscissa and ordinate, respectively. Fluorescence detection is observed to have the highest sensitivity among single-point CE detection schemes. Also shown in the plot is the estimated detection capability for fluorescence detection in a microfluidic system with an intensified 12-bit CCD camera.

Shown together with the CE detection limits summarized in Haber [26] is an estimate of the capability of fluorescence visualization in a typical chip-based system using a high sensitivity CCD camera and mercury arc lamp illumination. This estimate is based on an experiment [34] using a 60 pM concentration of fluorescein (in 20mM HEPES, pH 7.4) in an electrophoretic acrylic microchip (Aclara BioSciences, Mountain View, California). The microchannel has a 50 μm top width and a centerline depth of 20 μm. For the purposes of this estimate, the microchannel was filled with the dye and imaged using an epifluorescent microscope fitted with a 60X objective with a numerical aperture of 1.4. A 12 bit intensified CCD camera (Roper Scientific, Tucson, Arizona) was used to capture an image of this dye-filled intersection with a 10 ms exposure time. The signal-to-noise ratio (SNR) of the image (the difference between the average signal in the region of interrogation and average background noise divided by the standard deviation of the background noise) was 2.0. Although this simple imaging experiment does not demonstrate an actual separation, the SNR of the channel intersection image and the magnitude of the exposure time are consistent with the parameters required for a chip-based electrophoretic separation [35] and may be interpreted as the estimated range for on-chip electrophoresis with CCD-based detection and mercury arc lamp illumination. Approximating a sample plug volume on the order of the channel width along the axis of the channel, there are on the order of a thousand molecules of analyte detected in this experiment.

In summary, it may be said that with the increasingly smaller dimensions expected for CE applications on a chip, optical detection techniques and, more specifically, fluorescence-based techniques hold great promise for accurate measurements with high spatial and temporal resolutions. Electrochemical detection devices, although less sensitive and more difficult to fabricate, probably have the potential for being more compact and lower cost than optical-detection-based detection systems (e.g., as would be required for portable, single-use devices).

Weighing

The earliest electroosmotic microchannel measurements were made in free-standing fused-silica capillaries with inner diameters on the order of tens of microns [25]. A common and perhaps the simplest technique to measure electroosmotic flow is to measure the weight of the liquid pumped from one reservoir to another. A schematic of a typical weighing setup is shown in Figure 3.6. The configuration shown in the figure was applied by VanDeGoor [36] and we will mention some of their equipment as an example system. The grounded electrolyte reservoir is placed on an analytical balance (e.g., a Sartorius microbalance MP8-1). An electric field is applied using a high voltage power supply (Heinzinger 30000-1, Rosenheim, Germany) with special care taken to ensure that the electrode in the grounded reservoir does not influence the weighing. The weight of one electrode reservoir/vessel is monitored with the analytical micro-balance at time intervals ranging from 1 –10 s. Measurements were taken for flows in both directions by reversing the polarities of the electrodes, and a simple average was calculated to yield the electroosmotic flow rate. Weighing measurements have also been reported by Wanders et al. [37], Altria and Simpson [38], and VanDeGoor et al. [39].

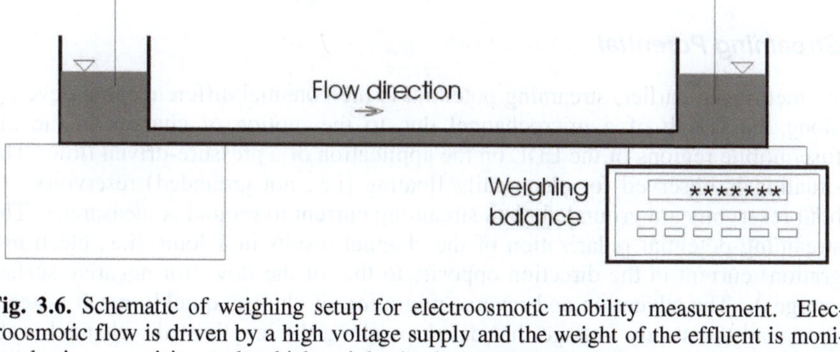

Fig. 3.6. Schematic of weighing setup for electroosmotic mobility measurement. Electroosmotic flow is driven by a high voltage supply and the weight of the effluent is monitored using a precision scale which weighs the downstream reservoir.

In all weighing experiments, losses due to evaporation are particularly critical and should minimized and estimated to quantify uncertainty. This is especially critical for the low volume flow rates (of order 100 nl/min) typically encountered in electrokinetic flows. Environmental parameter controls such as temperature and humidity may help to mitigate this effect. Another limitation to the resolution obtainable from this method is the sensitivity of the balance and the effects of room air currents on the balance.

The weighing method has been applied to measure flow rates of so-called electroosmotic nanopumps designed for volumetric nanotitrations [40]. The resolution of the balance used for the measurements, obtained at a sampling frequency of 1Hz, was 0.01 mg (Mettler-Toledo AE 240, Columbus, Ohio). Attempts to incorporate the technique in on-chip applications should take particular care into accounting for dead volume (particularly regions which can hold gas bubbles) in chip-to-external fluidic interconnects and the hydraulic resistances associated with the interconnects as these can introduce unwanted pressure gradients into the flow experiment. Methods for removing bubbles include outgassing working liquids (e.g., using a vacuum) before and after the liquid is introduced into the flow system.

Conductivity Cell

Conductivity cell measurements of electroosmotic flow monitor the development of the conductivity of the fluid in the downstream electrode vessel. The microchannel of interest and inlet (high voltage) reservoir are filled with a run buffer and the second, grounded downstream reservoir, referred to as the conductivity cell is filled with a diluted buffer [36]. On application of the driving potential, the bulk conductivity of the downstream cell increases due to the electroosmotic pumping of a fluid of higher conductivity. A stirrer mechanism, typically a magnetic stirrer or an air driven rotor is mounted within the cell to ensure that the fluids are well mixed.

Recently Liu et al. [41] investigated electroosmotic flow in hybrid poly(dimethyl-siloxane)/glass electrokinetic microchips using AC conductivity detection. Liu's experiments used microfabricated electrodes in direct contact with the working electrolyte and which were located upstream of the waste reservoir.

Streaming Potential

As mentioned earlier, streaming potential is the potential difference that develops along the length of a microchannel due to the motion of charges in the diffuse/mobile regions of the EDL on the application of a pressure-driven flow. This situation is observed for electrically floating (i.e., not grounded) reservoirs. (If both reservoirs are grounded, then streaming current to ground is measured). This streaming-potential polarization of the channel results in a Joule (i.e., electromigration) current in the direction opposite to that of the flow (for negative surface charges). The advection and reverse migration of charges quickly reach a steady state, and the steady voltage that develops along the length of the channel is the measurable streaming potential.

A schematic of a streaming potential measurement setup is shown in Figure 3.7. Pressure driven flow has been achieved, for example, by regulating nitrogen into the reservoirs through a series of magnetic valves [36]. The direction of the differential pressure forces is controlled from a computer, through an interface card (Perkin Elmer, Netherlands). A high input impedance electrometer (millivolt meter Philips PW9414, Netherlands) and a pair of platinum electrodes is used to measure the streaming potential. The electrometer is necessary to ensure that the streaming potential of the cell is not affected by the presence of the measurement device in the circuit (i.e., it is a high input impedance device capable of resolving low voltage readings). A reference measurement with no applied pressure was obtained to correct for possible contributions from gravity flow and asymmetry between the electrolyte/electrode systems (i.e., to account for the electric double layer potentials associated with the electrolyte/electrode interfaces).

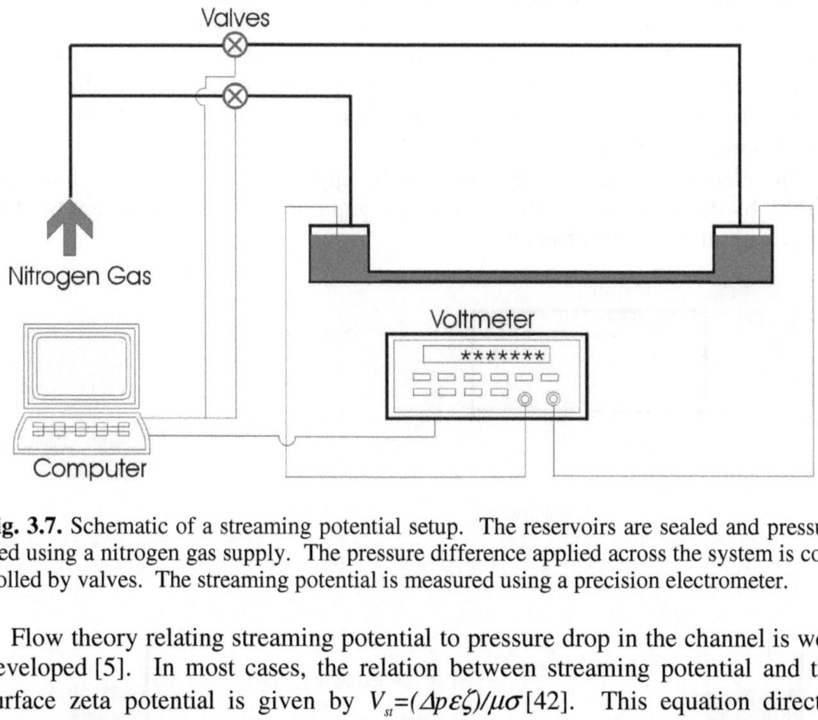

Fig. 3.7. Schematic of a streaming potential setup. The reservoirs are sealed and pressurized using a nitrogen gas supply. The pressure difference applied across the system is controlled by valves. The streaming potential is measured using a precision electrometer.

Flow theory relating streaming potential to pressure drop in the channel is well developed [5]. In most cases, the relation between streaming potential and the surface zeta potential is given by $V_{st}=(\Delta p \varepsilon \zeta)/\mu\sigma$ [42]. This equation directly yields the zeta potential, ζ, with a measurement of the streaming potential generated, V_{st}, and the conductivity of the fluid, σ, and applied pressure, Δp. This equation assumes a thin EDL. Streaming potential measurements have also been made by Reijenga et al. [42], and Van De Goor et al. [39].

The effect of surface conductance on streaming potential measurements can be important for small (order 50 µm and smaller) electrokinetic microchannels. Gu and Li [43] made simultaneous measurements of ζ and surface conductivity from streaming potential experiments in a parallel-plate microchannel (with a characteristic height of 50 µm). They showed that erroneous estimates of ζ are obtained by neglecting surface conductance in streaming potential measurements. The importance of surface conductance depends on the size of the microchannel and the (dimensional) ratio of the surface conductivity to the bulk conductivity of the electrolyte.

Current Monitoring

Current monitoring is a convenient and simple technique that can be used to measure the electroosmotic mobility of a channel of nearly uniform surface charge. The method was first demonstrated by Huang et al. [44] and determines the electroosmotic mobility of a capillary by measuring the conductance transients associated with the displacement of one buffer (working fluid) in a capillary with a second buffer of a measurably different electrical conductivity. The conductivity of the buffers can be tailored by either diluting one buffer or adding salt (e.g., KCl) to one or more of the buffers. A schematic of the setup is shown in Figure 3.8. The length of the channel between the two reservoirs, L is known. The time interval of interest, τ is the time for the trailing liquid to completely displace the leading liquid from the channel system. This time is determined from a current measurement of the cell as discussed below.

The electroosmotic velocity can then be approximated by L/τ, or more precisely, by the derivative of the current transient during the period where the front propagates through the channel.

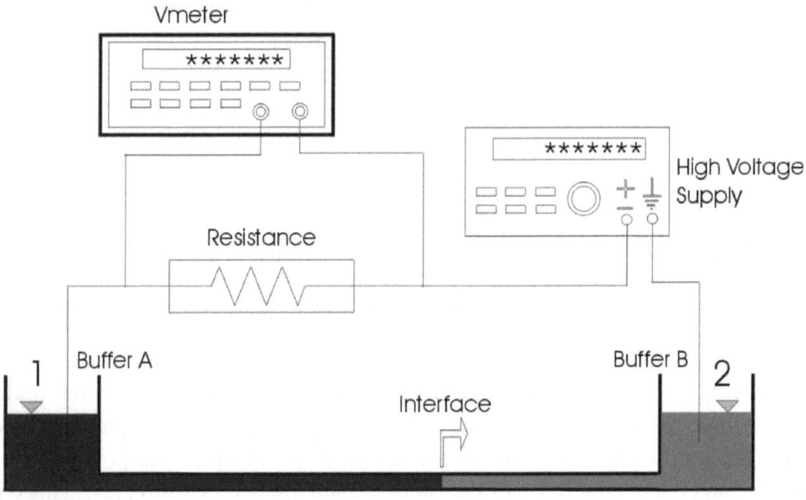

Fig. 3.8. Schematic of current monitoring setup. The motion of the interface (between buffers of two different conductivities) changes the effective resistance of the circuit. The current transients are captured by measuring voltage across a precision resistor placed in series with the channel system.

The instrumentation for this technique is simple. The channel system is placed in series with a precision resistor on the ground side of the circuit as shown in Figure 3.8. The polarity of the power supply is chosen such that electrolyte flows from reservoir 1 to reservoir 2. The current in the circuit is monitored as a voltage drop across the reference resistor. In the example shown in the figure, a high conductivity buffer is displaced by a low conductivity buffer. The maximum signal is the current difference of the initial, high conductivity cell and the final, low conductivity cell. Measurements are easily acquired with a computer using data acquisition cards and real time monitoring can be performed in conjunction with other flow (e.g., optical) diagnostics.

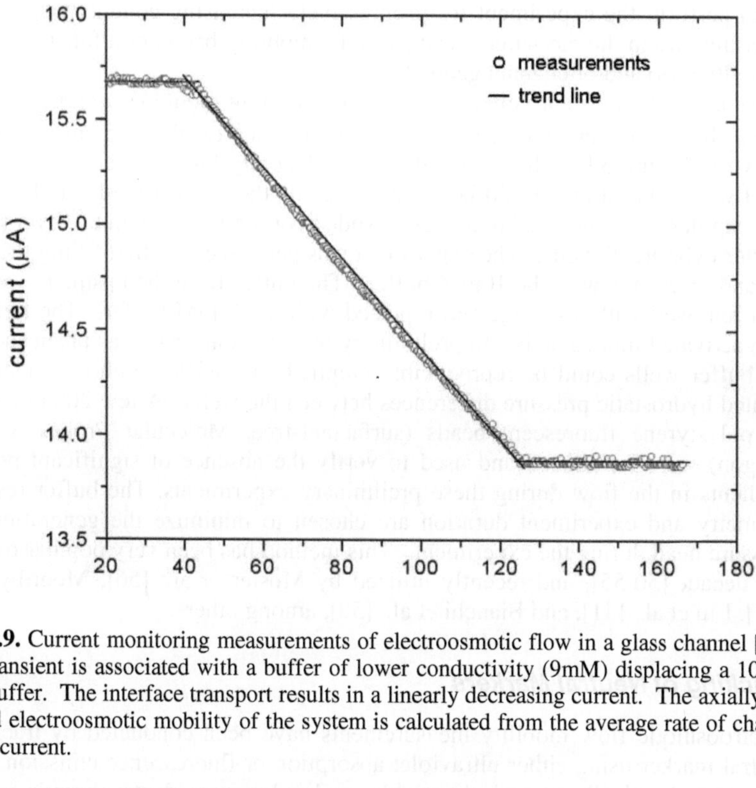

Fig. 3.9. Current monitoring measurements of electroosmotic flow in a glass channel [45]. The transient is associated with a buffer of lower conductivity (9mM) displacing a 10mM lead buffer. The interface transport results in a linearly decreasing current. The axially averaged electroosmotic mobility of the system is calculated from the average rate of change of the current.

There are constraints in optimizing the difference in concentrations of the leading and trailing fluids to yield unbiased results of the channel mobility. The most important factor to consider is the larger buffer conductivity differences yield larger signals but also disturb the flow. Flow disturbance is due to the fact that electroosmotic mobility of the channel walls is a function of the local buffer chemistry (particularly ionic concentrations). Electroosmotic mobility and zeta potential are well known to be functions of the ionic concentration [46]. A buffer/buffer interface with a mismatch in conductivity is known to result in internal pressure generation as demonstrated by the fluorescence visualizations of Bharadwaj and

Santiago [47]. This dispersion mechanism can be predicted by the theory of Anderson and Idol [48] for the case of non-uniform zeta potentials, and demonstrated by the measurements of Herr et al. [49]. For relatively large conductivity ratios, the pressure component of the flow can be large enough that pressure-driven flow advection causes non-negligible dispersion of the buffer / buffer interface. In a channel of significant internal pressure generation, the dynamics of the current transition is at least a function of channel geometry and the temporal response of the EDL to changes in local buffer concentrations [5]. To avoid the effects of mismatched velocity dispersion, we suggest a difference in buffer concentrations not exceeding ten percent for optimal results. One method for verifying that the measurements do not suffer from internal pressure-driven dispersion may be to perform the experiment for progressively increasing conductivity ratios to determine when the measured electroosmotic mobility becomes a function of conductivity ratio and/or channel geometry.

An example transient voltage signal from a current monitoring experiment in a 400×40 μm (rectangular cross section) fused-silica capillary, 5 cm in length is shown in Figure 3.9. The high and low conductivity buffers used in this experiment were 10 mM and 9 mM borate buffers, and the applied field was 100 V/cm. The capillary was mounted onto a glass slide between two 10 mm tall by 5 mm diameter cylindrical wells. The experiment was performed by first filling the channel and reservoirs with the 10mM buffer. The buffer from the upstream well was then removed with a syringe and replaced with the 9 mM buffer. The field was then activated immediately. In preliminary observations, care was taken such that the buffer wells could be reproducibly emptied and refilled without causing unwanted hydrostatic pressure differences between the wells. A few 200 nm diameter polystyrene fluorescent beads (surfactant-free, Molecular Probes, Eugene, Oregon) were introduced and used to verify the absence of significant pressure gradients in the flow during these preliminary experiments. The buffer reservoir geometry and experiment duration are chosen to minimize the generation of a pressure head during the experiment. This method has been very popular over the last decade [50-55], and recently utilized by Mosier et al. [56], Moorthy et al. [57], Liu et al. [41], and Bianchi et al. [58], among others.

Tracking of Neutral Markers

Electroosmotic flow mobility measurements have been conducted by tracking a neutral marker using either ultraviolet absorption or fluorescence emission detection. An electrically neutral, detectable marker has zero electrophoretic velocity and migrates at the electroosmotic flow velocity for systems with zero pressure gradient. In CE systems, this is just one more sample to be injected among several others. The electroosmotic mobility is then simply calculated from the migration time of a neutral marker, and is given by the relation $\mu_{eo} = Ll/Vt_{eo}$, where L is the total length of the channel, l is the distance from the marker injection position to the detector, V is the applied voltage, and t_{eo} is the migration time

A schematic of the experimental setup for marker tracing is given in Figure 3.10. This example system shows a pointwise fluorescence detection system with

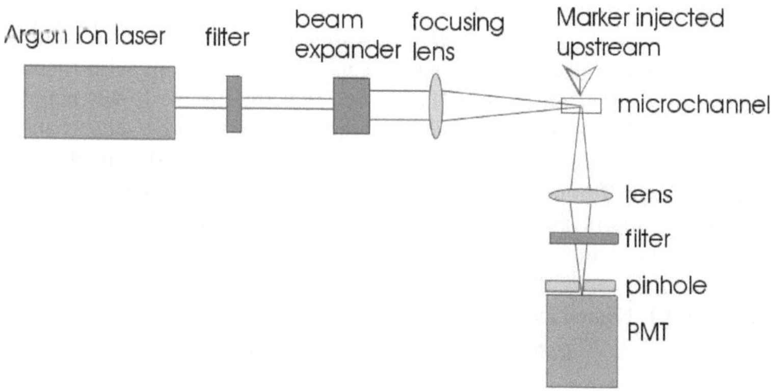

Fig. 3.10. Schematic of neutral marker experimental setup (view along the axis of the channel). This example system is applicable to coumarin, a fluorophore that can be excited by the 488 nm line of an argon ion laser.

a photomultiplier tube (PMT) applicable to on-chip systems, but commercial UV detection systems are prevalent in free-standing capillary systems. The marker is injected into the flow and migrates due to electroosmosis until it reaches the detection site. In the figure, marker fluorescence (e.g., coumarin) is excited at 488 nm using an argon ion laser.

Important criteria for a neutral marker are 1) fluorescence excitation should be near the wavelength of interest used in the experimental setup and the emission should be readily detectable, 2) marker should be soluble in the background buffer solution, 3) adsorption to the capillary wall should be negligible, and 4) the marker should not react with other species in the system. The neutrality of ionizable markers depends on solvent conditions and users should verify that the marker is applicable to their buffer (e.g., with an independent current monitoring experiment). One obvious drawback of this method is that extremely low electroosmotic mobility systems can result in unacceptably long elution times where the marker signal becomes small compared to the background noise (due to dispersion effects including molecular diffusion).

Several neutral marker chemistries have been reported for mostly traditional fused-silica capillary electrokinetic experiments. Tsuda et al. [59] and Walbroehl and Jorgenson [60] used pyridine and formamide, respectively, as neutral markers and employed UV absorption detectors. The dependence of electroosmotic mobility on the pH of the solution was investigated by Lambert and Middleton [61] with acetophonone as the marker, again with an UV absorption detector. Some other groups which have used UV-detectable neutral markers are Sandoval and Chen [62], Cross and Smairl [63], Liu et al. [64], Hayes and Ewing [65], and Hayes et al. [66,67]. Schutzner and Kenndler [68] used three different fluorescent markers (included in Table 1) to study the dependence of electroosmotic flow on pH. Fluorescence detection with coumarin 334 as the neutral marker was used by Preisler and Yeung [69] to characterize the electroosmotic mobility of nonbonded polyethylene oxide coatings for capillary electrophoresis. The sensitivity of fluorescence detection allows very low concentrations of fluorescent markers, typical in microfluidic systems, to measure electroosmotic velocities. Jacobson and Ramsey [70] have demonstrated electrokinetic focusing in microchips with rhodamine b as a neutral dye. Schrum et al. [71] showed that rhodamine b was neutral for pH's between 6 and 10.8 with independent comparisons with UV absorbance detection. Pittman et al. [72] have presented simultaneous measurements of electroosmotic flow with fluorescent marker and UV detection of analytes. A listing of some neutral markers showing detection methods and pH conditions for the reported experiments is shown in Table 3.1.

Table 3.1. Neutral markers used in electroosmotic flow measurements

Marker	Reference	pH	Detection
acetophonone	Lambert and Middleton, 1990	2 - 12	UV absorption
phenol	Hayes and Ewing,1992	6.3	UV absorption
dimethyl sulfoxide	Huang et al.,1993 Sandoval and Chen 1996	3, 7 3	UV absorption
mesityl oxide	Sandoval and Chen,1996 Cross and Smairl,2001	3 7	UV absorption
7-hydroxy-coumarin	Schutzner and Kenndler,1992	< 5.8	Fluorescence
riboflavin	Schutzner and Kenndler,1992	5.8 - 8	Fluorescence
coumarin 334	Preisler and Yeung,1996	7 – 8.2	Fluorescence
rhodamine b	Schutzner and Kenndler,1992 Jacobson and Ramsey,1997 Schrum et al.,2000 Pittman et al.,2001	> 8 > 8 6 – 10.8 9	Fluorescence

3.2.2 Simple Dye Visualization

UV and fluorescence tracking of neutral markers is typically accomplished using point measurement techniques. Full field imaging diagnostics for electroosmotic flow in capillaries were first demonstrated by Tsuda et al. [73]. Figure 3.11 shows the progress of a zone front of a fluorescent solution in a rectangular capillary (1mm × 50 μm, Wilmad, Buena, New Jersey). 0.05 mM rhodamine 590 in methanol is the working fluid, and the applied electric field is 330 V/cm. The electroosmotic flow is from left to right and a slight curvature of the sharp dye front is apparent. Taylor and Yeung [74] have imaged fluorescent plugs of riboflavin in circular capillaries (75 μm diameter) and have compared the transient dynamics of hydrodynamically and electrokinetically driven fronts. Kuhr et al. [75] studied the influence of ionic strength and applied electric fields on electrokinetic flow at a capillary junction by observing images of the dyed fluid (Congo Red). The setup consisted of two capillaries spaced by a gap (varied between 50 – 100 μm) and filled with the working phosphate buffer.

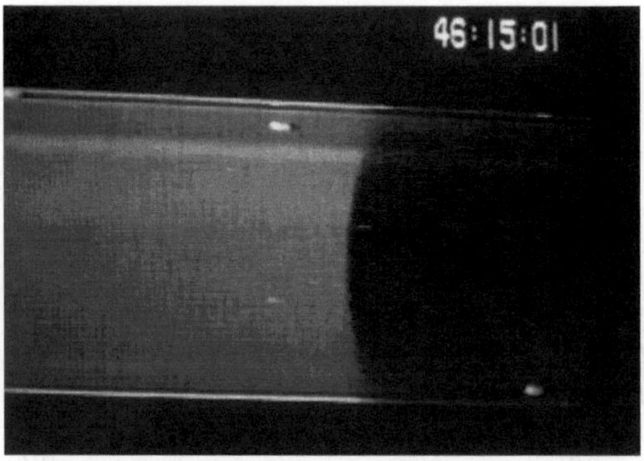

Fig. 3.11. Imaging of a fluorescent front driven electroosmotically in a capillary. This image was adapted from Tsuda [76] and the experimental setup used to obtain this image is described in Tsuda et al. [73]. The working electrolyte is 0.05 mM rhodamine 590 in methanol. The rectangular capillary inner dimensions are 1000 × 50 μm with a wall thickness of 50 μm. The applied electric field is 330 V/cm and the capillary is imaged through a side wall which is 1000 μm wide in the spanwise direction (in the plane of the image). Tsuda points out that this is the first visualization of a dye front in electroosmotic flow.

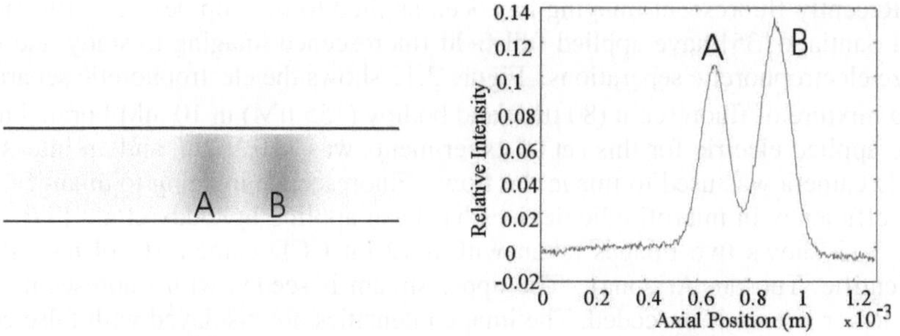

Fig. 3.12. Electrophoretic separation data for a mixture of (A) fluorescein (80 μM) and (B) bodipy (155 μM) dyes in 10 mM borate buffer. These data were obtained by the experimental setup described by Bharadwaj et al. [35]. (a) An image of the two separation bands. The separation electric field here was 100 V/cm. The channel length, width and centerline depth were 8 cm, 50 μm and 20 μm, respectively. An intensified CCD array (12 bit digitization, 512 x 512, 15 frames per second) was used for imaging the concentration field. A background image has been subtracted from the raw image data. The channel outline has been added and the image intensity has been inverted for clarity. (b) A plot of width-averaged intensity as a function of axial location along the separation channel. The plot shows the high signal-to-noise ratio provided by this simple CCD setup.

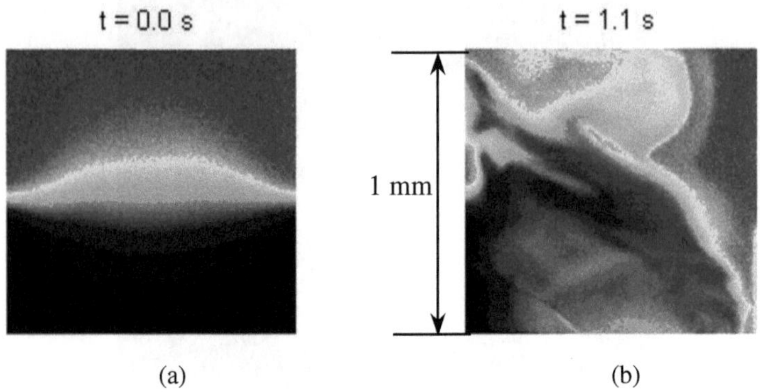

Fig. 3.13. Imaging of mixing dynamics of an electrokinetic instability micromixer [77]. The micromixer shown here is 100 µm deep and has a 1 × 1 mm footprint. Fluorescence images at two instances in time visualize the mixing process. A false color map has been applied to the images. On the left (a) is the initial, unmixed concentration profile with fluorescently tagged liquid shown as red and unseeded liquid as dark blue. The seeded and unseeded streams are flowing from left to right and some initial mixing has occurred due to diffusion. An electrokinetic flow instability is introduced into the flow field by an externally-applied transverse AC electric field. On the right (b), is an image of the concentration profiles 1.1 s after the initialization of the active mixing scheme.

Recently fluorescent imaging has been applied to on-chip devices. Bharadwaj and Santiago [35] have applied full field fluorescence imaging to study and optimize electrophoretic separations. Figure 3.12 shows the electrophoretic separation of a mixture of fluorescein (80 µM) and bodipy (155 µM) in 10 mM borate buffer. The applied electric for this set of experiments was 100 V/cm, and an intensified CCD camera was used to image the flow. Fluorescence imaging to quantify mixing efficiency in microfluidic devices has been applied by Oddy et al. [77]. Figure 3.13 shows two images taken with a 12 bit CCD camera (Coolsnap, Roper Scientific, Tucson, Arizona). The upper stream is seeded with fluorescein while the lower stream is unseeded. The image intensities are displayed with false color. Both streams are pressure driven with an external syringe pump (Harvard Apparatus, Holliston, Massachusetts). The mixing process on the application of a transverse AC electric field is captured using fluorescence imaging. Other groups who have used fluorescence visualization to study mixing in microfluidic geometries are Jacobson et al. [78], and He et al. [79]. Simple dye visualization can be a powerful tool in understanding the flow physics of electrokinetic injections [80].

One recent and interesting application of fluorescence visualization to electrokinetic flows is the temperature measurement method described by Ross et al. [81]. Ross et al. used the temperature dependence of fluorescein fluorescence intensity to map out temperature fields with spatial image resolutions of 1 µm and 33 ms temporal resolution. They suggest that temperature uncertainties of less than 0.1°C are possible for measurement profiles integrated over a 400 µm length and ensemble averaged over 30 realizations.

3.2.3 Photobleached Fluorescence Visualization

Photobleaching has been applied to study molecular diffusion of fluorescent dyes across cell membranes and within cells [82]. This technique is referred to as fluorescence recovery after photobleaching (FRAP). FRAP methods and analysis techniques include modulation FRAP [83], video FRAP [84] and spatial Fourier analysis FRAP [85]. Photobleaching velocimetry as demonstrated by Ricka [86] and later by Fiedler and Wang [87] relates the fluorescence intensity of the dye traversing through the laser-illuminated region to the flow velocity. Gated fluorescence techniques [88,89] have been applied in capillary zone electrophoresis. A disadvantage to the latter approach is the temporal and spatial resolution sacrificed in favor of a larger bleached region that is easier to detect. Also, the shape of the bleached region is dependent on the flow velocity profile and the bleaching time. More recently, photobleaching has been used as a line writing technique to monitor volume-averaged bulk electroosmotic flow velocities by Schrum et al. [71], and Pittman et al. [72]. Mosier et al. [56] have recently applied photobleached fluorescence visualization to simultaneously measure diffusivities and electrophoretic mobilities of fluorescein and fluorescein-dextran conjugates in microchannels. They have also used the technique to visualize two-dimensional advective dispersion effects for electrokinetic flows in channel turns.

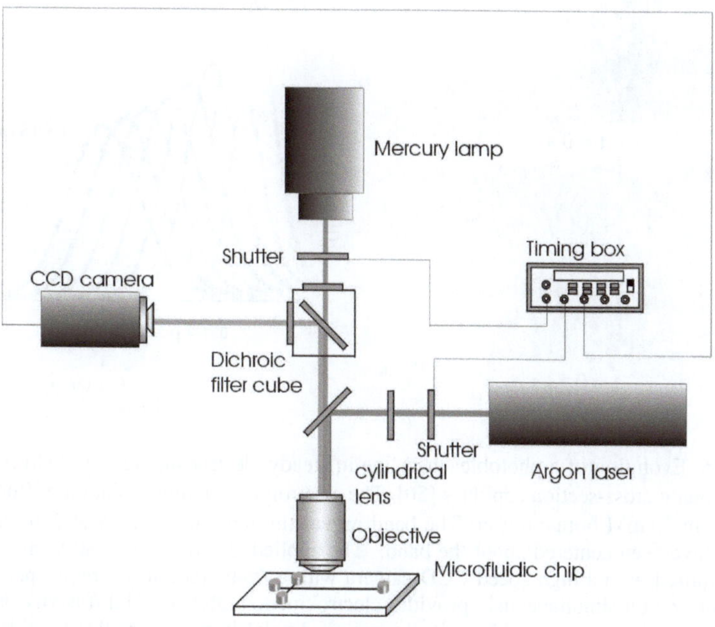

Fig. 3.14. Schematic of a photobleached-fluorescence imaging experimental setup. The 488 nm line from an argon ion laser is used to effect photobleaching process and a mercury lamp is used to image the unbleached dye field. Shutters for both the illumination sources and the CCD camera are controlled by timing electronics.

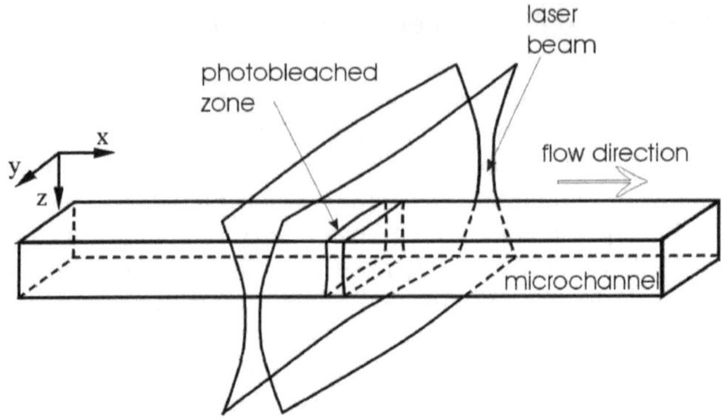

Fig. 3.15. Schematic of the micro laser sheet shape relative to the microchannel and the resulting photobleached region. The photobleached region has a Gaussian intensity profile along the capillary axis and negligible gradients in the y and z directions. Rapid shuttering of the bleaching pulse yields high resolution flow tagging.

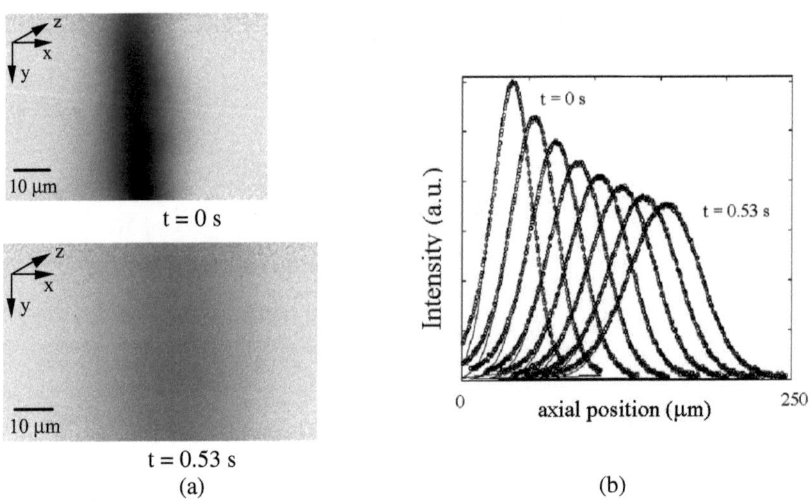

Fig. 3.16. Evolution of a photobleached line in steady electroosmotic flow field in a 50 × 50 μm square cross-section capillary [56]. The electrolyte is a dilute solution of fluorescein (<1mM) in 20 mM borate buffer. The band moves through the capillary at 220 μm/s, and images have been centered about the band. The applied electric field is 80 V/cm. Images were acquired with a high speed CCD camera with a frame rate of 53 frames per second. The visualization simultaneously provides electrokinetic mobility and diffusivity data. On the right is a time sequence of vertically-averaged axial intensity profiles for this simple straight-channel electroosmotic flow experiment. These profile intensities are of the form (I_o-I), where I is the intensity of the imaged, unbleached fluorophores and I_o is a normalization constant.

The method adopted by Mosier et al. [56], and described here is a photobleached fluorescence visualization technique for two- and, in some cases, three-dimensional flows. The visualization system is shown in Figure 3.14. The two light sources in this experiment are an argon ion laser and a broad spectrum mercury arc lamp. Both light sources are routed to the microfluidic section through an epifluorescent microscope (Olympus, Melville, New York) through which the fluid flow is imaged. The laser is used for photobleaching, and the mercury lamp is used to illuminate the field of view for image collection. Both light sources are electromechanically shuttered (two shutters from Uniblitz, Rochester, New York). A laser light sheet, formed by a combination of the microscope objective and a cylindrical lens, is used to optically write a photobleached line. The high intensity laser irradiation chemically changes the fluorophore in the fluid so that it no longer participates in the absorption/emission process. The photobleached zone then migrates due to fluid motion (e.g., electroosmotic or pressure-driven flow) and is detected by a CCD camera (or alternately by a PMT). The advective and diffusive development of the photobleached zone can then be used to determine flow field conditions and transport coefficients such as electrophoretic mobility and diffusivity.

A detailed view of the bleaching region is shown in Figure 3.15. The photobleached region has the Gaussian intensity profile along the axis of the capillary and its characteristic width is approximately uniform over the depth of the channel. To achieve uniform bleaching, the channel depth should be less than the Rayleigh range of the laser sheet. The temporal resolution of the shutter for the laser beam, which defines the time interval over which photobleaching occurs, is 2 ms. The 10 ms resolution of the mercury lamp's shutter is used to avoid unwanted photobleaching of the dye as a result of the low intensity, background illumination between the time of the high intensity bleaching pulse and imaging of the bleached band. A cube filter with excitation, dichroic and emission filters taylored for fluorescein excitation and emission wavelengths is applied. Image collection is achieved using a back-illuminated, 14 bit digitization CCD camera with 512 x 512 pixel array and a maximum frame speed of 40 Hz. Figure 3.16a shows a photobleached line in a rectangular cross-section capillary at t = 0 s (immediately after photobleaching) and at t = 0.53 s. The images are flat-field corrected using the following correction typical to quantitative scalar imaging.

$$I_{corr} = \frac{\left(I_{raw} - I_{background}\right)}{\left(I_{flatfield} - I_{background}\right)} \tag{3.14}$$

The background image ($I_{background}$) is subtracted from the raw image (I_{raw}) and normalized by the difference between a flatfield ($I_{flatfield}$) and the background image. The two images show the rapid decrease in signal-to-noise ratio of the image as the line diffuses while it advects electrokinetically through the channel. The motion with respect to the capillary can be characterized using the arithmetic sum of the electroosmotic mobility of the channel and the electrophoretic mobility of the dye. Figure 3.16b shows a time sequence of axial intensity profiles (averaged along columns) and fitted with Gaussian curves. As expected, the maximum intensity of these curves scales as $t^{-1/2}$, where t is the time of diffusion. Since charged dyes were used for the photo-bleaching experiments, the measurements were coupled with the current monitoring technique to yield a simultaneous measurement of electrophoretic mobility and diffusion coefficient of the fluorophore.

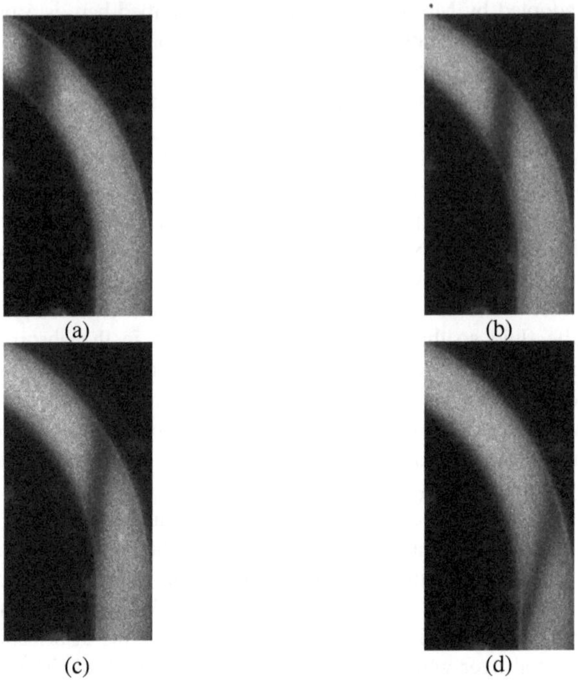

Fig. 3.17. Sequence of images showing a bleached zone, driven electrokinetically in a curved acrylic channel [56]. The channel has a trapezoidal cross-section with a bottom width of 32 μm, a top width of 97 μm and a centerline depth of 50 μm. The electric field in the straight-channel sections is 30 V/cm. The fluorophore is a 2 MD dextran fluoroscein conjugate in 20 mM borate buffer. A higher electric field and shorter pathlength along the inner wall of the curve compared to the outer curve stretches and tilts the initially vertical photobleached region.

The imaging field Peclet number can be tuned by using high and low molecular weight dyes. An example of this is shown in Figure 3.17. A two million Dalton molecular weight dye is used in this experiment [56] to visualize the effects of a microchannel turn on an initially vertical bleached region. The bleached region stretches and tilts as it electroosmotically travels around the microchannel turn. Such turns have also been visualized and studied by Molho et al. [1]. The achievable spatial resolution in simple velocity measurements is approximately 5 μm with this technique. The spatial image resolution is determined by the optics.

The rapid bleaching flow visualization technique described here is applicable to a range of flow velocities where the displacement of the fluid during the time of bleaching is less than the width of the bleaching laser sheet. As such, the imaging signal-to-noise ratio of the technique is limited by the bleaching sensitivity of the dye used. Another limit is the case of very low velocities where unbleached fluorophores diffuse into the bleached region of the flow in a time that is small compared to the timescale for the fluid to advect a distance w. These limits place a constraint on the addressable flow velocities which can be expressed as:

$$\frac{2D}{w} << U << \frac{w}{\delta t} \tag{3.15}$$

where w is the axial width of the laser sheet, δt is the photobleaching time, U is the characteristic velocity of the flow and D is the diffusivity of the fluorophore. In practise, these inequalities can be interpreted as "an order of magnitude less than". These relations assume that the minimum bleached region displacements of interest are at least an order of magnitude higher than the axial width of the bleached region, w. These constraints also apply to the caged-fluorescence line writing method described in the next section.

3.3 Caged-Fluorescence Visualization

Caged fluorescence was originally developed by Lempert et al. [90], as a flow visualization tool for studying high Reynolds number incompressible turbulent flows. They termed the method as photo-activated nonintrusive tracing of molecular motion (PHANTOMM). Paul et al. [91] first applied this diagnostic to image pressure driven and electrokinetically driven flows in capillaries. Since then several groups have used this technique to study the flow field conditions in electroosmotically driven flows (in both capillaries and microchannels) [21,49,92,93]. Caged fluorescence involves the irreversible conversion of a photoactive fluorescent dye, initially in a nonfluorescent caged state to a state that fluorescences. This conversion is achieved by exposing the dye molecules to ultraviolet (UV) light which photocleaves molecular bonds associated with the caging groups of the molecule that quench fluorescence. This photolysis process enables the recovering of the unmodified dye, which is then available for conventional fluorescence based tracking techniques [90]. After a time delay controlled by the timing electronics of the experimental setup, a short pulse of a laser excites the uncaged dye and the resulting fluorescence image is collected on a CCD camera. The convection and diffusion of the dye (a conserved scalar in the case of negligible photobleaching) is captured on successive images by the camera. Caged dyes are available with a range of molecular structure and charge and commonly used chemistries include DMNB caged fluorescein dextran, CMNCBZ- caged 5- and 6 carboxy Q rhodamine, CMNB caged fluorescein, among others.

Figure 3.18 shows the schematic of a typical caged fluorescence setup. A frequency tripled Nd:YAG laser ($\lambda = 355$ nm) is used to uncage the dye. A lens train in the laser path provides a laser sheet with a thickness of 25 μm and a width of 2000 μm. The blue wavelength from a broad spectrum mercury lamp is selectively routed by a dichroic filter assembly (similar to that described in the section on bleached fluorescence) and used to excite the uncaged dye. The emitted fluorescence is then routed through the same dichroic assembly onto a high speed CCD camera (PixelVision, Pluto CCD 14, Tigard, Oregon). A UV protection filter (Newport, Irvine, CA) protects the coated optics in the objective lens of the microscope from the UV laser pulses used for the uncaging process. The timing of the various events which include the uncaging of the dye and the fluorescence imaging are controlled through a digital delay generator (Berkeley Nucleonics, Berkeley, California). Figure 3.19 shows the temporal evolution of a line written into an electrokinetically driven flow. The dye used for this set of experiments was a caged fluorescein dye [1]. The plug-like profile demonstrated earlier by the bleached fluorescence technique, is shown by the caged fluorescence images. Figure 3.20 shows a sequence of images of an uncaged band entering a sudden expansion. The width of the larger channel is 1 mm and 9 μm deep. The flow is approximately two-dimensional. On close observation, a separation of distinct species resulting from the uncaging process (showing up as low intensity bands) is observed.

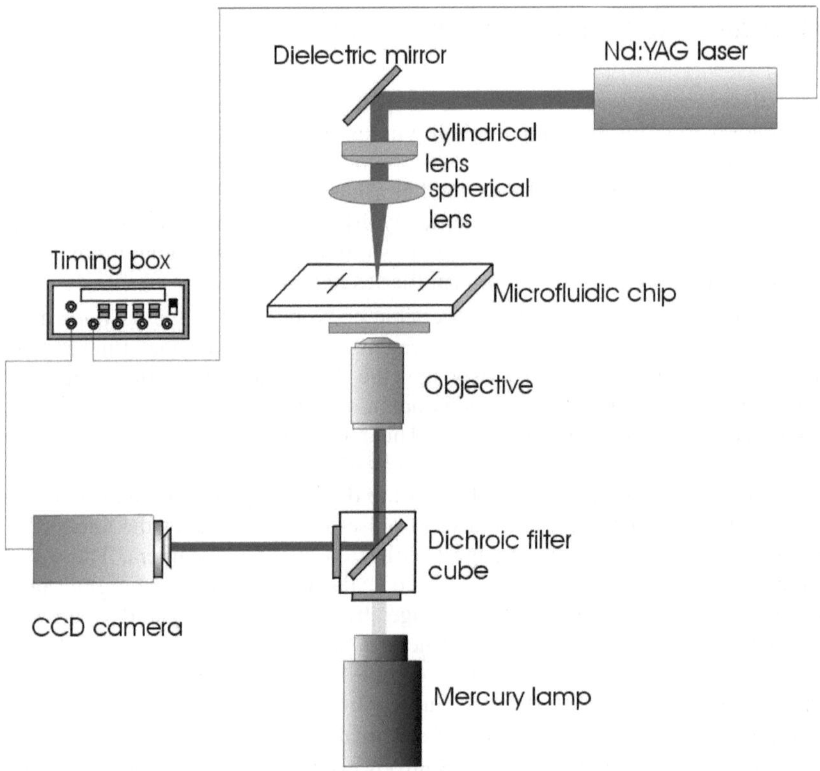

Fig. 3.18. Schematic of a caged-fluorescence visualization experimental setup. The two illumination sources are a frequency tripled Nd:YAG laser for uncaging the dye and a mercury lamp for the visualization of the uncaged dye.

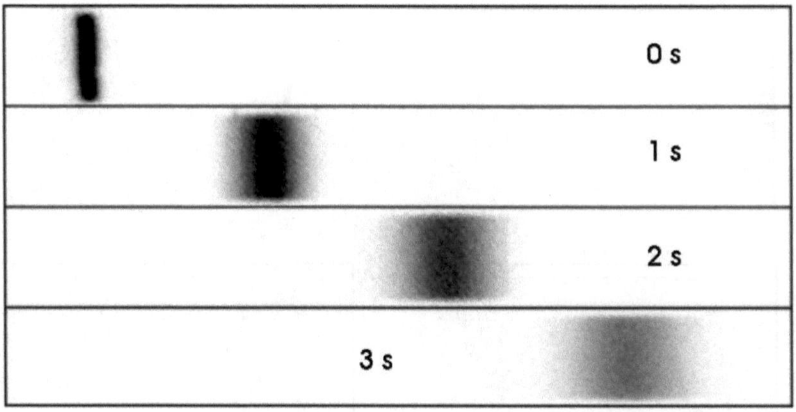

Fig. 3.19. Caged fluorescence images of electrokinetically driven flow in a microchannel [1]. The images have been inverted for clarity of presentation, and time stamps are shown for each image. The channel has a rectangular cross-section 120 μm wide (in the plane of the image) and 9 μm deep. The uncaged dye progresses at a velocity determined by the effects of both electrophoresis and electroosmosis. The width of the sample band increases due to the effects of diffusion.

The two techniques, bleached fluorescence and caged fluorescence, can be broadly defined as line-writing and/or molecular tagging techniques (a.k.a, molecular tagging velocimetry). The advantages that these line writing techniques have over conventional dye injection and dye front monitoring methods are that the initial shape of the line is dictated by the laser sheet thickness and can be finely tuned. Moreover the dye can be present in the entire fluid system and the band specifically written wherever optical access is available. The analysis for the range of measurable flow velocities with the caged fluorescence technique follows that described in the section on the bleached fluorescence technique; namely, $2D/w << U << w/t_c$ where w is the axial width of the laser sheet which approximately corresponds to the thickness of the line written into the flow field and t_c is the pulse duration of the laser beam used to uncage the dye. Typically the upper velocity limit due to 'blurring' of the line is unimportant in caged dye experiments since the pulse width using frequency tripled Nd:YAG lasers is of order 10 ns.

There are advantages to using either caged- or photo-bleached fluorescence visualization as line writing techniques. The signal intensities (in particular, the image signal-to-noise ratio) for the caged dye technique are typically as much as an order of magnitude higher than that of photobleached fluorescence. This difference is probably due to the efficiency of the uncaging process as compared to the photobleaching process. The difference may also be partly due to the fact that the work of Mosier et al. [56] used the gated beam of a continuous wave laser (488 nm line of an argon ion laser), rather than a high fluence pulsed laser, and kept the fluence and exposure times to a low level to avoid the effects of heating. An upper limit of the incident laser beam energy (to ensure that temperature rise is kept below a couple of °C) is dictated by the geometry of the light sheet shaping

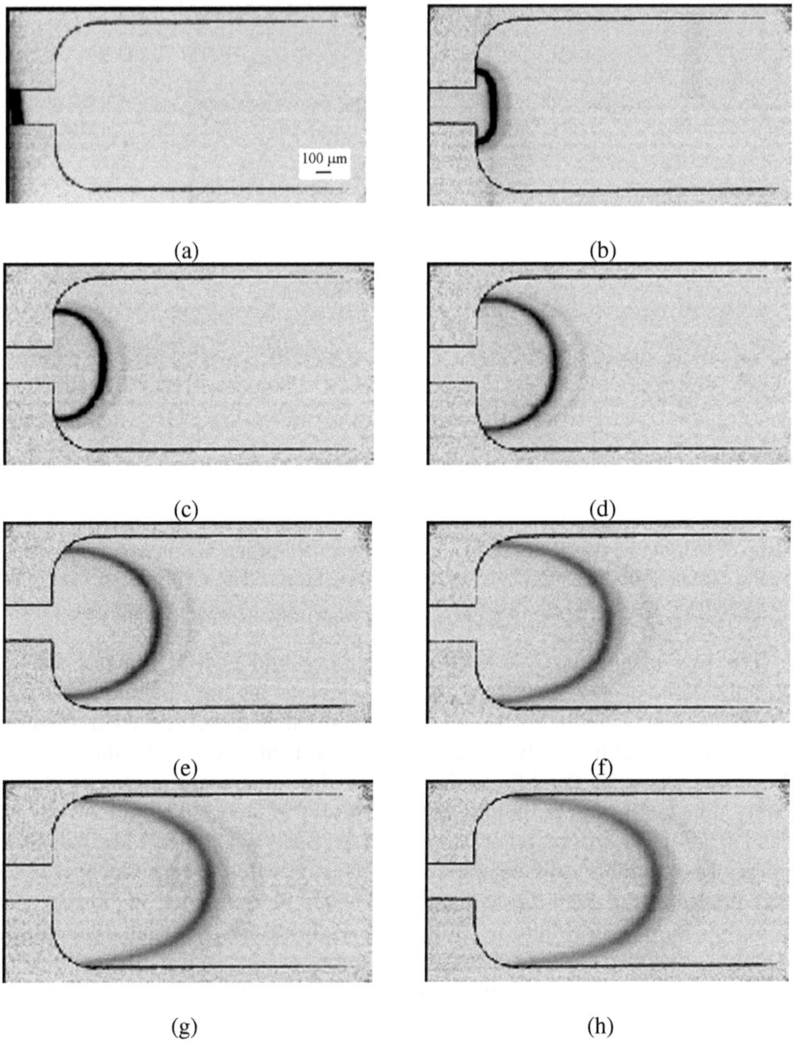

Fig. 3.20. A sequence of images showing an uncaged band entering a sudden expansion in a microfluidic system [94]. The flow is from left to right into the larger channel which has a width of 1000 μm and is 9 μm deep. This electrokinetic flow is approximately two dimensional, with an applied electric field of 200 V/cm (within the small channel). The channel outline has been highlighted for clarity.

optics and the concentration and type of the dye being used. Temperature non-uniformities lead to local changes in viscosity and also may denature the biological specimens under study. The incident power of the laser beam for the work reported by Mosier et al. was chosen to be 100 mW. On the other hand, a clear advantage of the bleached fluorescence technique is that it can be used to tag and track molecules in bioanalytical devices that already use fluorophores in their assays, such as fluorescein isothiocyanate-labeled proteins and amino acids. In such applications, the technique can be used to tag concentration fields and quantify the development of undisturbed (i.e., still fluorescent) dye molecules. For example, diffusivities and electrophoretic mobilities measured using bleached fluorescence are those of undisturbed molecules. Further, the current requirement for UV radiation in caged-fluorescence makes it difficult to apply the technique to microfluidic systems with UV-absorbing substrate materials (specifically, the optical access windows). Although possible in borosilicate glass substrates [1], the technique will be challenging to adopt in polymer-based microchannel systems given current uncaged-molecule chemistries.

3.4 Particle Imaging Techniques

Fluid mechanicians have used seed particles extensively to visualize and quantify fluid flow. An excellent review of particle imaging techniques is presented by Adrian [95]. The typical requirement for seed particles is that they faithfully follow the flow. In macroscale fluid mechanics applications, this includes the criteria that particles be neutrally buoyant and that the particle inertia be small enough such that particles can track the flow with negligible velocities relative to the fluid. The former criterion is certainly a consideration in electroosmotic microflows. Since electroosmotic flows are necessarily liquid flows, the former criterion is easily met as neutrally buoyant or nearly-neutrally buoyant particles are widely available [33]. Further, in electroosmotic flows, inertial particle lag effects are typically not important since flow accelerations are low enough that particle drag-to-inertial force ratios are typically much greater than unity.

Several new criteria arise in applying particle tracking to (liquid) electroosmotic microflows. First, the criterion that particle diameters be much smaller than the characteristic dimension of the flow channels can be stringent in microchannels. This criterion arises from the requirement that seed particle motion does not appreciably disturb the flow. An approximate practical limit is that the particle diameters should be at least two orders of magnitude smaller than the flow channel hydraulic diameter. Particle diameters of 0.5 μm have been shown to produce results consistent with theory of electroosmotic flows of aqueous solutions [96]. A related second criteria is that particle volume fraction be kept small enough such that the constitutive properties of the fluid (e.g., effective viscosity of the two-phase medium) are not affected [2]. Third, as in the case of pressure-driven microflows [97], the effects of Brownian motion are important. At typical length and velocity scales, Brownian motion becomes a key component of the total particle measured velocity and is not representative of the underlying "average" fluid motion (i.e., the continuum flow vector field). Unlike macroscale flow seed particles limited by particle inertia, the smaller the Brownian seed particle, the larger the random thermal motion of the particle and the worse the particle will follow the flow. Further discussion on the Brownian component of velocity measurement will be covered later on in this section.

A fourth consideration in seed particle selection for electroosmotic flows is that stability of colloidal suspensions of particles in liquids typically require that particles have some surface charge in order to prevent (mitigate the effects of) flocculation and adsorption to channel walls [11]. In electric field-driven flows, this surface charge results in significant electrophoretic drift velocities. This drift velocity is along the direction of the local electric field and its mean value (for some population of particles) can be interpreted as a fluid flow velocity measurement bias. In the case of electroosmotic fluid velocity fields with no similarity to the electric field, this drift component may not be in the same direction as the local flow. Examples of charged seed particles include fluorescent submicron polystyrene spheres (Molecular Probes, Eugene, Oregon) with carboxylate, amine, and sulfate surface groups which can be applied to cover a wide range of solution pH. As we will discuss, the particle electrophoretic drift velocity needs to be accounted for in studies of electroosmotic flow. Lastly, the optical detection of submicron seed particles can be a challenge in electroosmotic flows due to the high surface-to-volume ratio of the microchannels. This is because the light intensity of elastic scatter from microchannel walls is typically high compared to elastic scatter from submicron particles. A convenient and demonstrated solution to this is to use fluorescently labeled seed particles for high image signal-to-noise ratio [97].

With these features of electroosmotic flow particle seeding in perspective, we can examine various particle based techniques adopted by research groups over the years to visualize and quantify electroosmotic flows.

The use of streak images to estimate in-plane (i.e., within the measurement region corresponding to the imaged particle field) electroosmotic velocities was first reported by Taylor and Yeung [74]. They used carboxylate modified 300 nm latex microspheres to seed electroosmotic flow in a 75 μm diameter microchannel. The length of the streaks were manually estimated from a video monitor to estimate particle velocity. Taylor and Yeung pointed out that their measured streaks are a result of the superposition of electroosmotic and electrophoretic velocity components, and an estimate of the electrophoretic velocity was made from an independent measurement of the electroosmotic mobility of the capillary (using fluorescent band tracking measurements). An interesting application was reported by Stroock et al. [98], where the electroosmotic flow over a surface with patterned surface charges was estimated from particle trajectories. More recently McKnight et al. [99] used streak images of 1 μm diameter carboxylate modified latex particles to estimate particle velocities in an electroosmotic flow. These experiments were conducted in a microfluidic channel system, with electrodes patterned onto the glass cover plates.

As pointed out by Adrian [95], the difficulties in quantifying particle image streaks make it only an approximate measure of particle velocities. Streak images also have an inherent directional ambiguity. Quantification of unsteady flow phenomena is extremely difficult. Further, the long exposures associated with streak imaging can lead to associated image signal-to-noise ratio problems. Particle streak imaging is therefore a good tool in providing a qualitative understanding of the flow assuming that particles are indeed following the flow. A good example application is the case of electroosmotic flow devices which are expected to (or, preferably, known to) have velocity fields that are similar to the applied electric field. An example visualization is shown in Figure 3.21. This figure shows the particle streak visualization of flow through the intersection of two wet-etched channels with a top width of 120 μm and a centerline depth of 50 μm. 500 nm fluorescent particles are excited using the mercury arc lamp of an epifluorescent microscope and streaks are recorded with a 12 bit CCD camera (Roper Scientific, Tucson, Arizona). The image shows the right half of the intersection.

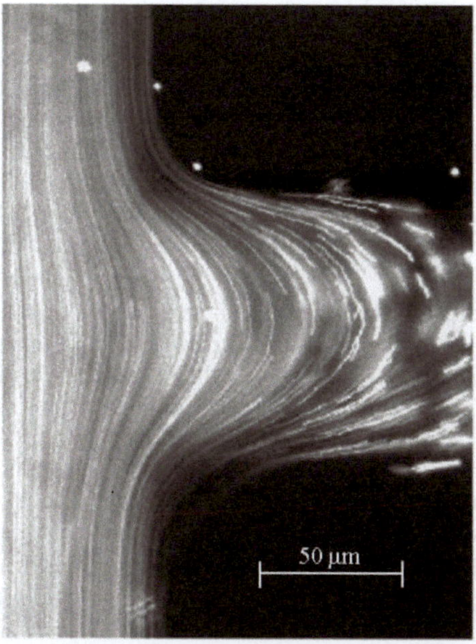

Fig. 3.21. Visualization of fluorescent particle pathlines for electrokinetic flow through an intersection. The experimental system used to obtain this image is described by Devasenathipathy et al. [96]. The two channels have a D-shaped cross-section characteristic of wet-etching fabrication with a top width of 120 μm and a centerline depth of 50 μm. The flow is from bottom to top and was generated with a 100 V/cm field (in the straight, fully-developed flow regions of the channel). The particles are fluorescently doped polystyrene microspheres and are 500 nm in diameter. The effects of Brownian motion is apparent for the slower moving particle streaks in the side-legs of the channel.

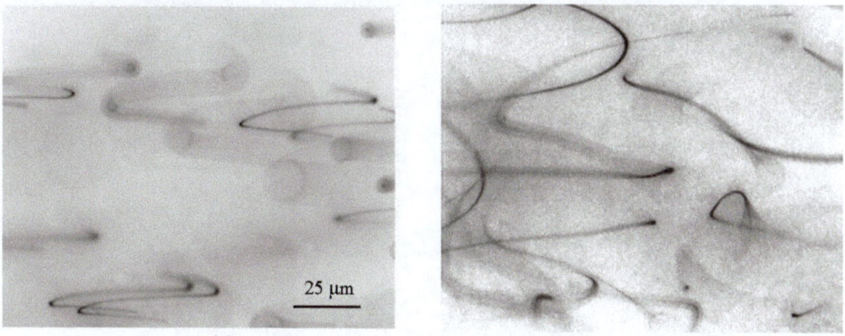

(a) (b)

Fig. 3.22. Visualization of particle pathlines in an unstable electrokinetic flow The experimental setup used in these experiments is described by Oddy et al. [77]. The microchannel has a 2000 × 200 μm cross-section and a 4 cm length. The applied AC field for (a) is 100 V/mm (RMS) and for (b) is 200 V/mm (RMS). Exposure time for the images were 50 ms, and images were binned to 4 × 4 pixel regions on chip. The base state for this flow results in simple reciprocal motions of the particles. The intermediate field strength case (a) has a significant vertical component of particle velocity. The high field case (b) has complex, three-dimensional trajectories.

The effect of Brownian motion associated with the slower moving particle streaks is apparent in the flow regions furthest from the centerline. Such visualizations have been used to compare streamline visualizations in a steady flow to predicted electric fields [19]. Another application of streak flow images has been the visualization of flow instabilities in electrokinetic flows [77], as shown in Figure 3.22. Although not yet demonstrated, this type of visualization may also be applicable to determining the degree of uniformity of wall mobility in electroosmotic systems. Presumably, significant non-uniformities in surface charge would result in measurably curved, complex streak patterns.

Another recent particle tracking work is an application of Fourier transform analysis to the detection of the motion of groups of particles [101]. These researchers measured particle velocities using a PMT to detect the fluorescence signal of particles moving under a slit array of detection windows. The emitted fluorescent signal of moving particles fluctuates at a frequency related to the particle velocity and the slit spacing. This method is analogous to laser Doppler velocimetry [102]. Application of this one-dimensional technique would be difficult in systems with multiple particle velocities (since signal strengths and spectral resolution depend on particle velocity), and the spatial resolution is limited to the size of the window array (40 μm slit width in the streamwise direction). One advantage is that only a point-wise detector is required.

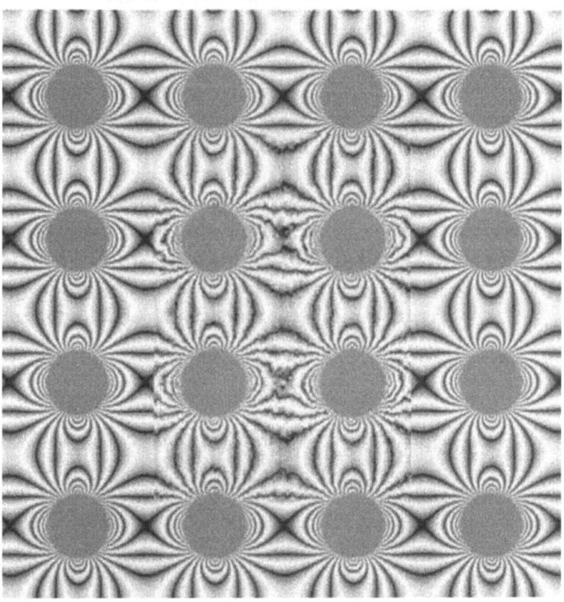

Fig. 3.23. Contours of electrokinetic velocity magnitudes (sum of electroosmotic and electrophoretic velocities) for a flow field through a circular post array [100]. The posts are 93 μm in diameter and the cell is 10 μm deep. The experimental data (shown in regions around the center four posts) is inlaid into contours determined using two-dimensional simulations (the regions around the 12 posts along the perimeter of the figure). The electric field of magnitude 2 V/mm is oriented from top to bottom. This magnitude visualization highlights small (order 2 μm/s) discrepancies between measured and predicted velocities.

Micron resolution particle image velocimetry (micro-PIV) [103], which applies depth-of-field techniques and fluorescent detection of particles, is a high-resolution, quantitative particle tracking technique applicable to microflows [97,104,105]. The application of PIV to electrokinetic flows is currently a developing field with contributions from Devasenathipathy et al. [96], and Cummings et al. [106]. Cummings [100] has studied the flow between square and circular posts in an electrokinetic Hele-Shaw cell with micro-PIV. Contours of the electrokinetic velocity field magnitudes measured by Cummings are shown in Figure 3.23 and compared to predicted values calculated with a two-dimensional flow model.

To date, nearly all reported particle-based electrokinetic flow fields are the effective particle velocity fields that result from the superposition of electroosmotic and electrophoretic components associated with raw particle velocity measurements. An effort by us to decouple these two velocity field components and obtain accurate liquid velocity measurements is summarized here [96]. The measured velocity of a particle, $\bar{u}_{meas}$, can be described simply as

$$\overline{\mathbf{u}}_{meas} = \overline{\mathbf{u}}_{eof}(\zeta) + \overline{\mathbf{u}}_{pres} + \overline{\mathbf{u}}_{eph}(\zeta_p) + \frac{\overline{\mathbf{d}}_{bm}}{\Delta t} \tag{3.16}$$

The total measured velocity of the seed particle is a linear superposition of the bulk liquid motion (both electroosmotic and pressure-driven components), electrophoretic motion of the particles and the Brownian displacement of particles. $\bar{u}_{eph}$ is the electrophoretic drift velocity of the seed particle and is a function of the zeta potential of the particle, ζ_p and the local electric field, $\bar{\mathbf{E}}$. A typical case is fluorescently tagged, polystyrene particles with a native surface charge which results in a significant electrophoretic drift velocity. For a wide range of cases where the particle diameter-to-Debye length is large enough for the ionic cloud near the particle surface to be approximated by the thin EDL limit, the drift velocity of an electrophoretic particle simplifies to the Helmholtz Smoluchowski equivalent relation, as described earlier. The fourth component on the RHS of the above equation is due to Brownian motion. d_{bm} is the displacement vector due to Brownian motion which occurs during the interval of observation, Δt. The magnitude of the standard deviation of d_{bm} is given by $\sqrt{4D\Delta t}$ for in-plane (i.e., imaged) particle displacements [96].

As demonstrated by Equation 3.16, the electrophoretic mobilities of seed particles need to be calibrated in order to determine fluid velocities from $\bar{u}_{meas}$. Several approaches have been adopted by research groups to measure mobilities of particles [107,108]. An approach adopted by us is outlined here. First, a microchannel or capillary is 'calibrated' using the current monitoring technique described earlier. The electrophoretic velocities of a sample of seed particles are then monitored in this channel of known electroosmotic mobility. Individual particle displacements can be obtained using an image analysis/velocimetry technique, micron-resolution particle tracking velocimetry (micro-PTV) [109]. An example result of particle displacements for this calibration experiment is shown in Figure 3.24 for data obtained from a single pair of images. Successive interrogations over several image pairs yield a distribution of particle displacements and, given the known applied electric field, the electrophoretic mobility distribution may be quantified [96]. The mean value and standard deviation of the electrophoretic mobility distribution of the particles experiment shown in Figure 3.24 are 4.29 μm cm/V s and 0.03 μm cm/V s, respectively. This particle-to-particle variability is important as it limits the accuracy of bulk liquid velocity measurements that can be deduced from raw particle velocity measurements. A particle calibration therefore helps quantify the number of image pairs required to achieve accurate velocity field measurements of the liquid motion. This knowledge is critical in the application of ensemble averaged PIV measurements in steady electrokinetic flow fields.

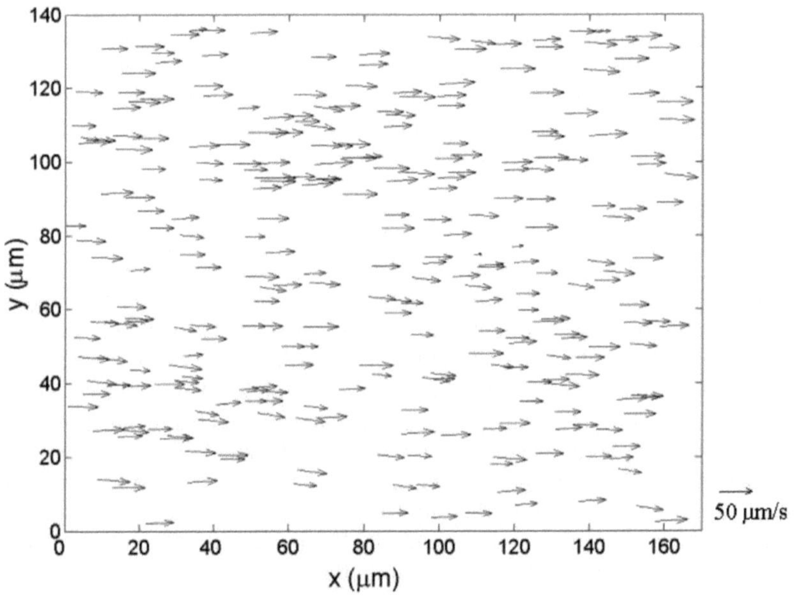

Fig. 3.24. Particle tracking velocimetry measurements (micro-PTV) of 0.5 μm polystyrene microspheres in an electrokinetic microchannel. The experimental setup is described by Devasenathipathy et al. [96]. The channel has a rectangular 400 × 40 μm cross-section and the applied field is 50 V/cm. The particle motion is a linear superposition of the electroosmotic profile and the drift velocity of the particles. The vectors display individual particle displacements for one pair of images. These 500 nm polystyrene seed particles are free of surfactants and have sulfate surface groups. The solution is a 10mM borate buffer at a pH of 9.2.

A micro-PIV experimental setup which has been used to study electroosmotic flows in several geometries [96] is shown schematically in Figure 3.25. The imaging system consists of a Nikon TE300 epifluorescent inverted microscope (Technical Instrument, San Francisco, California) with illumination provided by dual Nd:YAG lasers (New Wave, Minilase System, Fremont, California). The 532 nm laser pulse is transmitted through an optical fiber into a custom-built fluorescence color filter assembly. The optical fiber (Oriel Instruments, Stratford,

Connecticut) is a single fiber light guide with a liquid core and plastic cladding which flood illuminates the microchannel test sections. The optical fiber is convenient to use and lowers the coherence length of the laser illumination which helps avoid laser speckle in particle images. The pulse energy of the laser beam should be carefully chosen to minimize damage to the optical fiber and the objectives. Pulse energies less that one mJ is recommended. The microscope's color filter assembly consists of a 532 nm clean-up exciter filter, a dichroic beamsplitter with a cut-on wavelength of 545 nm, and a barrier emission filter transmitting wavelengths longer than 555 nm. A Nikon plan achromat oil immersion objectives ($M = 60$, nominal NA equal to 1.4) focuses the laser beam onto the fluid channel. The seed particles are 0.5 μm polystyrene latex microspheres with sulfate charge groups. A 0.6X demagnifying lens included in the optical path on the camera port enables a larger field of view to be captured by the CCD array with a negligible loss in image resolution. The images are recorded using a Princeton Instruments Micromax cooled inter-line transfer CCD camera (Roper Scientific, Tucson, Arizona) with a 1300 x 1036 pixel array and 12 bit read-out resolution. Synchronization of the camera with the laser pulses is achieved with a digital delay generator (Stanford Research Systems, Sunnyvale, California). A detailed description of micron-resolution PIV is given in this text's chapter on flow measurements for pressure driven microflows [103]. Two dimensional velocity field maps are obtained by cross-correlating interrogation regions from successive images of a seeded flow field.

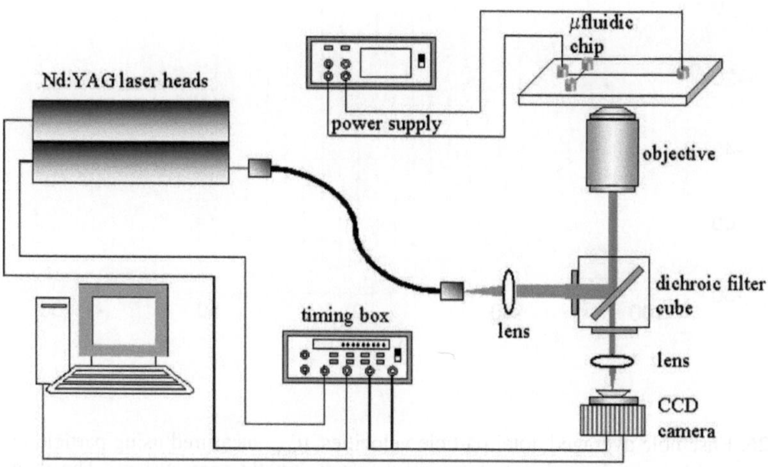

Fig. 3.25. Schematic of particle image velocimetry experimental setup. A liquid-filled optical fiber routes the two frequency doubled Nd:YAG laser beams into the microscope. A 12-bit interline CCD camera captures two successive images which are then transferred to a computer for post-processing. The triggering of the laser heads and camera is achieved through a timing box. Epifluorescence microscopy is used to obtain high signal-to-noise ratio particle images.

An example velocity vector field obtained at a cross-channel using micro-PIV is shown in Figure 3.26. There are several new publications associated with micro-PIV studies of pressure-driven flows that are applicable to electrokinetic particle tracking efforts. Specific algorithms have been implemented for extracting velocity fields for steady microflows with maximum spatial resolution [110,111]. Wereley and Meinhart [110] report an adaptive methodology which is second order accurate. Cummings [111] describes the application of a non-linear filter to separate the pressure driven and electrokinetic velocity components in a flow past an array of posts. Both Meinhart et al. [104] and Olsen and Adrian [112] present independent analyses of the effective measurement depth for micro-PIV setups. Devasenathipathy et al. [113] present an estimate of measurement depth for PTV measurements.

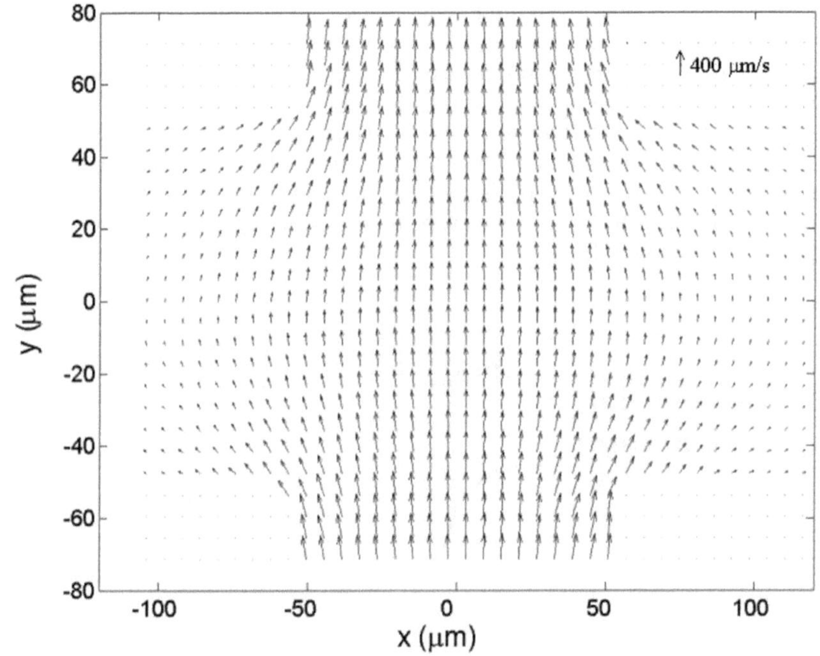

Fig. 3.26. Ensemble averaged, total particle velocities, u_{meas}, measured using particle image velocimetry at a cross-channel intersection of an electrokinetic microsystem. The channels are the same microfluidic system visualized in Figure 21. The particles are 500 nm in diameter and the field is 150 V/cm along the vertical, straight channel sections. The side channels are allowed to electrically float. These data were obtained using an experimental setup described by Devasenathipathy et al. [96].

Nuclear Magnetic Resonance Studies of Electroosmotic Flows

Flow field studies in pressure-driven and electroosmotic flows have been accomplished using spatially-resolved nuclear magnetic resonance (NMR) [114–118]. Since liquid molecules are directly tagged by altering their nuclear magnetic spin, additional tracer particles or labels need not be added. NMR studies in electroosmotic flows have traditionally focused on the study of flow in open and packed capillaries, with applications oriented towards capillary electrochromatography (CEC). Tallarek et al. [116] measured electroosmotic flow in a 250 μm id capillary. The spatial resolution of these measurements is of order > 10 μm and temporal resolutions range between 10 and 100 ms. This technique offers the ability to simultaneously measure diffusion and advection of the tagged molecules. Wu et al. [115] have demonstrated the application of a one-dimensional NMR system to measure electroosmotic flow profiles in simple geometries. More recently Locke et al. [118] have reported in-plane spatial resolutions of 78 μm for NMR measurements of electroosmotic flow in porous media.

3.5 Concluding Remarks

The field of electrokinetic flow diagnostics is developing rapidly. This development is largely due to a surge of interest in microfabricated electrokinetic systems with applications to bioanalytical devices. Earlier bulk flow methods of flow characterization include weighing of effluent, conductivity cell monitoring, streaming potential, and current monitoring. These relatively simple techniques are very important as they will probably always form the basis of initial characterizations of electrokinetic microsystems and, indeed, provide a reference for comparison with more than a century of electrokinetic measurements activity. The value of these techniques is being complemented by that of more complex flow diagnostics with higher spatial resolution, higher temporal resolution, and the ability to analyze two- and three-dimensional flow fields.

The simplest of the multi-dimensional, high temporal resolution techniques are simple visualization of the temporal development of fluorescent dye fields. These visualizations form the simple, initial thrust in the direction of field-based diagnostic techniques. In particular, experiments such as the tracking and imaging of sample plugs in electrophoretic systems are today shedding new light on sample band dispersion rates and the coupled problem of sensitivity in microfluidic systems. The application (and validation) of neutral marker imaging promises to yield further insight into the electroosmotic (i.e., bulk) liquid motion independent of the effects of tracer electromigration. Such visualizations are direct and relatively robust since they avoid problems of high intensity and short duration laser illumination, as well as the adsorption and/or flow disturbance problems associated with particle flow seeding. Further along the evolution of field-based flow diagnostic systems are the methods that provide more quantitative and/or spatially resolved flow field information. For example, scalar line writing techniques such as photobleached fluorescence and caged fluorescence imaging allow for the simultaneous measurement of advection and diffusion processes in microfluidic electrokinetic systems.

Although probably the most complex to implement, particle-based diagnostics offer measurements resolved in the depthwise direction which can be applied in three dimensional flow fields and which offer the highest available spatial and temporal resolutions. This feature is in sharp contrast to the line-of-sight averaged measurements provided by scalar techniques. Another contrast is that the particle tracking methods are not really model systems for scalar development visualizations where diffusion of molecular species is of primary interest. In the end, the choice of visualization should and often is determined by the phenomena of interest and, ultimately, the application of interest. Most diagnostics offer some relative set of advantages ranging from simplicity to resolution.

The future of electrokinetic diagnostics is tied to the future of electrokinetic systems. One key characteristic of their development is that electrokinetic systems and the applications which they target are inherently multiphysics oriented (i.e. multidisciplinary). This characteristic is unlike much of the development of modern fundamental fluid mechanics and, in particular, turbulence research where the major goals of diagnostics have been in providing higher spatial and temporal resolution measurements of the gradients of unsteady, three-dimensional velocity fields. In contrast, the development of electrokinetic systems is much more diverse in that the key issues are the interplay between electrostatics, electrodynamics, molecular and particle transport, fluid motion, reactive systems, and functionalities of biological systems. As such, an important area in the development of electrokinetic flow diagnostics will probably be the development of simultaneous measurements of scalar and vector fields of interest. The merits of, for instance, simultaneous measurements of temperature and concentration fields together with velocity fields in efforts to study fundamental flow/macromolecule interactions should be significant. Clearly, the multiphysics field of electrokinetics will need multiphysics measurements and our work has just begun.

References

[1] Molho, J. I. Electrokinetic Dispersion in Microfluidic Separation Systems. Ph.D.Thesis, Stanford University, 2001.

[2] Probstein, R. F. *Physicochemical Hydrodynamics : An Introduction*, 2nd ed.; John Wiley & Sons: New York, 1994.

[3] Jiang, L.; Koo, J.; Zeng, S.; Mikkelsen, J. C.; Zhang, L.; Zhou, P.; Santiago, J. G.; Kenny, T. W.; Goodson, K. E.; Maveety, J. G.; Tran, Q. A. "Two-phase Microchannel Heat Sinks for an Electrokinetic VLSI Chip Cooling System"; 17th Annual IEEE Semiconductor Thermal Measurement and Management Symposium, 2001, San Jose, CA.

[4] Yao, S.; Huber, D. E.; Mikkelsen, J. C.; Santiago, J. G. "A large flowrate electroosmotic pump with micron pores"; ASME International Mechanical Engineering Congress and Exposition, Sixth Micro-Fluidic Symposium, 2001, New York, NY.

[5] Hunter, R. J. *Zeta Potential in Colloid Science*; Academic Press: London, 1981.

[6] Sharp, K. V.; Adrian, R. J.; Santiago, J. G.; Molho, J. I. Liquid Flows in Microchannels. In *CRC Handbook on MEMS*; Gad-el-Hak, ed.; CRC, 2001.

[7] Scales, P. J.; Grieser, F.; Healy, T. W.; White, L. R.; Chan, D. Y. C. *Langmuir ;* **1992**, *8*, 965.

[8] Roberts, M. A.; Rossier, J. S.; Bercier, P.; Girault, H. *Analytical Chemistry ;* **1997**, *69*, 2035.

[9] Adamson, A. W., and A.P. Gast *Physical Chemistry of Surfaces*, Sixth ed.; John Wiley & Sons, Inc.: New York, 1997.

[10] Dukhin, S. S.; Zimmermann, R.; Werner, C. *Colloids and Surfaces A-Physicochemical and Engineering Aspects ;* **2001**, *195*, 103.

[11] Hiemenz, P. C.; Rajagopalan, R. *Principles of Colloid and Surface Chemistry*, Third ed.; Marcel Dekker, Inc.: New York, 1997.

[12] White, F. M. *Viscous Fluid Flow*, Second ed.; McGraw-Hill, Inc.: New York, 1991.

[13] Rice, C. L.; Whitehead, R. *Journal of Physical Chemistry* **1965**, *69*, 4017.

[14] Burgreen, D.; Nakache, F. R. *Journal of Physical Chemistry* **1964**, *68*, 1084.

[15] Patankar, N. A.; Hu, H. H. *Analytical Chemistry ;* **1998**, *70*, 1870.

[16] Chen, C. H.; Santiago, J. G. *Journal of Microelectromechanical Systems* **2002**, *11,* 672.

[17] Russel, W. B.; Saville, D. A.; Schowalter, W. R. *Colloidal Dispersions*; Cambridge University Press, 1999.

[18] Overbeek, J. T. G. Electrochemistry of the Double Layer. In *Colloid Science*; Kruyt, H. R., ed.; Elsevier: Amsterdam, Netherlands, 1952; pp 115.

[19] Santiago, J. G. *Analytical Chemistry ;* **2001**, *73*, 2353.

[20] Cummings, E. B.; Griffiths, S. K.; Nilson, R. H.; Paul, P. H. *Analytical Chemistry* **2000**, *72*, 2526.

[21] Molho, J. I.; Herr, A. E.; Mosier, B. P.; Santiago, J. G.; Kenny, T. W.; Brennen, R. A.; Gordon, G. B.; Mohammadi, B. *Analytical Chemistry ;* **2001**, *73*, 1350.

[22] Harrison, D. J.; Fluri, K.; Seiler, K.; Fan, Z. H.; Effenhauser, C. S.; Manz, A. *Science;* **1993**, *261*, 895.

[23] Harrison, D. J.; Glavina, P. G.; Manz, A. *Sensors and Actuators B-Chemical ;* **1993**, *10*, 107.

[24] Lauer, H. H.; McManigill, D. *Analytical Chemistry ;* **1986**, *58*, 166.

[25] Jorgenson, J. W.; Lukacs, K. D. *Science ;* **1983**, *222*, 266.

[26] Landers, J. P. *Handbook of Capillary Electrophoresis*, Second Edition ed.; CRC Press: Boca Raton, 1997.

[27] *Electrophoresis ;* **2000**, *21*, 3871.

[28] Altria, K. D. *Journal of Chromatography A ;* **1999**, *856*, 443.

[29] Baker, D. R. *Capillary Electrophoresis*; John Wiley & Sons, Inc.: New York, 1995.

[30] StClaire, R. L. *Analytical Chemistry ;* **1996**, *68*, R569.

[31] Krylov, S. N.; Dovichi, N. J. *Analytical Chemistry ;* **2000**, *72*, R111.

[32] SalimiMoosavi, H.; Jiang, Y. T.; Lester, L.; McKinnon, G.; Harrison, D. J. *Electrophoresis ;* **2000**, *21*, 1291.

[33] Haughland, R. P. *Handbook of Fluorescent Probes and Research Chemicals*; Molecular Probes, 1996.

[34] Jung, B. S.; Santiago, J. G. **2002**, *unpublished results.*

[35] Bharadwaj, R.; Santiago, J. G. *Electrophoresis* **2002**, *23,* 2729.

[36] VanDeGoor, A. A. A. M. Capillary Electrophoresis of Biomolecules; Theory, Instrumentation and Applications. Ph.D. thesis, Eindhoven University of Technolgy, 1992.
[37] Wanders, B. J.; Vandegoor, A.; Everaerts, F. M. *Journal of Chromatography ;* **1989**, *470*, 89.
[38] Altria, K. D.; Simpson, C. F. *Chromatographia ;* **1987**, *24*, 527.
[39] Vandegoor, A.; Wanders, B. J.; Everaerts, F. M. *Journal of Chromatography ;* **1989**, *470*, 95.
[40] Guenat, O. T.; Ghiglione, D.; Morf, W. E.; de Rooij, N. F. *Sensors and Actuators B-Chemical ;* **2001**, *72*, 273.
[41] Liu, Y.; Wipf, D. O.; Henry, C. S. *Analyst ;* **2001**, *126*, 1248.
[42] Reijenga, J. C.; Aben, G. V. A.; Verheggen, T.; Everaerts, F. M. *Journal of Chromatography ;* **1983**, *260*, 241.
[43] Gu, Y. G.; Li, D. Q. *Journal of Colloid and Interface Science ;* **2000**, *226*, 328.
[44] Huang, X., Gordon, M.J., and Zare, R.N. *Analytical Chemistry* **1988**, *60*, 1837.
[45] Devasenathipathy, S.; Santiago, J. G. **2002**, *unpublished results.*
[46] Scales, P. J; Grieser, F.; Healy, T. W.; White, L. R.; Chan, D. Y. C. *Langmuir* **1992**, *8*, 965.
[47] Bharadwaj, R.; Santiago, J. G. "Dynamics of field-amplified sample stacking"; ASME International Mechanical Engineering Congress and Exposition, 2001, New York, NY.
[48] Anderson, J. L.; Idol, W. K. *Chemical Engineering Communications* **1985**, *38*, 93.
[49] Herr, A. E.; Molho, J. I.; Santiago, J. G.; Mungal, M. G.; Kenny, T. W.; Garguilo, M. G. *Analytical Chemistry* **2000**, *72*, 1053.
[50] Lee, C. S.; McManigill, D.; Wu, C. T.; Patel, B. *Analytical Chemistry ;* **1991**, *63*, 1519.
[51] Chien, R. L.; Helmer, J. C. *Analytical Chemistry ;* **1991**, *63*, 1354.
[52] Tang, L.; Huber, C. O. *Talanta ;* **1994**, *41*, 1791.
[53] Tsuda, T.; Kitagawa, S.; Dadoo, R.; Zare, R. N. *Bunseki Kagaku ;* **1997**, *46*, 409.
[54] Locascio, L. E.; Perso, C. E.; Lee, C. S. *Journal of Chromatography A ;* **1999**, *857*, 275.
[55] Ocvirk, G.; Munroe, M.; Tang, T.; Oleschuk, R.; Westra, K.; Harrison, D. J. *Electrophoresis ;* **2000**, *21*, 107.
[56] Mosier, B. P.; Molho, J. I.; Santiago, J. G. *Experiments in Fluids* **2002**, *33*, 545.
[57] Moorthy, J.; Khoury, C.; Moore, J. S.; Beebe, D. J. *Sensors and Actuators B-Chemical ;* **2001**, *75*, 223.
[58] Bianchi, F.; Wagner, F.; Hoffmann, P.; Girault, H. H. *Analytical Chemistry ;* **2001**, *73*, 829.
[59] Tsuda, T.; Nomura, K.; Nakagawa, G. *Journal of Chromatography ;* **1982**, *248*, 241.
[60] Walbroehl, Y.; Jorgenson, J. W. *Analytical Chemistry ;* **1986**, *58*, 479.
[61] Lambert, W. J.; Middleton, D. L. *Analytical Chemistry ;* **1990**, *62*, 1585.
[62] Sandoval, J. E.; Chen, S. M. *Analytical Chemistry ;* **1996**, *68*, 2771.
[63] Cross, R. F.; Smairl, A. M. *Journal of Chromatography a ;* **2001**, *929*, 113.
[64] Liu, C. Y.; Ho, Y. W.; Pai, Y. F. *Journal of Chromatography A ;* **2000**, *897*, 383.
[65] Hayes, M., and Ewing, A. *Analytical Chemistry* **1992**, *64*, 512.
[66] Hayes, M., Kheterpal, I., and Ewing, A. *Analytical Chemistry* **1993**, *65*, 27.
[67] Hayes, M., Kheterpal, I., and Ewing, A. *Analytical Chemistry* **1993**, *65*, 2010.
[68] Schutzner, W.; Kenndler, E. *Analytical Chemistry ;* **1992**, *64*, 1991.

[69] Preisler, J.; Yeung, E. S. *Analytical Chemistry ;* **1996**, *68*, 2885.
[70] Jacobson, S. C.; Ramsey, J. M. *Analytical Chemistry ;* **1997**, *69*, 3212.
[71] Schrum, K. F.; Lancaster, J. M.; Johnston, S. E.; Gilman, S. D. *Analytical Chemistry;* **2000**, *72*, 4317.
[72] Pittman, J. L.; Schrum, K. F.; Gilman, S. D. *Analyst ;* **2001**, *126*, 1240.
[73] Tsuda, T.; Ikedo, M.; Jones, G.; Dadoo, R.; Zare, R. N. *Journal of Chromatography;* **1993**, *632*, 201.
[74] Taylor, J. A.; Yeung, E. S. *Analytical Chemistry ;* **1993**, *65*, 2928.
[75] Kuhr, W. G.; Licklider, L.; Amankwa, L. *Analytical Chemistry ;* **1993**, *65*, 277.
[76] Tsuda, T., Imaging of dye front in electroosmotic flow. *Personal Communications*
[77] Oddy, M. H.-H.; Santiago, J. G.; Mikkelsen, J. C. *Analytical Chemistry* **2001**, *73*, 5822.
[78] Jacobson, S. C.; McKnight, T. E.; Ramsey, J. M. *Analytical Chemistry ;* **1999**, *71*, 4455.
[79] He, B.; Burke, B. J.; Zhang, X.; Zhang, R.; Regnier, F. E. *Analytical Chemistry ;* **2001**, *73*, 1942.
[80] ShultzLockyear, L. L.; Colyer, C. L.; Fan, Z. H.; Roy, K. I.; Harrison, D. J. *Electrophoresis ;* **1999**, *20*, 529.
[81] Ross, D.; Gaitan, M.; Locascio, L. E. *Analytical Chemistry ;* **2001**, *73*, 4117.
[82] Axelrod, D.; Koppel, D. E.; Schlessinger, J.; Elson, E.; Webb, W. W. *Biophysical Journal ;* **1976**, *16*, 1055.
[83] Lanni, F.; Ware, B. R. *Review of Scientific Instruments ;* **1982**, *53*, 905.
[84] Salmon, E. D.; Saxton, W. M.; Leslie, R. J.; Karow, M. L.; McIntosh, J. R. *Journal of Cell Biology ;* **1984**, *99*, 2157.
[85] Tsay, T. T.; Jacobson, K. A. *Biophysical Journal ;* **1991**, *60*, 360.
[86] Ricka, J. *Experiments in Fluids ;* **1987**, *5*, 381.
[87] Fiedler, H. E.; Wang, G. R. Anemometer based on the effect of photobleaching. In *Deutsches Patent 19838344.4* Germany, 1998.
[88] Monnig, C. A.; Jorgenson, J. W. *Analytical Chemistry ;* **1991**, *63*, 802.
[89] Moore, A. W.; Jorgenson, J. W. *Analytical Chemistry ;* **1993**, *65*, 3550.
[90] Lempert, W. R.; Magee, K.; Ronney, P.; Gee, K. R.; Haugland, R. P. *Experiments in Fluids ;* **1995**, *18*, 249.
[91] Paul, P. H.; Garguilo, M. G.; Rakestraw, D. J. *Analytical Chemistry* **1998**, *70*, 2459.
[92] Ross, D.; Johnson, T. J.; Locascio, L. E. *Analytical Chemistry* **2001**, *73*, 2509.
[93] Johnson, T. J.; Ross, D.; Gaitan, M.; Locascio, L. E. *Analytical Chemistry ;* **2001**, *73*, 3656.
[94] Molho, J. I.; Santiago, J. G. **2001**, *unpublished results.*
[95] Adrian, R. J. *Annual Review of Fluid Mechanics* **1991**, *23*, 261.
[96] Devasenathipathy, S.; Santiago, J. G.; Takehara, K. *Analytical Chemistry* **2002**, *74*, 3704.
[97] Santiago, J. G.; Wereley, S. T.; Meinhart, C. D.; Beebe, D. J.; Adrian, R. J. *Experiments in Fluids* **1998**, *25*, 316.
[98] Stroock, A. D.; Weck, M.; Chiu, D. T.; Huck, W. T. S.; Kenis, P. J. A.; Ismagilov, R. F.; Whitesides, G. M. *Physical Review Letters ;* **2000**, *84*, 3314.
[99] McKnight, T. E.; Culbertson, C. T.; Jacobson, S. C.; Ramsey, J. M. *Analytical Chemistry ;* **2001**, *73*, 4045.
[100] Cummings, E. B. *AIAA Journal* **2001**, *2001-1163.*
[101] Kwok, Y. C.; Jeffery, N. T.; Manz, A. *Analytical Chemistry ;* **2001**, *73*, 1748.

[102] Goldstein, R. J. *Fluid mechanics measurements*, 2nd ed.; Taylor & Francis: Washington, DC, 1996.
[103] Meinhart, C. D.; Wereley, S. T. Micron-Resolution Particle Image Velocimetry. In *Micro- and Nano- Scale Diagnostic Techniques*; Breur, K., ed.; Springer Verlag, 2002.
[104] Meinhart, C. D.; Wereley, S. T.; Gray, M. H. B. *Measurement Science & Technology;* **2000**, *11*, 809.
[105] Meinhart, C. D.; Wereley, S. T.; Santiago, J. G. *Experiments in Fluids ;* **1999**, *27*, 414.
[106] Cummings, E. B.; Schefer, R. W.; Chung, J. N. "A PIV methodology for high-resolution measurement of flow statistics"; 2000 ASME International Mechanical Engineering Congress & Exposition, 2000, Orlando, FL.
[107] Minor, M.; vanderLinde, A. J.; vanLeeuwen, H. P.; Lyklema, J. *Journal of Colloid and Interface Science ;* **1997**, *189*, 370.
[108] ElGholabzouri, O.; Cabrerizo, M. A.; HidalgoAlvarez, R. *Colloids and Surfaces A-Physicochemical and Engineering Aspects ;* **1999**, *159*, 449.
[109] Takehara, K.; Adrian, R. J.; Etoh, G. T.; Christensen, K. T. *Experiments in Fluids ;* **2000**, *29*, S34.
[110] Wereley, S. T.; Meinhart, C. D. *Experiments in Fluids ;* **2001**, *31*, 258.
[111] Cummings, E. B. *Experiments in Fluids ;* **2000**, *29*, S42.
[112] Olsen, M. G.; Adrian, R. J. *Measurement Science & Technology ;* **2001**, *12*, N14.
[113] Devasenathipathy, S.; Santiago, J. G.; Meinhart, C. D.; Wereley, S. T.; Takehara, K. *Experiments in Fluids* **2003**, *34,* 504.
[114] Manz, B.; Stilbs, P.; Jonsson, B.; Soderman, O.; Callaghan, P. T. *Journal of Physical Chemistry ;* **1995**, *99*, 11297.
[115] Wu, D. H.; Chen, A.; Johnson, C. S. *Journal of Magnetic Resonance Series a ;* **1995**, *115*, 123.
[116] Tallarek, U.; Rapp, E.; Scheenen, T.; Bayer, E.; VanAs, H. *Analytical Chemistry ;* **2000**, *72*, 2292.
[117] Tallarek, U.; Scheenen, T. W. J.; de Jager, P. A.; Van As, H. *Magnetic Resonance Imaging ;* **2001**, *19*, 453.
[118] Locke, B. R.; Acton, M.; Gibbs, S. J. *Langmuir ;* **2001**, *17*, 6771.

4. Micro- and Nano-Scale Diagnostic Techniques for Thermometry and Thermal Imaging of Microelectronic and Data Storage Devices

M. Asheghi and Y. Yang

By all measures, the semiconductor and data storage industries are among the most important components of the Information Technology (IT) revolution. Thermally induced failure and reliability issues at the nanoscale are becoming increasingly important due to rapid device miniaturization in microelectronic and data storage applications. Additionally, many of the emerging technologies in the data storage area rely heavily on energy transport at extremely short time and length scales as a means to overcome the superparamagnetic limit--a serious impediment to the future advancement of storage technology. Further improvements in performance, design and reliability in high-technology semiconductor and data storage devices will be difficult, if not impossible, without high temporal and spatial thermal imaging, thermometry, and thermal characterization of their constituent components and materials. This manuscript describes the principles, characteristics and applications of electrical and optical thermometry techniques that measure the absolute or relative temperatures of microelectronics and data storage devices. The range of techniques includes conventional thermal imaging using scanning laser probing, near-field thermal microscopy, and scanning probe microscopy. This manuscript focuses on high spatial and temporal resolution thermometry of devices with dimensions in the range of ten to several hundred nanometers, and time scales in the range of several picoseconds to tens of nanoseconds, respectively.

4.1 Introduction

Advances in microfabrication processes have led to a continuous miniaturization of microelectronic and data storage devices as well as MicroElectroMechanical Systems (MEMS) (e.g., mechanical and chemical sensors) that contain semiconductor or metallic layers only a few nanometers thick (Asheghi, 1999). The performance and reliability of microelectronic and data storage devices (systems) are influenced by transport of thermal energy in multilayer structures. Because the thermal phenomena are not directly responsible for the electrical or optical functionality of these devices, they often receive only indirect consideration during system design. The situation is however changing rapidly as dimensions of these devices approach several nanometers and timescales of their operation gets closer to the nano- to picoseconds range. The thermal energy transport that governs the maximum temperature in semiconductors and data storage devices or structures includes macroscopic convection and conduction in the device packaging level, and *nanoscale* and/or *microscale* heat generation and transport within the ultra thin multilayer structures (Goodson et al., 1998). The maximum local temperature in the device and at its surface depends on numerous factors: the materials and their composition, the geometry, the layer sequence and internal topography, the thermal conductivity and heat capacity of the individual constituents, the electrical or optical dimensioning of individual components, etc. (Kölzer et al., 1996). Ever increasing demands on the most diverse applications have encouraged both the semiconductor and data storage industries to invent new materials and improved deposition techniques. Thin film geometry, microcrystalline or amorphous structure of thin films, and the large number of potential defects due to the microfabrication process lead to inhomogeneities and anisotropic physical properties on a microscopic scale (Kölzer et al., 1996; Asheghi et al., 1997). As a result, thermal properties of materials in thin-film form in many cases differ strongly from those in bulk materials (Goodson and Ju, 1999). In this context, *high-resolution thermometry* and *thin-film thermal characterization* play a central role in the design and optimization of transistors, data storage devices and nanostructures.

The term thermal characterization refers to diagnostic techniques that measure internal thermal resistance, thermal boundary resistance at the interfaces, the in-plane and out-of-plane thermal conductivities, and heat capacity of thin layers. A variety of thin-film thermal characterization techniques are available at the present time (Goodson and Flik, 1994; Cahill, 1998; Goodson and Ju, 1999), however it is not always clear which technique is most appropriate for a given application. The timescale of the measurements and the geometry of the experimental structures influence the measured thermal transport properties. If the film is nonhomogeneous, the region governing the signal can vary strongly depending on the measurement technique. For these reasons, it is possible to extract thermal property data for a given film that are substantially different from those governing the temperature distribution in a given device containing that particular film. It is therefore important that measurements be tailored to yield a specifically targeted property needed in the design process (Touzelbaev and Goodson, 2001).

There has been much progress in recent years on high-resolution thermometry by employing either electrical, near- and far-field optical, or scanning probe microscopy diagnostic techniques. Electrical thermometry techniques have been widely used in the past to measure the local or average temperature rise during the steady-state and/or transient operation of microelectronic devices with spatial resolution limited by the physical or nominal dimension of the patterned bridge, junction or temperature sensitive semiconductor component. Optical diagnostic techniques, in general, have enjoyed a tremendous success in the failure analysis of electronic and data storage devices mainly due to their unique advantages over competitive techniques. They are fast down to the femtosecond regime, nondestructive, and possess spectroscopic capabilities. While the conventional optical microscope belongs to the most easily usable tools, nevertheless, their spatial resolution is limited by diffraction. This limitation is currently imposing a key obstacle for a further application in semiconductor analyses, as structure sizes move on beyond the diffraction limit of visible light. The solution to this problem is brought by near-field optical (Goodson and Asheghi, 1997) and scanning near-filed (Majumdar, 1999) thermometry techniques.

Recently, several outstanding review papers have been published on *thermal characterization techniques* at micro- and nanoscales (e.g., Goodson and Flik, 1994;

Goodson et al., 1998; Cahill, 1998; Touzelbaev and Goodson, 2001). As a result, the present manuscript only focuses on diagnostic techniques for high-resolution thermometry of transistors, interconnects, data storage devices and thin film micro- and nanostructures. Sections 4.2 and 4.3 provides an overview of the state-of-art technologies and relevant thermal phenomena in semiconductor devices, interconnects and data storage devices at nanoscales. Section 4.4 reviews the high-resolution thermometry techniques.

4.2 State-Of-Art Technologies and Relevant Thermal Phenomenon in Semiconductor Devices

Field Effect Transistors (FETs) are the building blocks of most digital electronic circuits made on a silicon substrate. One way to chart the course of microelectronic development is by the minimum feature size, such as the channel length, that can be made at a given time (e.g., Sze, 1998). In 2002, the minimum feature size of a transistor in an integrated circuit is roughly 130 nm, and the operation frequency of commercial circuits exceeds 1 GHz. According to the latest estimates, the minimum feature size achievable with good electrical performance is around 35-50 nm. Even recently, researchers from ST Microelectronics (Boeuf et al., 2001) have introduced the smallest manufactured FET with a 16 nm gate using the complementary metal-oxide semiconductor (CMOS) process. Ever increasing demand for faster microprocessors and the continuous trend to pack more transistors on a single chip result in an unprecedented level of power dissipation, which yields higher temperatures at the chip level (Fig. 4.1).

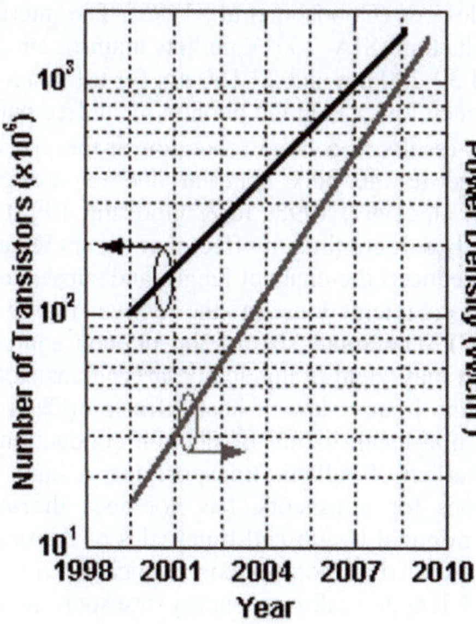

Fig. 4.1. Road map for the number of transistors and the level power density on the lead microprocessor (2001 ITRS road map).

Thermal phenomena are not directly responsible for the electrical functionality of semiconductor devices, but adversely affect their reliability. Three major thermally-induced reliability concerns for transistors are: a) failure due to a large electrical stress during short timescales, i.e. the electrostatic discharge phenomenon (Amerasekera et al., 1992; Raha et al., 1977); b) stresses due to different thermal expansion of transistor constituents; and c) failure of metallic interconnects due to the diffusion or flow of atoms along a metal interconnect in the presence of a bias current, known as the electromigration phenomenon. Self-heating of the device reduces electron mobility and results in a poor or, at best non-optimal, performance of the transistor. This is particularly important for transistors in Silicon-on-insulator (SOI) circuitry.

Silicon-on-insulator circuits promise advantages in speed and processing cost compared to circuits made from bulk silicon (e.g., Peters, 1993). Around the year 2000, IBM built and tested SOI-based microprocessors that had 20 to 25% faster circuit speed compared to CMOS technology made on bulk silicon substrates. The source of increased SOI performance is the elimination of area junction capacitance and the "body effect" in bulk CMOS technology. As microelectronics technology enters the deep sub-micron arena, fully depleted SOI (FDSOI) technology assumes a prominent position as a potential solution to the problems associated with continued device scaling. Some of the possible benefits of using FDSOI are improved control of the transistor threshold voltage, lower junction capacitance, higher device packing density, and latchup immunity (Maiti et al., 1998). However, the buried silicon-dioxide layer in SOI circuits has a very low thermal conductivity (~1 W m^{-1} K^{-1}) compared to the silicon device layer. This results in a relatively large thermal resistance between the device and the chip packaging. The thermal conduction in the silicon device layer strongly influences the peak temperature rise in SOI devices (Goodson et al., 1995). The international technology roadmap for semiconductors (SIA, 2001) predicts mainstream devices with silicon overlayer thickness of 30-200 nm and 20-100 nm for the years 2001 and 2005, respectively, which is much lower than the phonon mean free path at room temperature, Λ~300 nm. This results in a large reduction in thermal conductivity of the silicon layer compared to the bulk material due to strong phonon-boundary scattering (Asheghi et al., 1997, 1998; Ju & Goodson 1999). Phonon boundary scattering is not the only sub-continuum effect that occurs in nanoscales. The scaling of transistors has reduced the channel length and subsequently the size of the intense phonon-electron interactions in the active region of the transistor (Sverdrup et al., 1998). The small size of the phonon source compared to the phonon mean free path may yield dramatically larger transistor temperatures than those predicted using the Fourier law of heat diffusion (Chen 1996). This results from the ballistic, or non-local, nature of phonon conduction near a small heat source. However, the effect of ballistic transport near a small heat source, which has greater implications for transistors, has not been thoroughly investigated. Figure 4.2 shows the nominal length and timescales of the operation of bulk and SOI field effect transistors (right-bottom axis), which provide some indication of the relevant time and length scales of energy transport in these devices. The relevant time and length scales associated with ESD failure and localized heating effect in transistors are also depicted in Fig. 4.2 (left-top axis).

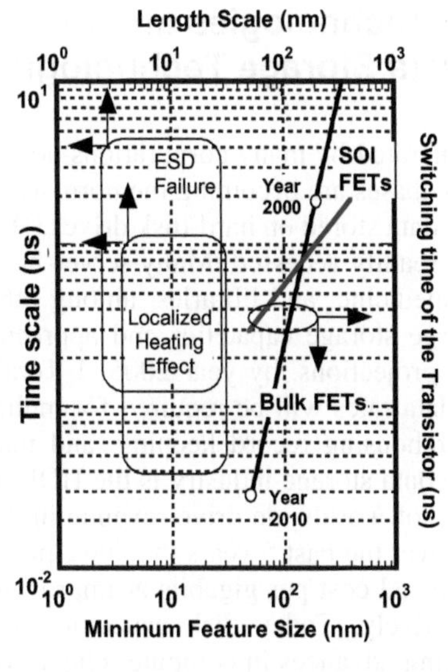

Fig. 4.2. Time and length scales associated with ESD failure and localized heating effect in transistors (left-top axis). Switching time of a transistor and relevant minimum feature size (right-bottom axis).

High-resolution thermometry techniques are urgently needed for both temperature measurements and the fundamental study of energy transport at *nano* and/or *microscales*.

The trend for miniaturization is likely to be sustained in the future by the introduction of a number of advanced yet exploratory technologies such as single electron transistors (SET) and Carbon Nanotube FETs. Inokawa et al. (2001) have successfully merged single electron transistors (SET) and MOS technology and as a result have opened up the possibility that a new class of multiple-valued logic and single-electron transistors can be constructed with half the number of elements needed in conventional implementations. For years, the carbon nanotube transistors have been looked at as a possible solution to the limits of silicon MOSFETs, but have been limited because of a lack of known technology to make electrical contact with them. IBM scientists (Martel et al., 2001) have proposed a theory that, in terms of logic applications, carbon nanotube FETs may compete with Si MOSFETs due to key device characteristics and advancements in contacts. These improvements are significant because the use of carbon nanotubes has the potential to make transistors up to ten times smaller than current existing silicon transistors. The emergence of these new technologies further motivates the experimental investigation of electron and phonon transport and heat dissipation phenomena in carbon nanotubes, silicon nanowires, and semiconductor/metal nanocrystals. The ability to locate hot spots and measure temperature at such extreme length and timescales will not be possible without near-field optical and scanning probe microscopy techniques.

4.3 State-Of-Art Technologies and Relevant Thermal Phenomena in Data Storage Technologies

The volume of data generated by many corporations doubles every year such that several terabyte size databases are becoming the norm as companies begin to keep more and more of their data stored on hard-disk drives (HDDs) and on-line, where the information can be readily accessed. Many server-based applications, such as electronic commerce, medicine, and libraries, among others, require modest access times but very large storage capacities and appreciable data transfer rates. Based on conservative projections, by year 2005, 1 Terabits/in^2 storage capacity and 10-100 MBytes/s data rates will be required for multimedia archiving, delivery and authoring, warehousing record keeping, and medical applications. The dominant branch of the data storage industry is the HDD, representing 50% of all drives shipped and 66% of worldwide drive revenue in 2000. The HDD industry has delivered products over the past 5 years that have provided increased capacity per disk platter and reduced cost per gigabits at improvement rates of 100% and ~60% per year, respectively. Today disk capacities are doubling every nine months, quickly outpacing advances in computer chips, which obey Moore's Law (doubling every 18 months). These improvements have been driven by the industry's incredible ability to improve the areal density (AD) of HDD storage at a compounded annual growth rate of >100% per year over this period. The industry shipped 145 million hard-disk drives in 1998 and nearly 170 million in 1999. That number is expected to surge to about 250 million in 2002, representing revenues of $50 billion.

However, whether the industry can maintain this pace is questionable in light of the *superparamagnetic effect* (Toigo, 2000). The problem facing the HDD industry is due to the continued shrinkage of the dimensions of the bit cells on the disk. Each of these individual magnetic data bit cells is comprised of a collection of smaller crystalline grains of a thin magnetic film, each of which is uniformly magnetized. In order to maintain adequate signal-to-noise ratio for reliable data recording and retrieval, it is necessary to keep the number of such grains per bit cell adequately large. This has required the size of the grains to be reduced with increasing AD. The superparamagnetic effect becomes important when the grain volume V is so small that the inequality $K_uV/k_BT > 40$ can no longer be met. Here K_u is the material's magnetic crystalline anisotropy energy density, k_B is Boltzmann's constant, and T is absolute temperature. When the above inequality is not satisfied, thermal energy demagnetizes the individual grains and the stored data bits will not be stable. Therefore, as we make the grain diameter smaller with increasing AD, we reach a regime for a given material K_u and temperature T, such that reliable data storage is no longer feasible. With the current pace of miniaturization, some experts believe the industry could reach this barrier as early as 2005 (Fig. 4.3).

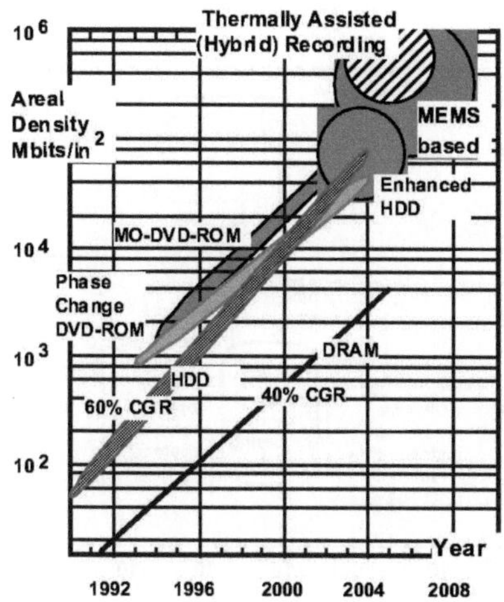

Fig. 4.3. Roadmap describing past performance and speculations on future performance of magnetic, optical and alternative data storage systems and technologies.

Data storage opportunities using nanoscale thermal effects arise within system architectures that overcome the *superparamagnetic effect* by using thermally assisted magnetic or nonmanetic writing schemes (e.g., hybrid thermomagnetic disk recording systems, thermally assisted scanned probe magnetic recording systems, and cantilever probe based thermomechanical recording systems). The data storage industry's ambition to improve AD (see Fig. 4.3) and data rates has pushed the characteristic length and timescales of these devices and processes down to the *nanometer* and *picosecond* range, respectively. If a small quantity of heat is generated over a period of time less than the thermal time constant of the magnetic element or device, then heat travels only a few nanometers away during the heating pulse. The energy must therefore be absorbed by a very small volume, which dramatically increases the temperature in the device, structure, or system. Such heating phenomena will be vastly underestimated by continuum theory and could melt or damage the magnetic element, or, at the very least, cause long-term reliability concerns for magnetic devices and/or data storage systems. The read and write elements in giant magnetoresistive (GMR) heads (Wallash, 2000), interconnects (Goodson et al., 1998) and Magnetic Random Access Memory (MRAM) are particularly susceptible to failure and/or degradation due to short timescale heating events.

The small-scale transport processes in data storage devices and systems occur within timescales and regions of dimensions varying by orders of magnitude in a given data storage device or system, as indicated in Fig 4.4. Both high temporal and spatial resolution thermometry techniques are needed to probe the thermal events in these devices. Ironically, near-field optical thermometry research and techniques can tremendously benefit from research efforts in the area of near-field optical data storage systems.

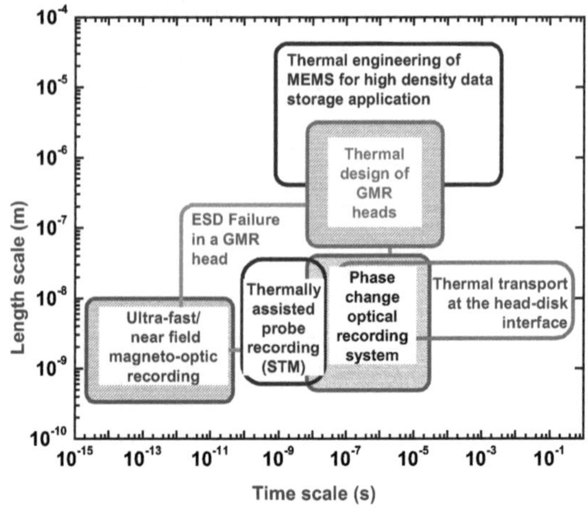

Fig. 4.4. Time and length scales associated with the heat transport process in data storage devices and systems.

4.4 Thermometry

High-resolution thermometry techniques have been classified in a number of ways. It is very common to categorize these techniques depending on whether they employ electrical or optical signals for diagnostic measurements (Goodson et al., 1998). It is also common to categorize the thermometry techniques based on near- or far field applications (Kölzer et al., 1996). For example, scanning thermal microscopy (SThM) can be either classified as the electrical (Goodson et al., 1998) or near-field (Kölzer et al., 1996) thermometry technique. In the end, what really matters is a clear understanding of the advantages and disadvantages of these techniques along with the proper selection of diagnostic tools to achieve desired spatial, temporal and temperature resolutions. This section reviews the electrical (4.1), far-field optical (4.2) and near-field (4.3) thermometry techniques, which are commonly used as diagnostic tools to probe thermal phenomena in semicondutor and data storage devices.

4.4.1 Electrical Thermometry

Electrical thermometry techniques have been widely used in the past to measure the local or average temperature rise during the steady-state and/or transient operation of transistors or GMR heads. Either the electrical-resistance thermometry in patterned bridges or temperature dependence of the electrical operating characteristics of a semiconductor component can be used to monitor the temperature of the device under electrical stress or normal operating conditions. A patterned thermocouple can also be used to measure localized temperature in micro- or nano- devices, with spatial resolution limited by the nano- devices, with spatial resolution limited by the dimensions of the patterned junction, as shown in Figure 4.5. While these techniques can yield superior spatial resolution, they can only measure temperature at a fixed point. To address this problem a new class of SThM techniques have emerged that can provide thermal images of a region as large as 8000 μm^2 and with spatial resolution better than 100 nm.

Electrical-Resistance Thermometry

Patterned metallic or semiconducting bridges (Fig. 4.5) have been extensively used in the past for high-resolution thermometry of transistors, interconnects, GMR heads, and microdevices (e.g., Wallesh, 2000; Goodson et al., 1995; Maloney and Khurana, 1985; Banerjee et al., 1996). The temperature dependent electrical resistance of the bridges can be precisely calibrated using a hot-chuck, which significantly reduces the uncertainty in the measurements. Various sources of error inherent in resistance thermometry make it difficult to achieve high level of accuracy in the order of 10 mK. For instance, lead resistance in some cases can cause errors of several tenths of a degree. Problems also arise from sources such as thermoelectric effects, reactance, and leakage. Some of the techniques apply an AC driving current and use sensing circuits that detect only the AC signal, rejecting the DC thermoelectric effects. However, the use of an AC driving current often causes errors in resistance thermometry because sensors and their lead wires have inductance and capacitance that cannot be entirely eliminated. Another source of trouble in electrical-resistance thermometry is the self-heating of the sensor. This results from power being dissipated in the sensor by the driving current. It causes the temperature of the sensor to be higher than it should be. This is particularly relevant in the thermometry of suspended MEMS structures.

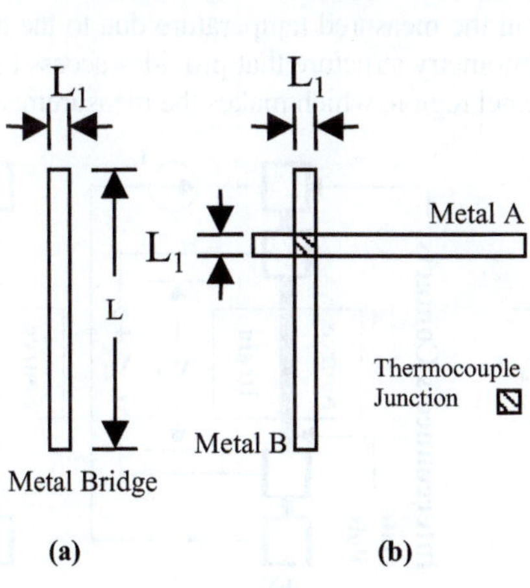

Fig. 4.5. Spatial resolution of patterned electrical resistance thermometer and thermocouple junction.

Either a modified gate structure (Estreich, 1989; Mautry and Trager, 1990; Goodson et al., 1995) or additional pattered bridge (Leung et al., 1995; Goodson et al., 1996) can be used as a sensing element in the electrical-resistance thermometry of transistors. Steady-state thermometry of the high-power SOI transistor was performed by Leung et al. (1995) using a polysilicon bridge patterned above the drift region of the device. However, the thermal resistances due to the silicon substrate and interface between the substrate-package can significantly contribute to device temperature rise during the steady-state thermometry of large area devices or interconnects (500 μm × 500 μm). The transient thermometry can partially overcome this problem because it significantly reduces the contribution from substrate and package level thermal boundary resistances. While the steady-state measurements may not be appropriate for large area devices, it can provide accurate results for the thermometry of compact SOI FETs. This is due to the fact that the large thermal resistance of the buried oxide layer and the two dimensional heat conduction spreading effect in the substrate render the contributions of the substrate and external thermal resistances insignificant compared to the device level SOI FET thermal resistance.

Goodson et al. (1995) used a modified transistor gate structure (Fig. 4.6b) as a thermometer to study self-heating of compact FETs made from SOI wafers. They experimentally measured the thermal resistances of several SOI FETs as a function of buried silicon dioxide and silicon over layer thicknesses. The results agreed very well with the predictions of a multi-fin one dimensional heat transfer model that accounts for heat conduction by source, drain, gate and interconnects. The spatial resolution of a patterned electrical-resistance thermometer could be on the order of tens of nanometers in one dimension, L_l, while only an averaged temperature can be measured along the other direction, L (Fig. 4.5). As a result, the test structure in Fig. (4.6b) effectively measures the average temperature over the length w_l, which is not equal to the length of the gate thermometer over the channel region, w_d. Goodson et al. (1995) performed a careful analysis of the temperature distribution in the gate thermometer to find the upper and lower bounds for error in the measured temperature due to the above design. Fig. 4.3b depicts a modified thermometry structure that provides access for the voltage measurement only over the channel region, which makes the measurements even more accurate.

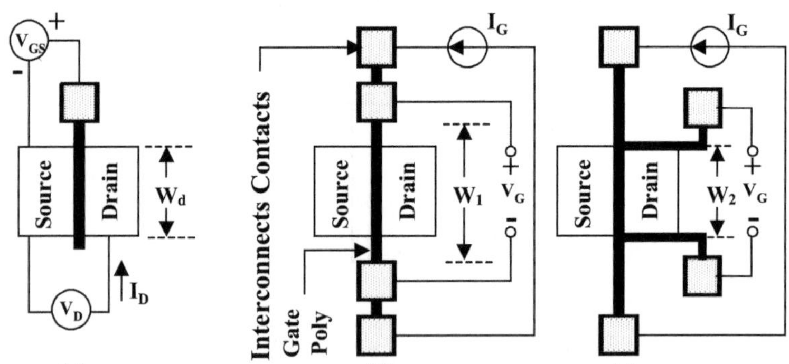

Fig. 4.6. (a) FET device, (b) test structure (Goodson *et al.*, 1995) that yields the average temperature over the distance $w_1 \neq w_d$, and (c) modified structure that yields the average temperature over the distance $w_1 = w_d$.

The lower limit for the timescale of transient thermometry of the transistor is determined by (a) the thermal diffusion time in the passivation layer that separates the thermometer from the channel region and (b) the time constant for voltage reflections and capacitive coupling in the thermometry circuit. In the electrical-resistance thermometry technique using the patterned bridges, the semiconductor device must be modified. The introduction of an additional structure at best influences the very short transient thermal behavior of the device and at worst can alter the device's performance during the steady-state or transient thermometry of the device. For example, the sensing current applied to a modified polysilicon gate structure can alter the device performance due to the voltage drop along the gate resulting in a spatially non-uniform electrical conductance in the transistor. While, this error may not be important for devices with smaller widths, it can cause significant error for wide transistors. In order to minimize this effect the sensing current should be reduced as much as possible, which incidentally helps to minimize the self-heating of the sensing element.

Thermometry Using Temperature-Sensitive Electrical Parameters

The thermometry techniques that use temperature-sensitive electrical parameters such as: mobility, threshold voltage, and saturation velocity (e.g., in SOI FETs or power devices), and base/emitter or turn-on voltages (e.g., in bipolar devices), allow thermometry of transistors without any addition or modification (e.g., Blackburn, 1988; Cain et al., 1992; Su et al., 1994; Arnold et al. 1994; Liu and Yuksel, 1995). Tenbroek et al. (1996) developed a measurement technique based on the small-signal drain conductance in saturation regime. This method is particularly appealing because it provides both the thermal and electrical characteristics of the SOI device as a function of frequency. The thermal response of the device was extracted by developing an analytical model that considers the temperature dependencies of three physical parameters: the carrier mobility, the threshold voltage, and the carrier saturation velocity. In these approaches no calibration for temperature dependent parameters was required. Su et al. (1994) and Jomaah et al. (1994) used similar temperature dependent parameters to extract the device thermal resistance by fitting experiments to the predicted current-voltage characteristics of a device.

Alternatively, the temperature-sensitive electrical parameter is calibrated using a hot-chuck and a small sensing current to avoid self-heating. The thermometry is performed using a large electrical current, usually comparable to the device bias conditions, which results in the self-heating of the device. Subsequently, the device electrical operation is interrupted and the temperature-sensitive electrical parameter is monitored using a small sensing current (Arnold et al., 1994).

The thermometry techniques that use temperature-sensitive electrical parameters can be performed on fully packaged devices, which require no addition or modification to the device structure. The spatial resolution of this technique is not entirely clear and depends on the spatial distribution of the temperature sensitive electrical parameter of the device. If an average value is used for the prediction of the temperature sensitive device parameter, then the spatial resolution will be limited by the relevant length scale of the transistor (e.g., channel length). In this measurement technique, the temperature is measured directly within the transistor rather than at the surface of a sample. As a result, the temporal resolution is not limited by the thermal diffusion time of any device component. One complication associated with this method is the impact of a nonisothermal temperature distribution in the device on the measured electrical parameter, which is typically calibrated under isothermal conditions (Goodson et al., 1998). Table I summarizes the advantages and disadvantages of various electrical thermometry techniques.

Table 4.1 Summary: Advantages and disadvantages of electrical thermometry techniques

Types	*Applications*	*Advantages and Disadvantages*
Electrical-resistance thermometry (4.1.1)	Local or average temperature measurements in transistors,nanostructures, GMR head and microdevices	Precise temperature calibration is possible. The spatial resolution in one dimension could be on the order of ~ 25 nm while the other dimension only yields an averaged temperature over the length of the bridge (Fig. 4.5). The thermometer is separated from the active region of the device limiting access to the device at very short timescales. Additional fabrication effort is required. Voltage reflections and capacitive coupling limits the timescale for transient thermometry of the device.
Thermometry using temperature-sensitive electrical parameters (4.1.2)	Temperature measurements of transistors	The thermometry can be performed on fully packaged devices. The spatial resolution of this technique is not entirely clear. The temperature is measured directly within the transistor and therefore the temporal resolution is not limited by the thermal diffusion time. A non-isothermal temperature distribution in the device during measurement of the electrical parameter and isothermal conditions during calibration will introduce an error in the temperature measurements.

4.4.2 Far-Field Optical Thermometry

In general, thermometry on a transistor, interconnect, nanostructure or microdevice can be performed by monitoring those properties of the solid layer that depend in a predictable way on their temperatures. The optical techniques are noncontact and often nondestructive. In many cases no special consideration or modification to the device under test is necessary to perform these measurements. The optical phenomena such as reflection, deflection, interference, and birefringence as well as fluorescence, absorption, and thermal emission can be exploited for measurement (Kölzer et al., 1996). The detection signal contains information about amplitude and phase, or frequency and polarization, which is different from the incident light due to its interaction with a solid layer. The optical techniques are truly versatile. A light beam can be used either as an excitation, detection, or reference signal. The intensity and frequency of light can also be modulated or controlled. The laser source can operate in CW, modulated, or pulsed modes, and, depending on a particular application, can be polarized, deflected, focused, or defocused. Optical techniques also provide superior spatial and temporal resolution, with additional imaging and/or scanning capabilities. Optical thermometry can be performed in near-field (see section 4.3.1) or designed in a manner to provide access to information from the depths of an object. The optical techniques can be classified as *active* or *passive*, depending on the mechanism of energy delivery to the device or surface. In the *passive* mode, a low power light source can be used to probe the surface of the functioning device or structure. In *active* measurement techniques, also known as *photothermal techniques*, energy is supplied to the structure by absorption of a laser beam and the resulting thermal relaxation processes are monitored. The optical energy conversion/dissipation process can occur either by radiationless relaxation (common in solids) or secondary radiant (fluorescence, phosphorescence) processes (Kölzer et al., 1996). A limited number of optical techniques are suitable for *direct* measurements of temperature in interconnects and transistors. For example, infrared (IR) thermometry requires an exact knowledge of the emissivity of the surface materials, or extensive calibration procedures are required for the internal IR laser deflection, thermoreflectance and liquid crystal thermography techniques. A wide range of optical diagnostic tools for high-resolution thermometry are readily available to the research community (*from* conventional mapping methods up to scanning microscopic and near-field techniques). The selection of the appropriate technique not only depends on the required temperature accuracy and sensitivity, and spatial and temporal resolution, but also is a function of the device's operating condition and physics, as well as its geometry and structure.

Thermal imaging or mapping techniques, such as liquid crystal thermography, fluorescence microthermography, and IR thermography techniques, have been extensively used for failure analysis and chip verification, as well as qualitative detection of hotspot temperatures in integrated circuits. The hot spots usually indicate technology defects (e.g., short circuits in interconnects, current leakage, gate-oxide breakdowns, etc.) or design weaknesses (e.g., increased current paths and faults in the layout, etc.). The measurement techniques previous work, along with a brief discussion of the temporal, spatial and temperature resolutions for these techniques will be outlined in this section.

The interferometry and thermoreflectance techniques utilize the *reflected* light that provides information about the local heating state of the device or structure. These techniques can be classified as optical beam displacement (reflected light). Laser-reflectance thermometry detects temperature changes near a surface using the dependence of the optical reflectance on temperature (e.g., Miklos and Lorincz, 1988). The optical interferometry techniques have been used both in active (Oesterschulze et al., 1993,) and passive modes (Claeys et al., 1994). Several variations of these techniques (e.g., Michelson, Mach-Zehnder and Fabry-Perot type the interferometers) are not only used for local probing, but also as a scanning procedure for measuring the surface topography or the thermal expansion.

The techniques such as the photothermal deflection spectroscopy and internal IR laser deflection that exploit the temperature dependence of the refractive index for making measurements are often classified as optical beam deflection techniques. Localized temperature gradients within a transistor, or between the device and the surrounding air, are characterized by a refractive index gradient, which can deflect an optical beam that is guided in parallel through such a region.

The spatial, temporal and temperature resolutions, as well as the common applications for the different far-field optical thermometry techniques will be also considered in this section.

Liquid Crystal Thermography (LCT)

In this technique, a thin layer of a liquid crystal (LC) is deposited onto the surface, where its optical properties are dependent on the temperature. The polarized light from a white-light source illuminates the surface and the reflected radiation is collected by a microscope with a reticulated analyzer. The LC liquid is crystalline (nematic LCs) just below the clearing-point temperature, T_c, resulting in a bright image field. If the temperature of the device is locally raised above T_c, the LC undergoes a transformation into the optically isotropic phase. Since the plane of polarized light remains unchanged, the hot spots appear dark in the polarization microscope. In this technique only a *relative* temperature mapping is possible. The use of the nematic/isotropic phase transition suffers from the drawback that only one isotherm can be obtained (Goodson et al., 1998). However, it is suggested that extensive isothermal plots can be made by means of LC crystals with different clearing-point temperatures and equidistant regulation of the chuck temperature (Kölzer et al., 1996). Detectable temperatures in the range 50 mK to 0.5 K and even 1 mK (e.g., Burgess and Tan, 1984) are reported in the literature. Temporal resolution as high as 20 ns is reported using LC voltage contrast (Picart and Minguez, 1992), but in general the resolution of conventional systems are in the range of 10 μs to 1 ms (Soref and Rafuse, 1972; Labrunie and Robert, 1973; Picart and Petit 1990; Picart and Minguez 1992). Spatial resolution of a few micrometers is reported using the nematic LCs (Aszodi et al., 1981). More common techniques use the temperature dependency of either phase sensitive (e.g., Beck, 1986) or peak wavelength reflectivity (Fergason, 1968) of LC to map the temperature distribution in a device. Spatial and temporal resolutions near 25 μm and 0.1 K, respectively, are achieved using the latter technique.

Fluorescent Microthermography (FMT)

In this technique, a thin-film fluorescing coating of europium thenoyl-trifluoroacetonate (EuTTA) dissolved in acetone is deposited onto the surface. The surface is illumined with ultraviolet light (340-380 nm) (Kolodner and Tyson 1983, 1984; Barton 1994), which stimulates fluorescence mainly at the bright 612-nm line. The fluorescence quantum efficiency of EuTTA decreases exponentially with temperature, so the measurement of the fluorescence intensity provides information about the temperature behavior of the device during operation (Barton and Tangyunyong, 1996). The proper design of the optical configuration is rather crucial in order to limit the intensity of the excitation light in a defined way and to focus the beam onto the specimen (UV light), and, at the same time, to guide the fluorescent light to a CCD camera. Spatial resolutions on the order of 0.3 μm (Barton, 1994; Barton and Tangyunyong, 1996), and 0.7 μm on a flat surface (Kolodner and Tyson, 1983), have been demonstrated. A temporal resolution is not yet implemented in FMT, although in principle it might be done performing fluorescence lifetime measurements, which is on the order of 200 μs for EuTTA (Barton and Tangyunyong, 1996), and in the picosecond regime for substituted anthroscenes (Kölzer et al., 1996). The bleaching or degradation of the fluorescence properties of the EuTTA films during lengthy exposure to ultraviolet radiation is one of the disadvantages of this technique.

Infrared Thermography

The spectral power density of the electromagnetic radiation emitted from a black body (Planck's distribution) depends on its temperature, whose maximum shifts to lower wavelengths with increasing temperature (Wien 's displacement law). The maximum wavelength at room temperature is about 10 μm. The real (gray) surfaces partially reflect the incident radiation that depends on the wavelength and spectral emissivity. The total emitted radiation power is given by the Stefan-Boltzmann law, $W=\sigma \varepsilon T^4$ ($\sigma = 5.7\times10^{-8}$ W m^{-2} K^{-1}), which depends both on temperature, T, and the material-dependent emissivity, ε. As a result, IR thermography of real surfaces is not possible without careful calibration of the emissivity (e.g., Bennett and Briles, 1989). Practically all the commercially available IR microscopes utilize this procedure, which have temperature sensitivities in the range of 0.1 to 1 K. Cooled detectors are able to provide sensitivities in the wavelength interval of 5 to 30 μm, which also corresponds to the bandwidth of the attainable lateral resolution (Kölzer et al., 1996). Temporal resolution near 100 μs can be obtained by using the lock-in technique. The IR thermography is regarded as a passive measurement technology.

Photothermal Radiometry

Photothermal radiometry, an active variation of the IR thermography measurement technique, uses a modulated laser beam to generate thermal waves that subsequently lead to fluctuations in the detected IR emission. Its advantages are that it provides deeper probing, and the results are less influenced by surface infrared and optical characteristics (Bison et al., 2000). The measured phase over the range of modulated probing frequency can be used to extract thermal properties of thin layers.

Optical Interferometry

The optical interferometer technique can provide extremely accurate measurements of thermal expansion or deformation of a surface (Oesterschulze et al., 1993, 1994, 1995; Claeys et al., 1994, Sodnik and Tiziani, 1988). The spatial and temperature resolutions of this technique are ~ 1 μm and 1 μK, respectively, for the passive mode. The spatial resolutions of the measurements in the active mode are limited by thermal diffusion length, $(\alpha\, t)^{1/2}$, where α is the thermal diffusivity of the solid layer. Thermal diffusivity measurements of dielectric, metallic, and semiconducting substrates, as well as metallic films on a glass substrate, have been performed in the past (Oesterschulze et al., 1995). Claeys et al. (1993, 1994) performed a short-pulse dilation analysis of a power MOS transistor and a compact FET using the optical interferometry technique. However, for complicated multilayer structures and devices, the spatial resolution is poor due to the strong coupling of the thermal expansion and the temperature field.

Thermoreflectance Laser Probing

The reflectance of a material at a given wavelength depends upon its temperature (Opsal and Rosencwaig, 1985). When a material undergoes a small temperature change, ΔT, its surface reflectance also undergoes a corresponding change, ΔR, which can be expressed as $\Delta R/R = \kappa T$. The thermoreflectance coefficient, κ, is on the order of 10^{-4} to 10^{-5} K^{-1} for metals and semiconductors, depending on the wavelength (Paddock and Eesley, 1986). In the laser reflectance thermometry technique, a low power probe laser beam is used to detect the temperature-induced changes in the optical reflectance of a surface. The local temperature change, at the position of the probe beam, can be induced by either optical or electrical pulse (or periodic) heating. The spatial resolution of the laser reflectance thermometry is limited by diffraction of the probing laser beam, which is on the order of its wavelength.

The thermoreflectance technique using ultra-short pulse laser heating has been widely used for the thin film thermophysical property measurements (Goodson et al., 1995a, 1995b). Ultra-short duration laser pulses, particularly those in the femto- and picoseconds time scale, are ideal tools to investigate the non-equilibrium thermal transport process in metallic thin films (Miklos and Lorincz, 1987; Hohlfeld et al., 1997, Naoyuki et al., 1997). In addition, they can provide important information concerning the thermal properties of the carriers, and lattice vibrations, of semiconductors, metal, and superconductors (Eesley, 1986; Brorson et al., 1987; Schoenlein et al., 1987; Doll et al., 1989). The limited bandwidth of the current optical detectors for ultra-short time scale laser heating motivates the use of the pump-probe setup. In this method, the laser output is split into two beam paths, a "pump" beam to heat the sample surface and a probe beam to measure the resulting change in reflectivity as shown in Fig. 4.7.

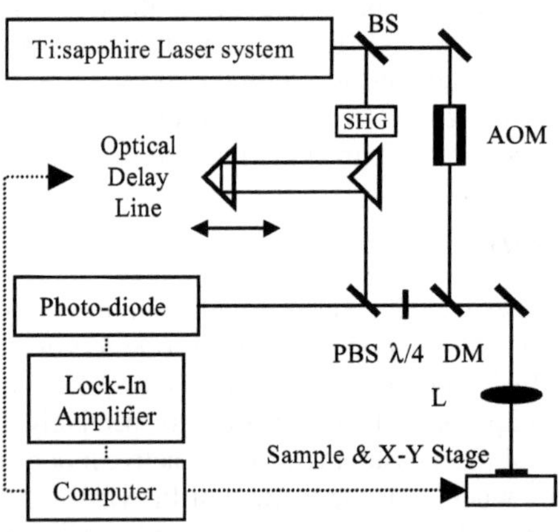

Fig. 4.7. Setup for picosecond transient thermorefectance thermometry. BS: beam splitter; PBS: polarized beam splitter; DM: dichroic mirror; SHG: second harmonic generator; L: lens; AOM: acoustic-optic modulator

Delay between the heating and probe pulses is controlled by passing the probe laser through a variable optical delay line. The heating pulse is modulated by an electro-optic modulator, in which the modulating frequency is much lower than the repetition rate of the heating pulse itself. The probe laser passes through the optical delay line, a polarization beam splitter, and a $\lambda/4$ plate, prior to being focused onto the sample surface. After passing through the $\lambda/4$ again, the retroreflected probe laser polarization is rotated by 90°, relative to the incoming light, and exited through the orthogonal port of the beam splitter. The heating-induced modulation of probe pulse intensity is measured by a lock-in-amplifier turned to the same modulation frequency as the heating pulse. The repetitive measurement of the probe response to many identical heating pulses, while varying the delay time between heating and probe beams, can greatly improve the signal to noise ratio. For the nanosecond thermoreflectance, the temporal temperature response can be directly measured with fast photodiode detectors (Roberts and Gustafson, 1986). The temperature variation generated by a single pulse is captured - but averaging of many pulses is needed to reduce the noise. In this situation, one can use a one nanosecond laser pulse to heat the material, while using another continuous He-Ne probe laser to get the time evolution of the thermoreflectance signals.

The modulated thermoreflectance technique is widely used for thermal diffusivities measurements (e.g., Langer and Hartmann, 1997), and thermal characterization of microdevices (Alomnd et al., 2000). For a modulated laser heating source, the solution of the heat diffusion equation yields thermal waves with one dimensional decay length on the order of $L_{th}=(\alpha/\pi f)^{1/2}$, where α and f are the thermal diffusivity of the layer and the modulation frequency, respectively. The thermal wave propagation can be utilized for conductivity measurements by locally heating the surface with a harmonically modulated excitation, and monitoring the surface temperature variation as a function of the distance from the heat source. Due to the propagation of the thermal wave, the phase lag between the heat deposition and the temperature oscillation at a given point on the surface is a linear function of the distance from the heat source. Scanning over a sample surface yields a straight line for the phase with a slope equal to the inverse of the L_{th}. Given the specific heat, ρC_p, and the thermal diffusivity, α, the thermal conductivity value, k, can be extracted. The experimental arrangement is schematically depicted in Fig 4.8.

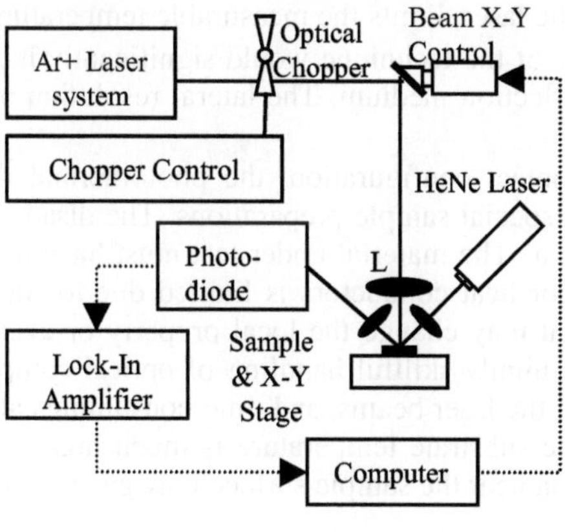

Fig. 4.8. Setup for modulated laser thermorefectance thermometry.

The modulated heat source is a mechanically chopped beam from a continuous laser that can be positioned by a computer-controlled X-Y translation stage. The reflectance is probed by a He-Ne laser beam focused on the same location as the heating beam. The harmonic component of the modulated reflectivity is detected by a two-phase lock-in amplifier that directly measures amplitude and phase of the sample surface temperature oscillation. The thermal profiles can be obtained by moving the heating beam with respect to probe beam.

The electrical heating method combines electrical heating and probe laser reflectance detection. The heat is generated by an electrical pulse/wave and the thermoreflectance signal is detected by a continuous laser. This setup allows simultaneous investigation of the thermal and electrical behavior of the materials and can be carried out both in transient (Ju and Goodson, 1997) and modulated mode (Quintard and Claeys, 1996).

Photothermal Deflection Spectroscopy

In this technique, a modulated argon-ion laser is used to generate a periodic localized heat source at the sample surface, while the temporal and spatial variations of the index of refraction of the air in proximity to the heated film surface are detected using a He-Ne probing laser (Roger et al., 1987; Skumanich et al., 1987; Boccara et al., 1980; Negus et al., 1989; Kölzer and Otto, 1991; Gorlich, 1992; Kölzer et al., 1992; Rantala et al., 1993; Solkner, 1994). A position-sensitive photodetector is used to monitor the magnitude and phase of both the normal and transverse components of the refracted probe beam. This method has a wide range of applications in the characterization of thin films, particularly for polycrystalline materials (Busse and Rosencwaig, 1980), whose heterogeneous structure can be mapped out as a function of local changes of their thermal properties. The thermal diffusivity can be obtained from fitting the solution to a three-dimensional heat diffusion equation for the relevant system (e.g., air, film, and substrate) to the experimental data. Fournier et al. (1987) estimated the theoretical limit of 10^{-7} $K/(Hz)^{1/2}$ for the thermal resolution of this technique - however, the noise level of the mirage cell induced by mechanical shocks, the shot noise of the detector, and the photon noise of the laser, limits the measurable temperature changes to around 1 μK. The sensitivity of the technique would significantly increase using a transparent liquid as a deflection medium. The lateral resolution of the technique is ~ 1μm.

Due to its non-contact configuration, the photothermal deflection technique does not require any special sample preparations. The disadvantages of this technique are as follows: a) The material under test must have a plane surface; b) Its application to the poor heat conductors is limited due to significant temperature rise in the system that may change the local property or even damage the specimen; c) It requires a highly skillful handling of optical components to achieve a precise positioning of the laser beams, and time-consuming calculations to analyze the data; d) When the substrate temperature is much higher than room temperature, the air convection near the sample surface may generate large noise signals.

Internal Infrared-Laser Deflection

In connection with thermally induced stress analysis of power transistors, Deboy et al. (1996) developed a non-contacting infrared laser detection technique that relates the internal carrier-density and temperature distributions. Due to the strong correlation of the internal refractive index of silicon and the carrier density, the gradients of the temperature and the carrier distribution normal to the direction of the infrared laser beam produce an angular deflection of the beam along the path. At the same time, the intensity of the irradiated beam along the path in the silicon substrate is reduced due to the absorption by free carriers. The imaginary and real part of the refractive index provides the gradients of carrier-density and temperature ~100 μK/μm (Deboy et al., 1996), as well as the absolute value of the carrier density. Simultaneous vertical and horizontal scanning of the beams allows the mapping of the transient temperature and carrier-density. Spatial and temporal resolutions in the range of 10 to 30 μm (Deboy et al., 1996) and 300 ns are reported, respectively. This technique requires a great deal of care in sample preparation (parallel milling and optical polishing of the lateral faces) and lengthy individual measurement. The electrical and thermal behavior of a 1600-V power diode (Soref and Bennett, 1987), and the insulated gate bipolar transistor (Deboy et al., 1996), were investigated using the internal infrared-laser deflection technique. The results were compared with corresponding numerical modeling (MEDICI device simulator). Furbock et al. (1998, 1999) used the noninvasive infrared backside laser beam (λ=1.3 μm) to study thermal effects in smart power electrostatic discharge (ESD) protection structures. The spatial and temporal resolutions of the measurements were ~5 μm and several nanoseconds, respectively.

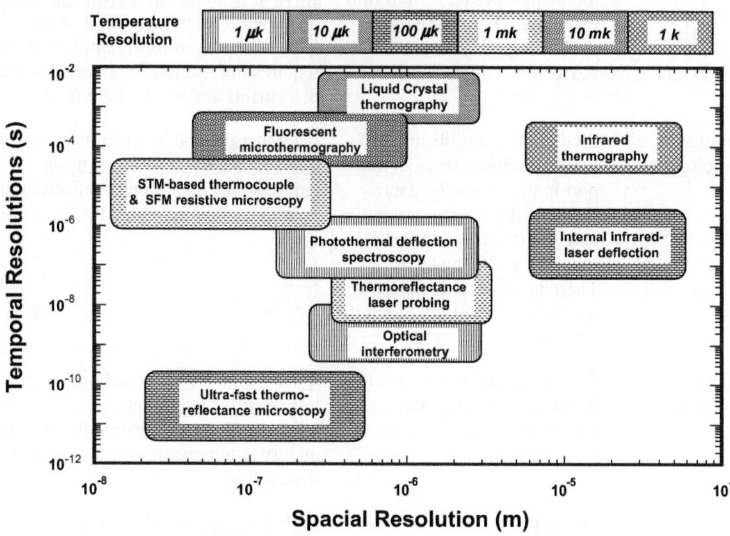

Fig. 4.9. The spatial, and temporal resolutions and temperature sensitivities of the far-field optical and near-field thermometry techniques.

Summary

The spatial, and temporal resolutions and temperature sensitivities of the far-field optical thermometry techniques described in this manuscript are illustrated in Fig. 4.9.

Table 4.2 summarizes the advantages, disadvantages, and general application of the far-field optical thermometry techniques.

Table 4.2 Summary of the advantages, disadvantages, and general application of the far-field optical thermometry techniques.

Types	*Applications*	*Advantages and Disadvantages*
Liquid Crystal Thermography	Failure analysis of the integrated circuits. Micro-thermography of electrical packaging and devices, hot-spot localization.	High-resolution automated measurement and can provide a visual temperature profile. However, it needs thin-film preparation over the sample and specific experience.
Fluorescence Microthermography	Thermal imaging of electronic devices, hot-spot localization; Integrated circuit testing and failure analysis.	It has a higher spatial and temporal resolution compared with LCT. Specific optical configuration and operation experience is need.
Infrared Thermography	Temperature mapping and thermal characterization of electronic components and devices.	It provides temperature image profile of the surface. However, it has a relatively low spatial and thermal resolutions. A careful emissivity calibration is required.
Optical Interferometry	Quantitative characterization of thermal properties of thin film materials; Thermal analysis and testing of semiconductor device.	Very high thermal resolution, extremely sensitive to local thermal expansion. It can be disrupted from heating ambient air and requires flat and uniform sample surface. It also requires the relationship between surface displacements and temperature field.
Thermoreflectance Laser Probing	Study of the equilibrium and non-equilibrium thermal transport in thin-films. Measurements of the thermal properties and resistance in semiconductor and metallic materials. Thermal characterization and temperature mapping of micro-devices.	High thermal and temporal resolution. Both quantitative and qualitative measurement. It requires the calibration of reflectivity index. Spatial resolution limited by the diffraction limit.
Photothermal Deflection Spectroscopy	Thermal characterization of thin-film materials. Surface temperature measurements of semiconductors.	It has a high thermal resolution and is usually less sensitive to environment. It is difficult to align the probe and heating beams. Optical quality requirements of the sample are more demanding.
Internal Infrared-Laser Deflection	Thermal and electrical characterizations for power devices. Measurement of carrier concentration in power devices.	Both investigation of dynamic current distribution and heat dissipation. It requires extensive sample preparation (parallel milling and optically polished)

4.4.3 Near-Field Thermometry Techniques

Optical diagnostic techniques, in general, have over the last years enjoyed a tremendous success in the failure analysis of electronic devices mainly due to their unique advantages over competitive techniques. They are fast down to the femtosecond regime, non-destructive, and possess spectroscopic capabilities - while the conventional optical microscope belongs to the most easily usable tools. Nevertheless, their spatial resolution is limited by diffraction to the theoretical value of $d = \lambda / (2\ NA)$, where λ is the wavelength of light, and NA is the numerical aperture of the lens. This limitation is currently imposing a key obstacle for a further application in semiconductor analyses, as structure sizes move on beyond the diffraction limit of visible light. The solution to this problem is brought by: (a) near-field optical (4.3.1), and (b) scanning near-filed (4.3.2) thermometry techniques.

Near-Field Optical Thermometry

Near-field optics, which enables optical imaging with spatial resolution significantly better than the diffraction limit, has recently found application in many diverse fields (Paesler and Moyer, 1996). The invention of the tapered fiber probe with its much improved transmission efficiency has enabled this recent period of growth (Betzig et al., 1991). In this technique, a metal-coated tapered optical fiber with a small aperture of diameter d at the tip is brought in close proximity (~1-10 nm) of a surface. Radiation interacts with a surface region of a diameter comparable to that of the probe optical orifice, which can be smaller than aperture size, d. An optical image can be obtained by scanning the probe across the sample surface, which requires control of the tip-surface separation using atomic-scale normal or shear forces, in a manner similar to that used by the atomic force microscope (AFM). Goodson and Asheghi (1997) used a tapered single-mode optical fiber to perform the first near-field optical thermometry (NFOT) measurements. This study showed that the radiation collected in reflection-mode can be used to map temperature distributions at interconnect surfaces in VLSI circuits, with spatial resolution better than 50 nm at frequencies up to 30 KHz.

The tapered optical fiber in near-field applications provides superior spatial resolution, however, its efficiency is still orders of magnitude smaller than unity. For example a probe of diameter $\lambda/10$ has a transmission efficiency of order 10^{-5} (Novotny and Pohl, 1995). This low efficiency limits use of the tapered fiber probe to applications with either large photon fluxes or slow acquisition rates. Many important applications in spectroscopy, photolithography, and data storage use the contrast obtained from absorption, reflection, or Kerr and Faraday polarization rotation of light. These applications require the interaction of a sufficiently strong light source with the sample. In particular, the slow acquisition rates limits the transient thermometry measurements to the bandwidths less than 100 KHz, which may not be appropriate for rapid thermal events relevant to semiconductor and data storage devices. A probe with unity efficiency would make near-field optics more generally applicable. Realizing such a probe remains one of the major challenges for near-field optics. Perhaps the most promising approach to the creation of high efficiency, very small optical spots is the use of an "optical antenna" structure (Grober et al., 1997). The very small aperture lasers (VSALs) can be used, with very little modification, for the near-field thermometry of semiconductor and data storage devices with reflective and smooth surfaces. For the near-field thermometry of surfaces with topography, however, a small tip size VSAL – or, alternatively, a cantilever based VSAL - must be fabricated. The latter approach gave birth to the concept of Near-field thermometry using vertical cavity surface emitting laser (VCSEL) scanning probe. Several interesting applications exist for microfabricated solid immersion lens (SIL), high-index lens waveguide at different wavelengths such as: infrared and reflectance thermometry, data storage, and surface thermal processing, which will be discussed in this section.

Near-Field Thermometry Using Tapered Optical Fiber

Goodson and Asheghi (1997) used a near-field scanning optical microscope, shown in figure 4.10, to perform near-field frequency domain thermometry of microelectronic structures heated by sinusoidal bias currents. The microfabricated structures, including doped silicon and aluminum interconnect bridges, were mounted on a chip carrier and electrically accessed by 50 μm-in-diameter gold wire bonds. An argon-ion laser was coupled into the metal-coated optical fiber, which delivers ~10^{-9} W of energy to the surface through the 50 nm orifice at the tip. The apparatus was capable of operating in two modes, *i.e.*, the reflected or transmitted light could be collected at a photomultiplier tube (PMT) using one of two far-field optical paths depicted in Figure 4.10. The collected radiation along either of these paths depended on the temperature dependent thermal reflectance of the sample and aluminum coated tip; thermal expansion of the probe tip and sample; separation distance between fiber tip and surface, δ; and orifice diameter, *d*. The frequency domain measurements allowed qualitative understanding and/or explanation of the contribution of the above parameters to the reflected radiation from the surface.

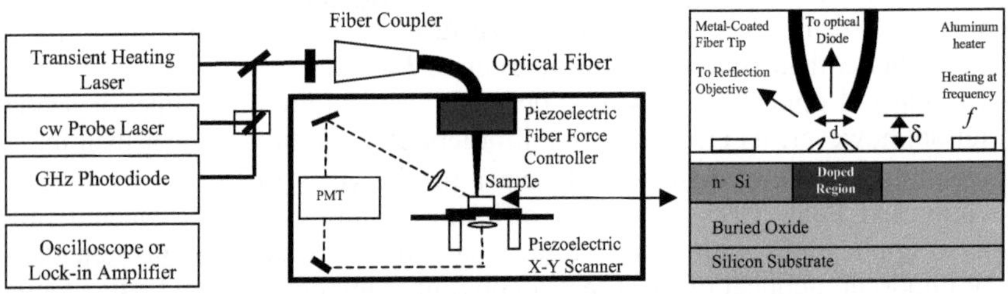

Fig. 4.10. Schematic of the near-field thermometry setup and the experimental structure (Goodson and Asheghi, 1997)

The near-field experiments were performed by collecting radiation within the optical enclosure using far-field objective. Two sets of experimental data were collected by performing transient NFOT above the doped silicon region at two separations distances, δ_1=5 nm and δ_2=3 μm. In these measurements a lock-in amplifier was used to detect the amplitude and phase of the collected radiation intensity at the heating frequency, that was twice the frequency, *f*, of the bias current applied to the aluminum interconnect. The third set of data was obtained by electrical measurements of the voltage across the doped region at frequency *f*, using the lock-in-amplifier. The phase lag of the thermistor (doped region) temperature, with respect to the heating intensity, approached zero for low frequencies, and increases with increasing frequency. The two sets of optical thermometry data agreed reasonably well in the frequency range 8-50 kHz. This suggests that surface-tip heat diffusion, which must be absent in the case of the large separation, is not important for near-field measurements at high frequencies. At high frequencies, the qualitative agreement between the optical and thermistor data indicates that the temperature dependence of the tip-surface separation, for which these two data sets should differ by 180°, was not important. Based on a more detailed analysis given in the original manuscript it was concluded that the temperature dependence of the optical constants dominated the measurement at high frequencies. Surface-tip heat diffusion and thermal expansion of the tip grow in importance at low frequencies, which may account for the disagreement between the optical and thermistor phase data below about 8 kHz. These two phenomena also grow in importance with decreasing tip-surface separation, which explains the disagreement of the two sets of optical data at these frequencies.

The authors also suggested the possibility of extending near-field thermometry technique to the infrared wavelengths. Boudreau et al. (1997) extended the near field optical thermometry technique to the infrared regime by developing an infrared microscope capable of imaging the thermal emissions in collection mode from micron scale conductors and an infrared laser source, with spatial resolutions near 2 μm. Goodson and Asheghi (1997) also discussed the merits of different probes and mechanisms of tip-surface distance control during the scanning process. While a straight optical fiber preserves the polarization state of the transmitted-radiation, and thereby allows the reflected-radiation to be routed back to the detector via a polarizing beam splitter, it has the disadvantage that only the tip-surface shear force can be used for controlling the tip-surface separation. Controlling the tip-surface separation using the normal forces are by far more sensitive compared to the shear force control approach. Alternatively, a bent optical fiber (Ben-Ami et al., 1996), AFM cantilever with a hollowed tip (Radmacher et al., 1994) or microfabricated cantilevered probes- consisting of solid quartz tips on silicon levers - can be used for this purpose (Eckert et al., 2000).

Near-Field Thermometry Using an Optical Antenna Structure

Grober et al. (1997) demonstrated that at microwave frequencies a planar bow-tie antenna with open circuited terminals functions as a near-field optical probe with transmission efficiency of order unity (Fig. 4.11). The radiating device is simply the open circuited terminal of the antenna. The terminals are truncated such that the antenna has a gap of width $d_{gap} \ll \lambda$. When illuminated with an optical field, currents induced in the arms of the antenna are guided towards and subsequently accumulated at the terminals, resulting in displacement current across the gap, which radiates like a dipole of length d_{gap} (Ramo et al., 1984). This field is concentrated in the gap and hence generates an output field whose source size (or spot size) is comparable to the size of the gap (50 nm or less).

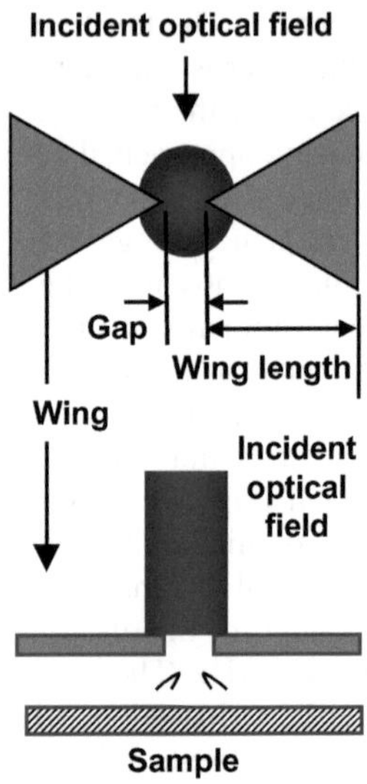

Fig. 4.11. The top and side view of a "bow tie" antenna. This incident optical field is concentrated in the gap and hence generates an output field whose source size (or spot size) is comparable to the size of the gap (Grober et al. , 1997).

The near-field probe described above is essentially an electric dipole coupled to free space via an antenna, which is more efficient. However, the traditional near-field optical probes, such as the tapered fiber probe, are effectively magnetic dipoles coupled to free space via a metal plane (Bethe, 1944). For an antenna placed at $\lambda/4$ and $\lambda/2$ away from the source, Grober et al. (1997) achieved optical efficiencies of near 2% and 30% (resonance), respectively. This concept has been proven to work at microwave frequencies but much work remains to be done both from a modeling and from a fabrication point of view, to demonstrate the feasibility of this device at optical frequencies. These antennas could be fabricated on the bottom of a solid immersion lens, or on the pyramidal walls of a conventional atomic force microscope probe for flat or rough surfaces, respectively. The bow-tie antenna structure can potentially make it feasible to perform near-field thermoreflectance thermometry with spatial resolution near 50 nm at timescales in the range of pico- to nanoseconds.

Near-Field Thermometry Using Very Small Aperture Lasers (VSALs)

An alternative method of focusing a small spot on a surface with a high throughput efficiency is to create very small apertures through which the light is transmitted in close proximity to the medium. VSALs with an output power exceeding 1 mW, and with small output beam size (50×50-300×300 nm^2), were first reported by Partovi et al. (1999). The measured far-field powers from VSALs are over 10^4 times the power measured from tapered fibers of similar aperture sizes. In a tapered source, much of the power is lost in the waveguide region where the width is reduced below the waveguide cutoff, while with an apertured flat screen this taper loss does not exist. In addition, a VSAL performs as an active source, where the photons not transmitted through the aperture can be recycled in the resonator (Partovi et al., 1999; Grober et al., 1997). The optical power throughput from an apertured metallic screen is highly dependent on the wavelength of the light, the size of the aperture, and the metal coating thickness (Durig et al., 1986). The smallest beam size and resolution achievable from a VSAL source, as well as any other apertured near-field source, is given by the penetration depth of the electromagnetic field into the screening metal. Betzig and Trautman (1992) suggested that the penetration depth limits the beam size to around 30 full widths at half maximum (FWHM). The reflection from the surface can be detected using "reflectivity modulation" for readback of optical disks with a laser diode in the far field (Mitsuhashi et al., 1981), and near field (Katagiri and Ukita, 1989; Goto et al., 1993). Partovi et al. (1999) used a 250×250 nm^2 VSAL to make 250-nm-diameter marks on a phase change media. Chen et al. (2001) used a focused ion beam etching process to form a 100 nm× 200 nm slit aperture on a laser, which is shown in Fig. 4.12. Goto (1998) proposed the fabrication of an array of vertical cavity surface emitting lasers (VCSEL) for optical data storage application.

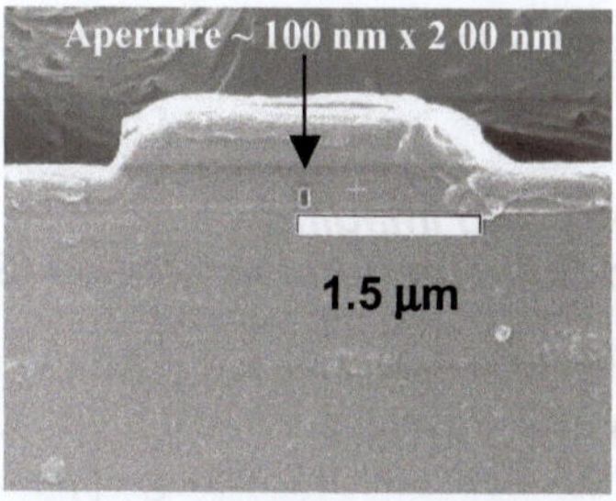

Fig. 4.12. 100 nm × 200 nm slit Apertures, which is etched across the active region of the laser (Chen et al., 2001).

VSALs can be used with very little modification for the near-field thermometry of semiconductor and data storage devices with reflective surfaces. For the near-field thermometry of surfaces with topography, however, a small tip size VSAL must be fabricated using etching or polishing of the VSAL substrate. This will be discussed in the following section.

Near-Field Thermometry Using a VCSEL Scanning Probe

Heisig et al. (2000) combined the SFM and scanning near-field optical microscopy by integrating an InGaAs vertical cavity surface emitting laser light (VCSEL) source into a galliumarsenide (GaAs) cantilever probe with a metallized tip, as shown in Fig. 4.13. The 8-µm-diameter VCSEL is centered with respect to the metalized GaAs tip and illuminates (λ~ 980 nm) a small near-field aperture at its apex. GaAs as substrate material is translucent at this wavelength. Its high refractive index of $n = 3.53$ significantly reduces the cut-off induced transmission losses in the tapered tip. From this point of view, GaAs could also be used for solid immersion lenses. Optical scans on triangular 15 nm thin aluminum islands with 200 nm side lengths, deposited on a thick glass cover slide, revealed a contrast of 10% and an edge resolution of about 80 nm. From these measurements a near-field resolution of near λ/10 was estimated.

Similar to the VSALs, the near field thermoreflectance thermometry should be feasible using VCSEL if the reflection from the surface can be detected using the "reflectivity modulation" of the same laser. This probe setup could be easily extended into an array arrangement for faster thermal imaging.

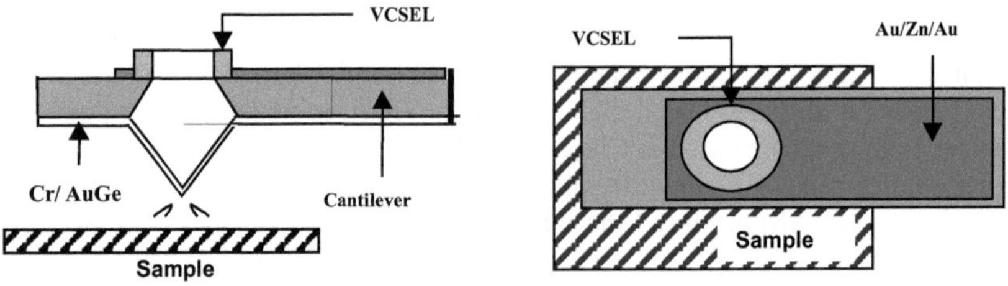

Fig. 4.13. The top and side view of the AFM based "VCSEL" (Heisig et al., 2000).

Near-Field Thermometry and Imaging Using Microfabricated Solid Immersion Lenses (SILs)

Solid immersion lens (SIL) systems offer the potential of smaller optical spots based on the decreased optical wavelength in the high index lens material (Mansfield and G. S. Kino, 1990). Several interesting applications have emerged for microfabricated SILs at infrared, visible, and ultraviolet wavelengths (e.g., optical data storage, high-resolution microscopy, and photolithography at visible and UV wavelengths). This section describes the capabilities of the SILs, Super SILs (SSIL), and integrated SILs (ISILs), as well as the mode index lens (MIL) structures, to form smaller optical spots for data storage and thermometry applications. In addition, the recent advances in high-resolution and high optical throughput infrared thermometry (using microfabricated Si SIL) and its application to high-resolution infrared spectroscopy and thermal processing (Fletcher et al., 2000, 2001) of surfaces are reviewed and discussed.

Near-Field Diagnostics Using SILs, SSIL, ISILs, and MIL Structures

In the first attempt to modify a liquid immersion microscope for near-field application, Mansfield and Kino (1990) replaced the liquid with a solid lens of high refractive index (n=2) material. They successfully resolved 100 nm lines and spaces (436 nm illumination) and demonstrated a factor of two improvements in the edge response over a confocal microscope. In optical disk storage devices, data bits are typically written and read using a laser beam focused to a small spot on the surface of a rapidly spinning recording medium. The SIL systems offer the potential of smaller optical spots for data storage application, which largely determines the attainable data density. Terris et al. (1996) fabricated and tested an optical assembly consisting of an objective lens (NA=0.5) and a truncated spherical super-SIL with an index of refraction near 1.86. A 360 nm optical spot size on a spinning magneto-optical disk was obtained at 830 nm illumination. Recently, Tang et al. (2001) used the combination of an aperture-probe and SIL to produces spot sizes below 100 nm (FWHM) with a 488 nm wavelength illumination. This fabricated probe has a special cone-like shape that funnels the light into a small opening at the base of the lens (Fig. 4.14). The opening is about 200 nm in diameter. Currently, research is under way for development of an ISIL that does not require an objective lens. This configuration would eliminate the need for alignment of the incident laser beam. The numerical aperture of the ISIL only depends on the refractive index of the material, *n* (Rausch et al., 2001). Karns et al. (2000) fabricated an optical assembly consisting of a 0.55 NA objective lens and a truncated spherical super-SIL (effective *NA* of 1.8), which was capable of producing an optical spot of less than 180 nm. The SILs technology developed in connection with data storage applications can be directly applied for near-field thermoreflectance thermometry with comparable spatial and temporal resolutions. Fletcher et al. (2000) used this same concept to develop the first cantilever based SIL for near-field infrared application, which will be discussed in this section.

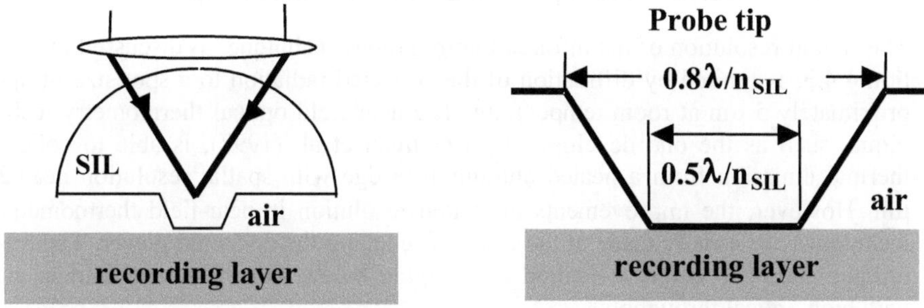

Fig. 4.14. (Top) Schematic of the combination aperture-ISL and (Bottom) the enlarged ISL probe tip (Tang et al., 2001).

Current hard drive technologies can barely accommodate SILs that are large on the scale of thin film sliders. In an attempt to overcome this problem, Rausch et al. (2001) proposed a design that implements a mode index waveguide lens, rather than a three dimensional objective lens. The $SiO_2/SiN_x/SiO_2$ waveguide lens takes advantage of the difference in mode index when the thickness of the waveguide is changed to focus light within the waveguide. The light is focused to the bottom of the waveguide where it is evanescently coupled to the media. Figure 4.15 shows a drawing of a mode index waveguide. Figure 4.6a depicts the optical spot at the focal plane where the narrow dimension is the diffraction limited spot size. The longer dimension is the thickness of the waveguide at the lens. Fabrication of SILs is rather involved, so, in connection with the near-field thermometry application, the mode index waveguide lens can significantly simplify the fabrication process of SILs. The coupling of the mode index waveguide with the light source is an area of active research.

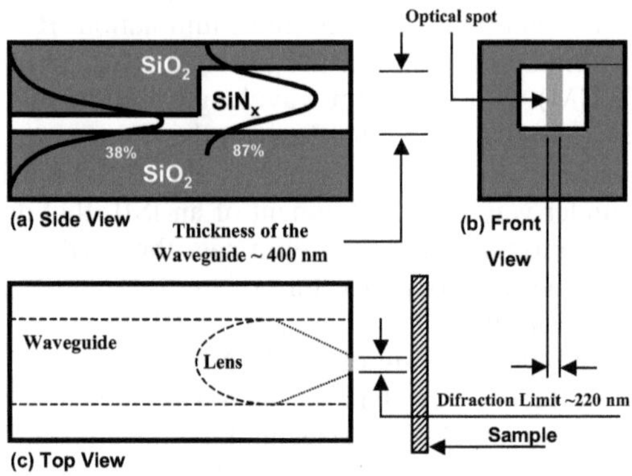

Fig. 4.15. A schematic of the (a) side, (b) front and (c) top views of a mode index waveguide lens (Rausch *et al.*, 2001)

Near-Field Infrared Imaging Using Cantilever Based SILs

The spatial resolution of the infrared thermography technique, as discussed in section 4.4.3, is limited by diffraction of the collected radiation to a spot size of approximately 5 μm at room temperature. The near field optical thermometry technique, such as the one developed by Boudreau et al. (1997), is able to collect thermal emission from a heated aluminum bridge with spatial resolution near 2 μm. However, the improvements in spatial resolution in near-field thermometry techniques are usually made at the price of reducing the collected power. The microfabricated SIL offers a method for imaging below the diffraction limit in air with high optical throughput.

Fletcher et al. (2000) reported fabrication and thermal microscopy using a microfabricated cantilever-based solid immersion lens (Fig. 4.16). In their experiment, a CO_2 laser light (λ=9.3 μm) was focused by a reflecting objective (NA=0.45) on the Si lens, transmitted through a 1.0-μm-diameter circular hole in a metal layer, then collected by a second reflecting objective (NA=0.45) and measured with a liquid nitrogen-cooled HgCdTe detector. The circular hole, fabricated in a 100 nm thick metal layer on a GaP substrate is scanned under the Si SIL, while the lens was kept at a fixed position. The measured normalized transmitted powers through the hole scanned at the focus of a CO_2 laser with and without the Si SIL, had the FWHMs of 2.1 μm and 10.6 μm, respectively. The optical throughput of the SI SIL was measured to be ~ $5x10^3$ greater than that of a 1.8-μm-diameter aperture with equivalent spatial resolution at λ=9.3 μm.

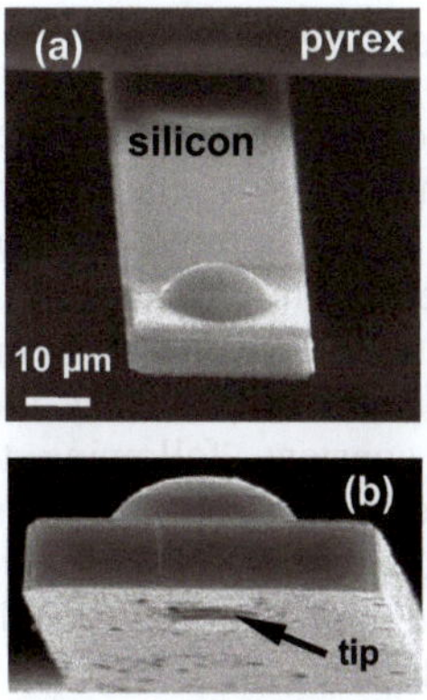

Fig. 4.16. Integrated solid immersion lens and Si cantilever (Fletcher et al., 2000).

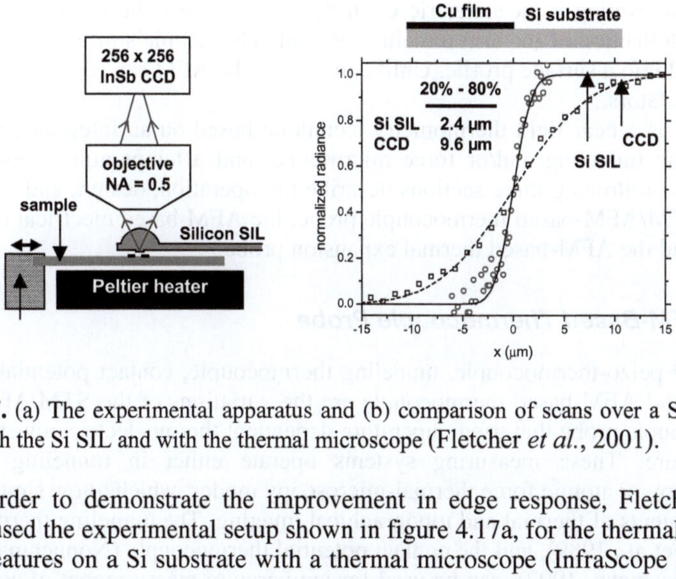

Fig. 4.17. (a) The experimental apparatus and (b) comparison of scans over a Si/Cu edge taken with the Si SIL and with the thermal microscope (Fletcher *et al.*, 2001).

In order to demonstrate the improvement in edge response, Fletcher et al. (2001) used the experimental setup shown in figure 4.17a, for the thermal imaging of Cu features on a Si substrate with a thermal microscope (InfraScope II, Quantum Focus Instruments) and a 15-µm-diameter microfabricated SIL. In this setup the SIL is fixed at the focus of a Si/Ge collection objective, and the sample is scanned below the SIL. A Peltier heater uniformly heats a sample held on a piezoelectric scanning stage. The emitted radiance from the Peltier heater is transmitted through the Si but is blocked by the Cu pattern. As a result, the emissivity and reflectivity differences between the two materials create a sharp radiance contrast. Figure 4.17b shows a comparison of scans over a Si/Cu edge taken with the microfabricated Si SIL and with the thermal microscope. The improvement in edge response with the microfabricated Si SIL is a factor of 4 over the thermal microscope without the SIL.

Scanning Thermal Microscopy (SThM)

The Scanning Tunneling Microscope (STM) senses atomic-scale topography by means of electrons that "tunnel" across the gap between probe and surface. A voltage is applied to the tip, and it is moved toward the conducting or semiconducting surface until a tunneling current starts to flow. The tip is then scanned back and forth in a raster pattern. The tunneling current tends to vary with the topography. A feedback mechanism responds by moving the tip up and down to keep the tunneling current constant, following the surface profile. The tip's movements are then translated into an image of the surface.

The Atomic Force Microscope (AFM) is based upon a measurement of the Van Der Waal's force between the atoms on the tip and the sample surface. The electron cloud of the AFM tip interacts with the clouds of the individual atoms on the surface, generating a repulsive force that varies with the surface profile. The force deflects the tip, whose movements are monitored by a laser beam reflected from the top of the arm. A feedback mechanism responds to the change in the beam's path by activating a piezoelectric control, which adjusts the sample's height so that the deflection of the arm remains constant. The sample's movements are then translated into a surface profile. Unlike the STM, the AFM can readily image electrical insulators.

SThM is a near field thermometry technique based on an integrated design of the atomic tunneling and/or force microscope, and a temperature sensitive element. The following three sections describe the operation, design, and limitations of the STM/AFM-based thermocouple probe, the AFM-based electrical resistance probe, and the AFM-based thermal expansion probe.

STM/AFM-Based Thermocouple Probe

Scanning peizo-thermocouple, tunneling thermocouple, contact potential thermocouple, and AFM-based thermocouple are the variations of the STM/AFM based thermocouple probe that use temperature dependent thermoelectric power to sense temperature. These measuring systems operate either in tunneling thermal-microscopy or atomic force thermal-microscopy modes, which allow simultaneous measurements of thermal and topographical imaging. The tunneling thermocouple (Weaver et al., 1989), and the contact potential thermocouple (Nonnenmacher and Wickramasinghe, 1992), can be used for temperature measurement of conductive (e.g., metallic) surfaces with spatial resolution better than 10-20 nm. Spatial resolution on the order of 100 nm can be achieved using the scanning peizo-thermocouple (Williams and Wickramasinghe, 1986, 1988) with temperature resolution on the order of 1 mK at 100 KHz bandwidth. Figure 4.18 depicts the schematic setup of the STM/AFM-based thermocouple (Majumdar et al., 1993, 1995, 1998) that can be used for thermometry of dielectric surfaces. The thermocouple junction is formed by two dissimilar inner and outer conductors that are separated by an insulator in all areas remote from the tip. A 100 nm thermocouple junction can be formed using the advanced microfabrication process, but the spatial resolution is a strong function of the heat conduction mechanism between the tip and surface. For dry surfaces, heat conduction by gas molecules can degrade the spatial resolution of the probe to values between 300 to 500 nm. However, sub 100 nm spatial resolutions can be achieved if the surface of the sample is covered with a thin layer of moisture. Heating the thermal probe with a laser beam results in a temperature gradient and thus a heat flux between tip and sample surface. In the constant height mode STM/AFM microscope, the amount of heat flux depends only on the local thermal properties of the sample. The junction temperature is obtained by keeping another junction at a reference temperature and measuring the thermoelectric voltage generated due to the temperature difference. The tip is raster-scanned across the surface to obtain a thermal profile. The minimum detectable change in tip temperature is less than 0.1 mK. However, the improper thermal design of the probe leads to large uncertainty, topography-related artifacts, and poor spatial resolution in thermal imaging (Kwok et al., 1987). Thermal probes with improved thermal characteristics based on thermal modeling (Majumdar et al., 2000) provide a better spatial resolution around 50 nm.

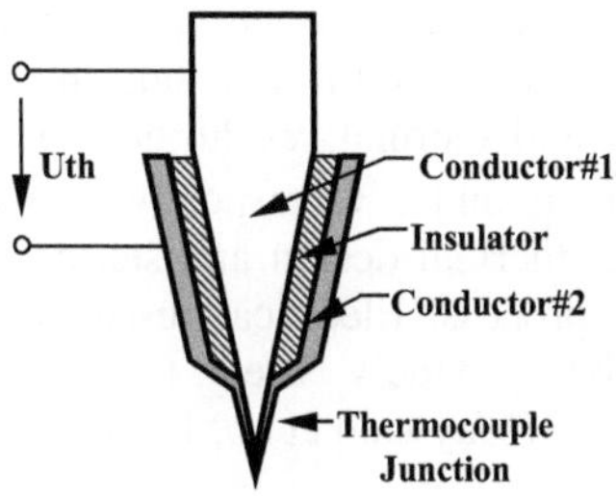

Fig. 4.18. Schematic of the thermal probe.

Scanning Thermal Microscopy (SThM)

The Scanning Tunneling Microscope (STM) senses atomic-scale topography by means of electrons that "tunnel" across the gap between probe and surface. A voltage is applied to the tip, and it is moved toward the conducting or semiconducting surface until a tunneling current starts to flow. The tip is then scanned back and forth in a raster pattern. The tunneling current tends to vary with the topography. A feedback mechanism responds by moving the tip up and down to keep the tunneling current constant, following the surface profile. The tip's movements are then translated into an image of the surface.

The Atomic Force Microscope (AFM) is based upon a measurement of the Van Der Waal's force between the atoms on the tip and the sample surface. The electron cloud of the AFM tip interacts with the clouds of the individual atoms on the surface, generating a repulsive force that varies with the surface profile. The force deflects the tip, whose movements are monitored by a laser beam reflected from the top of the arm. A feedback mechanism responds to the change in the beam's path by activating a piezoelectric control, which adjusts the sample's height so that the deflection of the arm remains constant. The sample's movements are then translated into a surface profile. Unlike the STM, the AFM can readily image electrical insulators.

AFM-Based Electrical Resistance Probe

The concept of using temperature dependent electrical resistance to develop a SThM probe was first introduced by Pylkki et al. (1994), who used a silver Wollaston wire with an encapsulated 5 μm Pt core as a sensing or heating element (Fig. 4.19). The probe is formed into an AFM cantilever probe. The distance between the resistance probe tip and the specimen is kept constant by a reflected laser controlled feedback loop. The resistance probes can be operated in two modes: *passive* or *active*. In passive mode, a very small constant current is passed through the resistor with negligible Joule heating compared with the heat flux between tip and sample. The temperature is estimated by measuring the probe resistance via voltage drop across the bridge. In active mode, a large current is passed through the probe resistor to induce Joule heating. The heat flow between tip and sample cools down the resistor probe, thus the voltage signal can be correlated directly with the thermal conductivity of the sample provided that the tip-sample distance is constant. The active mode can be operated at a constant temperature mode in which a feedback loop is used to maintain the constant resistance of the resistor probe. The spatial and thermal resolutions for the system designed by Pylkki et al. (1994) are ~ 1 μm and 1 °C, respectively, which can be significantly improved by more rigorous thermal design and sensor miniaturization using the advanced microfabrication process. Electrical resistance thermometry using the SThM arrangment has been widely used for thermal imaging, property measurement, and calorimetry (Maywald et al., 1994; Hammiche et al., 1996).

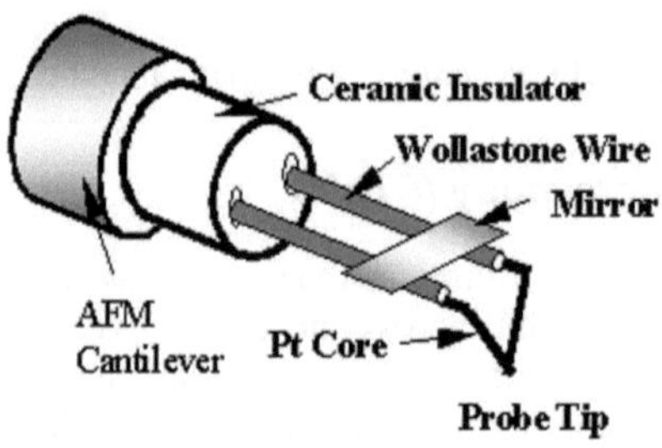

Fig. 4.19. Schematic of the AFM-based Electrical Resistance Probe.

AFM-Based Thermal Expansion Probe

The Bimaterial Cantilever (Nakabeppu et al., 1994) and Scanning Joule Expansion Microscopy (SJEM) (Majumdar and Varesi, 1998) techniques have been developed based on the measurement of thermal expansion in materials. The Bimaterial Cantilever thermometry technique uses a metal-coated AFM cantilever as a temperature sensor. Due to the mismatch in the thermal expansion coefficients of the two-layer cantilever system, any variation in temperature induces a bending moment (deflection) in the cantilever. The magnitude of the cantilever deflection can be measured and correlated to temperature with resolutions near 10^{-5} K (Majumdar, 1999). The spatial resolution of the Bimaterial Cantilever thermometry is rather poor because the thermal conduction is not restricted to the tip-surface region. In contrast, the SJEM thermometry technique provides high spatial resolution because it does not rely on the tip-sample heat transfer. In the SJEM thermometry technique, a sinusoidal or pulsed electrical current is applied to the metal interconnect or device under testing. Non-uniform temperature gradients in the system (due to the Joule heating effect) induce a non-uniform thermal expansion pattern that can be measured using an AFM feedback loop. The AFM topographical image is therefore a combination of both sample thermal expansion and sample surface topography. The local thermal expansion signal can be isolated from that of the surface topography by turning the lock-in amplifier to the Joule heating frequency. The accuracy of the systems relies on minimizing the heat conduction from the surface to the AFM cantilever, which cannot be eliminated all together except by working in a low-pressure environment. Another approach is to cover the surface with a high thermal expansion coefficient polymer layer, which would significantly increase the contribution due to the thermal expansion. Sub 100 nm features have been resolved using the SJEM thermometry technique (Majumdar and Varesi, 1998). However, the frequency dependence of the thermal expansion signal due to the Joule heating has not been well understood so far (Majumdar, 1998).

Summary

Table 4.3 summarizes the advantages, disadvantages, and general application of the near-field thermometry techniques.

Table 4.3a. Summary of the advantages, disadvantages, and general application of near-field optical thermometry techniques

Types	*Applications*	***Advantages and Disadvantages***
Tapered optical fiber	High spatial resolution thermometry, processing and thermal characterization.	It has a High spatial resolution but suffers from low optical transmission efficiency and slow acquisition rates.
Optical antenna Structure	Near-field thermometry of microelectronic structures. Data storage application.	High spatial resolution and transmission efficiencies. Remaining work to be done for feasibility at optical frequencies.
Very small aperture lasers (VSALs)	Near-field thermometry of microelectronic structures. Data storage application.	High spatial resolution, moderate transmission efficiencies, ease of fabrication and low cost. Can be applied to smooth surfaces.
VCSEL scanning probe	Thermometry of microelectronic structures. Data storage application.	High spatial resolution, moderate transmission efficiencies. Complicated microfabrication process.
Solid immersion lenses	Near-field diagnostics, infrared imaging and thermometry. Data storage application	High spatial resolution, moderate transmission efficiencies and can be used for surfaces with topographic features.

Table 4.3b. Summary of the advantages, disadvantages, and general application of the near-field STM/AFM thermometry techniques

STM-based thermal probe	Failure and thermal characterization of sub-micrometer electronic devices. Thermal properties measurements of materials in small length scales. Study of dynamic transport phenomena of the heat carriers.	High spatial resolution. Both measurements of surface topography and temperature profiles. It requires conducting surface for "tunneling" the electrons and relies on the tip-sample heat transfer. Complicated microfabrication process.
AFM-based thermal probe		High spatial resolution. Both measurements of surface topography and temperature profiles. Both conducting and non-conducting surface, material independent. The probe relies on the tip-sample heat transfer and requires careful thermal design of the probe. Complicated microfabrication process.
AFM-based resistive probe	Thermal imaging, thermal properties Measurement, and calorimetry	High spatial resolution comparable to STM or AFM thermal probe. Passive and active modes of operation. A resistor sensor must be fabricated at the end of tip. Thorough analysis of the signals is lacking.
Bimaterial cantilever	Temperature and topographical imaging.	High temperature sensitivity. Low spatial resolution. Careful thermal design is required in order to restrict the heat flow to the tip region. Experiments must be operated in vacuum.
Scanning Joule Expansion Microscopy	Thermal expansion and topographical imaging. Temperature mapping of sub-micron electronic devices.	It does not rely on tip-sample heat transfer, no need to fabricate the complicated tip sensor and require only standard AFM system. Reasonable spatial resolution with high temperature sensitivity. It requires calibration of the local temperature coefficient to extract temperature profile. Unresolved frequency dependence of joule heating expansion signal.

4.4.4 Summary and Recommendations

This manuscript describes the principles, characteristics and applications of electrical and optical thermometry techniques that are tailored for the research and development in micro- and nanoscales. Particular attention is made to the near-field thermometry techniques, which enable imaging with spatial resolution significantly better than the diffraction limit. The majority of the ongoing research and development in the area of high-density data storage systems and devices are relevant to the research in near field thermometry area. In this sense, the present manuscript provides a road map for research and development and a comprehensive review of the previous work in this area. The state-of-art technologies and relevant research efforts in the semiconductor and data storage industry that would benefit form the *high-resolution thermometry* and *thin-film thermal characterization* diagnostic tools are also presented in this manuscript.

This work was sponsored by National Science Foundation (NSF) under contract CTS-0103082. Many of the concepts in near field optical thermometry presented here developed during research-related discussions with Professors James Bain and Ed Schlesinger of Data Storage System Center (DSSC) at Carnegie Mellon University (CMU). Mehdi Asheghi appreciates support from the Institute for Complex Engineered Systems (ICES), DSSC and Berkman Foundation at CMU. Shu Zhang, Wenjun Liu, and Michael Scampone of CMU assisted us in schematic preparation and editorial work.

References

Almond, D.P., Nokrach, P., Stokes, E.W.R., Porch, A., Foulds, S.A.L., Wellhofer, F., Powell, J.R., and Abell, J.S., 2000, "Modulated optical reflectance characterization of high temperature superconducting thin film microwave devices," *Journal of Applied Physics*, Vol. 87, No. 12, pp. 8628-8635.

Amerasekera, A., Van den Abeelen, W., Van Roozendaal, L., Hannemann, M., and Schofield, P., 1992, "ESD failure modes: characteristics mechanisms, and process influences," *IEEE Transactions on Electron Devices*, Vol. 39, No. 2, pp. 430-436.

Arnold, E., Pein, H., and Herko, S.P., 1994, "Comparison of self-heating effects in bulk-silicon and SOI high-voltage devices," *International Electron Devices Meeting 1994. Technical Digest*, pp. 947, 813-816.

Asheghi, M., 1999, "Thermal Transport Properties of Silicon Films," *Ph.D. Thesis*, Stanford University, Stanford, CA.

Asheghi, M., Leung, Y.K., Wong, S.S., and Goodson, K.E., 1997, "Phonon-boundary scattering in thin silicon layers," *Applied Physics Letters*, Vol. 71, pp. 1798-1800.

Asheghi, M., Touzelbaev, M.N., Goodson, K.E., Leung, Y.K., and Wong, S.S., 1998, "Temperature dependent thermal conductivity of single-crystal silicon layers in SOI substrates," *Journal of Heat Transfer*, Vol. 120, pp. 30-36.

Aszodi, G., Szabon, J., Janossy, I., and Szekely, V., 1981, "High resolution thermal mapping of microcircuits using nematic liquid crystals," *Solid-State Electronics*, Vol. 24, No. 12, pp. 1127-1133.

Banerjee, K., Ting, L., Cheung, N., and Hu, C.-M., 1996, "Impact of high current stress conditions on VLSI interconnect electromigration reliability evaluation," *Proceedings Thirteenth International VLSI Multilevel Interconnection Conference (VMIC)*, pp. 628, 289-294.

Barton, D.L., 1994, "Fluorescent microthermographic imaging (IC failure analysis)," *ISTFA '94. Proceedings of the 20th International Symposium for Testing and Failure Analysis*, pp. 87-95.

Barton, D.L., and Tangyunyong, P., 1996, "Fluorescent microthermal imaging-theory and methodology for achieving high thermal resolution images," *Microelectronic Engineering*, Vol. 31, No. 1-4, pp. 271-279.

Beck, F., 1986, "Liquid crystal thermography localizes faults on a chip," *Elektronik*, Vol. 35, No. 13, pp. 82-84, 86-88, 91-92.

Ben-Ami, U., Tessler, N., Ben-Ami, N., Nagar, R., Fish, G., Lieberman, K., Eisenstein, G., Lewis, A., Nielsen, J.M., and Moeller-Larsen, A., 1996, "Near-infrared contact mode collection near-field optical and normal force microscopy of modulated multiple quantum well lasers," *Applied Physics Letters*, Vol. 68, No. 17, pp. 2337-2339.

Bennett, G.A. and Briles, S.D., 1989, "Calibration procedure developed for IR surface-temperature measurements," *IEEE Transactions on Components, Hybrids, and Manufacturing Technology*, Vol. 12, No. 4, pp. 690-695.

Bethe H. A., 1944, "Theory of diffraction by small holes," *Physical Review*, No. 66, pp. 163-182.

Betzig, E. and Trautman, J.K., 1992, "Near-field optics: microscopy, spectroscopy, and surface modification beyond the diffraction limit," *Science*, Vol. 257, No. 5067, pp. 189-195.

Betzig, E., Trautman, J.K., Harris, T.D., Weiner, J.S., and Kostelak, R.L., 1991, "Breaking the diffraction barrier: optical microscopy on a nanometric scale," *Science*, Vol. 251, No. 5000, pp. 1468-1470.

Bison, P.G., Grinzato, E., Marinetti, S., and Muscio, A., 2000, "Diffusivity measurement of thick samples by thermography and heating-cooling technique," *Proc. SPIE*, Vol. 4020, pp. 137-142.

Blackburn, D.L., 1988, "A review of thermal characterization of power transistors," *Fourth Annual IEEE Semiconductor Thermal and Temperature Measurement Symposium*, pp. 151-157.

Boccara, A.C., Fournier, D., and Badoz, J., 1980, "Thermo-optical spectroscopy: detection by the mirage effect," *Applied Physics Letters*, Vol. 36, No. 2, pp. 130-132.

Boeuf, F., Skotnicki, T., Monfray, S., Julien, C., Dutartre, D., Martins, J., Mazoyer, P., Palla, R., Tavel, B., f, Ribot, P., Sondergard, E., and Sanquer, M., 2001, "16 nm planar NMOSFET manufacturable within state-of-the-art CMOS process thanks to specific design and optimization," *Electron Devices Meeting, IEDM '01 Technical Digest., International*, pp.637-640.

Boudreau, B.D., Raja, J., Hocken, R.J., Patterson, and S.R., Patten, J., 1997, "Thermal imaging with near-field microscopy," *Review of Scientific Instruments*, Vol. 68, No. 8, pp. 3096-3098.

Brorson, S.D., Fujimoto, J.G., and Ippen, E.P., 1987, "Femtosecond electronic heat-transport dynamics in thin gold films," *Physical Review Letters*, Vol. 59, No. 17, pp. 1962-1965.

Burgess, D., and Tan, P., 1984, "Improved sensitivity for hot spot detection using liquid crystals," *22nd Annual Proceedings on Reliability Physics*, pp.119-121.

Busse, G., and Rosencwaig, A., 1980, "Subsurface imaging with photoacoustics," *Applied Physics Letters*, Vol. 36, No. 10, pp. 815-816.

Cahill, D.G., 1998, "Heat transfer in dielectric lthin films and at solid-solid interfaces," in *Microscale Energy Transport*, C.L. Tien et al., eds., Taylor & Francis, New York, NY, pp. 95-117.

Cain, B.M., Goud, P.A., and Englefield, C.G., 1992, "Electrical measurement of the junction temperature of an RF power transistor," *IEEE Transactions on Instrumentation and Measurement*, Vol. 41, No. 5, pp. 663-665.

Chen, F., Zhai, J., Stancil, D.D., and Schlesinger, T.E., 2001, "Fabrication of very small aperture laser (VSAL) from a commercial edge emitting laser," *Japanese Journal of Applied Physics, Part 1*, Vol. 40, No. 3B, pp. 1794-1795.

Chen, G., 1996, "Nonlocal and Nonequilibrium Heat Conduction in the Vicinity of Nanoparticles," *Journal of Heat Transfer*, Vol. 118, pp. 539-545.

Claeys, W., Dilhaire, S., and Quintard, V., 1994, "Laser probing of thermal behavior of electronic components and its application in quality and reliability testing," *Microelectronic Engineering*, Vol. 24, pp. 411-420.

Claeys, W., Dilhaire, S., Quintard, V., Dom, J.P., and Danto, Y., 1993, "Thermoreflectance optical test probe for the measurement of current-induced temperature changes in microelectronic components," *Quality and Reliability Engineering International*, Vol. 9, No. 4, pp. 303-308.

Deboy, G., Solkner, G., Wolfgang, E., and Claeys, W., 1996, "Absolute measurement of transient carrier concentration and temperature gradients in power semiconductor devices by internal IR-laser deflection," *Microelectronic Engineering*, Vol. 31, No. 1-4, pp. 299-307.

Doll, G.L., Eesley, G.L., Dresselhaus, M.S., Dresselhaus, G., Cassanho, A., Jenssen, H.P., and Gabbe, D.R., 1989, "Transient-thermoreflectance study of single-crystal lanthanum cuprate," *Physical Review B*, Vol. 40, No. 13, pp. 9354-9357.

Durig, U., Pohl, D.W., and Rohner, F., 1986, "Near-field optical-scanning microscopy", *Journal of Applied Physics*, Vol.59, No.10, pp. 3318-3327.

Eckert, R., Freyland, J.M., Gersen, H., Heinzelmann, H., Schurmann, G., Noell, W., Staufer, U., and de Rooij, N.F., 2000, "Near-field fluorescence imaging with 32 nm resolution based on microfabricated cantilevered probes," *Applied Physics Letters*, Vol. 77, No. 23, pp. 3695-3697.

Eesley, G.L., 1986, "Generation of nonequilibrium electron and lattice temperatures in copper by picosecond laser pulses," *Physical Review B*, Vol. 33, No. 4, pp. 2144-2151.

Estreich, D.B., 1989, "A DC technique for determining GaAs MESFET thermal resistance," *IEEE Trans. Compon. Hybrids Manuf. Technol. (USA), IEEE Transactions on Components, Hybrids, and Manufacturing Technology*, Vol. 12, No. 4, pp. 675-679.

Fergason, J. L., "Liquid crystals in nondestructive testing," *Applied Optics*, Vol. 7, No. 9, pp. 1729-1737.

Fletcher, D.A., Crozier, K.B., Quate, C.F., Kino, K.S., Goodson, K.E., Simanovskii, D., and Palanker, D.V., 2000, "Near-field infrared imaging with a microfabricated solid immersion lens," *Applied Physics Letters*, Vol. 77, pp. 2109-2111.

Fletcher, D.A., Webb, N.U., Kino, G.S., Quate, C.F., and Goodson K.E., 2001, "Thermal Microscopy with a Microfabricated Solid Immersion Lens," Proc. IEEE/LEOS International Conference on Optical MEMS, Okinawa, Japan.

Fournier, D., and Boccara, A.C., 1987, *Phatoacoustic and Thermal Wave Phenomena in Semiconductors*, A. Mandelis (ed.), Elsevier North-Holland, New York.

Furbock, C., Pogany, D., Litzenberger, M., Gornik, E., Seliger, N., Gossner, H., Muller-Lynch, T., Stecher, M., and Werner, W., 1999, "Interferometric temperature mapping during ESD stress and failure analysis of smart power technology ESD protection devices," *Electrical Overstress/Electrostatic Discharge Symposium Proceedings. 1999*, pp. 241-250.

Furbock, C., Seliger, N., Pogany, D., Litzenberger, M., Gornik, E., Stecher, M., Gosser, H., and Werner, W., 1998, "Backside laserprober characterization of thermal effects during high current stress in smart power ESD protection devices," *International Electron Devices Meeting 1998. Technical Digest*, pp. 1080, 691-694.

Goodson, K.E. and Asheghi, M., 1997, "Near-Field optical thermometry," *Microscale Thermophysical Engineering*, Vol. 1, pp. 225-235.

Goodson, K.E. and Flik, M.I., 1994, "Solid-Layer thermal-conductivity measurement techniques," *Applied Mechanics Reviews*, Vol. 47, pp. 101-112.

Goodson, K.E., Flik, M.I., Su, L.T., and Antoniadis, D.A., 1994, "Prediction and measurement of the thermal conductivity of amorphous dielectric layers," *Transactions of the ASME. Journal of Heat Transfer*, Vol. 116, No. 2, pp. 317-324.

Goodson, K.E., Flik, M.I., Su, L.T., and Antoniadis, D.A., 1995, "Prediction and measurement of temperature fields in silicon-on-insulator electronic circuits," *ASME Journal of Heat Transfer*, Vol. 117, pp. 574-581.

Goodson, K.E., Ju, Y.S., and Asheghi, M., 1998, "Thermal phenomena in semiconductor devices and interconnects," in *Microscale Energy Transport*, C.L. Tien et al., eds., Taylor & Francis, New York, NY, pp. 229-293.

Goodson, K.E., Käding, O.W., Rösler, M., and Zachai, R., 1995a, "Thermal conduction normal to diamond-silicon boundaries, " *Applied Physics Letters*, Vol. 66, pp. 3134-3136.

Goodson, K.E., Käding, O.W., Rösler, M., and Zachai, R., 1995b, "Experimental investigation of thermal conduction normal to diamond-Silicon boundaries," *Journal of Applied Physics*, Vol. 77, pp. 385-392.

Goodson, K.E. and Ju, Y.S., 1999, "Heat conduction in novel electronic films," in the *Annual Review of Materials Science*, E.N. Kaufmann et al., eds., Annual Reviews, Palo Alto, CA, Vol. 29, pp. 261-293.

Gorlich, S., 1992, "Electron beam testing versus laser beam testing," *Microelectronic Engineering*, Vol. 16, No. 1-4, pp. 349-366.

Goto, K., Sato, T., and Mita, S., 1993, "Proposal of optical floppy disk head and preliminary spacing experiment between lensless head and disk," *Japanese Journal of Applied Physics,* Vol. 32, No. 11B, pp. 5459-5460.

Goto, N., 1998, "Plasma density control in a low-pressure RF resonant field," *Journal of Physics D (Applied Physics),* Vol. 31, No. 4, pp. 428-433.

Grober, R.D., Schoelkopf, R.J., and Prober, D.E, 1997, "Optical antenna: towards a unity efficiency near-field optical probe," *Applied Physics Letters*, Vol. 70, No. 11, pp. 1354-1356.

Hammiche, A., Hourston, D.J., Pollock, H.M., Reading, M., and Song, M., 1996, "Scanning thermal microscopy: subsurface imaging, thermal mapping of polymer blends, and localized calorimetry," *Journal of Vacuum Science & Technology B (Microelectronics and Nanometer Structures)*, Vol. 14, No. 2, pp. 1486-1491.

Heisig, S., Rudow, O., and Oesterschulze, E., 2000, "Scanning near-field optical microscopy in the near-infrared region using light emitting cantilever probes," *Applied Physics Letters*, Vol. 77, No. 8, pp. 1071-1073.

Hohlfeld J., Muller J.G., Wellershoff S.S., and Matthias E., 1997, "Time-resolved thermoreflectivity of thin gold films and its dependence on film thickness," *Applied Physics*, Vol. B64, pp. 387-390.

Inokawa, H., Fujiwara., A., and Takahashi, Y., 2001, "A multiple-valued logic with merged single-electron and MOS transistors", *Electron Devices Meeting, IEDM '01 Technical Digest., International* , pp.147-150.

Jomaah, J., Ghibaudo, G., and Balestra, F., 1995, "Analysis and modeling of self-heating effects in thin-film SOI MOSFETs as a function of temperature," *Solid-State Electronics*, Vol. 38, No.3, pp. 615-618.

Ju, Y.S., Käding, O.W., Leung, Y.K., Wong, S.S., and Goodson, K.E., 1997, "Short-timescale thermal mapping of semiconductor devices," *IEEE Electron Device Letters*, Vol. 18, No. 5, pp. 169-171.

Ju, Y.S. and Goodson, K.E., 1999, "Phonon scattering in silicon films with thickness of order 100 nm," *Applied Physics Letters*, Vol. 74, pp. 3005-3007.

Karns, D., Zhai, J., Herget, P., Song, H., Gamble, A., Stancil, D.D., Vijaya Kumar, B.V.K., and Schlesinger, T.E., 2000, "To 100 Gb/in/sup 2/ and beyond in magneto-optic recording," *Proc. SPIE*, Vol. 4090, pp. 238-245.

Katagiri, Y. and Ukita, H., 1989, "Improvement in signal-to-noise ratio of a longitudinally coupled cavity laser by internal facet reflectivity reduction," *Japanese Journal of Applied Physics*, Vol. 28, Suppl. 28-3, pp. 177-182.

Kolodner, p. and Tyson, J.A., 1983, "Remote thermal imaging with 0.7 μm spatial resolution using temperature-dependent fluorescent thin films," *Applied Physics Letters*, Vol. 42, No. 1, pp. 117-119.

Kolodner, p. and Tyson, J.A., 1984, "Microscopic fluorescent imaging of surface temperature profiles with 0.01 degrees C resolution," *Applied Physics Letters*, Vol. 40, No. 9, pp. 782-784.

Kölzer, J. and Otto, J., 1991, "Electrical characterization of megabit DRAMs. 11. Internal testing," *IEEE Design & Test of Computers*, Vol. 8, No. 4, pp. 39-51.

Kölzer, J., Oesterschulze, E., and Deboy, G., 1996, "Thermal imaging and measurement techniques for electronic materials and devices," *Microelectronic Engineering*, Vol. 31, pp. 251-270.

Kölzer, J., Boit, C., Dallmann, A., Deboy, G., Otto, J., and Weinmann, D., 1992, "Quantitative emission microscopy," *Journal of Applied Physics*, Vol. 71, No. 11, pp. 23-41.

Kwok, T., Nguyen, T., Ho, P., and Yip, S., 1987, "Current density and temperature distributions in multilevel interconnection with studs and vias," *25th Annual Proceedings: Reliability Physics* pp. viii+279, 130-135.

Labrunie, G. and Robert, J., 1973, "Transient behaviour of the electrically controlled birefringence in a nematic liquid crystal," *Journal of Applied Physics*, Vol. 44, No. 11, pp. 4869-4874.

Langer, G., Hartmann, J., and Reichling, M., 1997, "Thermal conductivity of thin metallic films measured by photothermal profile analysis," *Review of Scientific Instruments*, Vol. 68, No.3, pp. 1510-1513.

Leung, Y.K., Suzuki, Y., Goodson, K.E., and Wong, S.S., 1995, "Self-heating effect in lateral DMOS on SOI," *Proceedings of the 7th International Symposium on Power Semiconductor Devices and Ics*, pp. 136-140.

Liu, W., and Yuksel, A., 1995, "Measurement of junction temperature of an AIGaAs/GaAs heterojunction bip transistor operating at large power densities," *IEEE Transaction Electron Device*, Vol. 42, pp. 358-360.

Maiti, B., Tobin, P.J., Hobbs, C., Hegde, R.I., Huang, F., O'Meara, D.L., Jovanovic, D., Mendicino, M., Chen, J., Connelly, D., Adetutu, O., Mogab, J., Candelaria, J., and La, L.B., 1998, "PVD TiN metal gate MOSFETs on bulk silicon and fully depleted silicon-on-insulator (FDSOI) substrates for deep sub-quarter micron CMOS technology," *Electron Devices Meeting, IEDM '98 Technical Digest., International*, p.781-784.

Majumdar, A. and Varesi, J., 1998, "Nanoscale temperature distributions measured by scanning Joule expansion microscopy," *Journal of Heat Transfer*, Vol. 120, No. 2 pp. 297-305.

Majumdar, A., Carrejo, J.P., and Lai, J., 1993, "Thermal imaging using the atomic force microscope," *Applied Physics Letters*, Vol. 62, No. 20, pp. 2501-2503.

Majumdar, A., Lai, J., Chandrachood, M., Nakabeppu, O., Wu, Y., and Shi, Z., 1995, "Thermal imaging by atomic force microscopy using thermocouple cantilever probes," *Review of Scientific Instruments*, Vol. 66, No. 6, pp. 3584-3592.

Majumdar, A., 1999, "Scanning thermal microscopy," *Annual Review of Materials Science*, Vol. 29, pp. 505-585.

Majumdar, A., Mao, M., Perazzo, T., Zhao, Y., Kwon, O., Varesi, J., and Norton, P., 2000, "Infrared vision using uncooled optomechanical camera," *Proc. SPIE*, Vol. 3948, pp. 74-79.

Mansfield, S.M. and Kino, G.S., 1990, "Solid immersion microscope," *Applied Physics Letters*, Vol. 57, No. 24, pp. 2615-2616.

Martel R., Wong, P., Chan, K., and Avouris, P., 2001, "Carbon nanotube field effect transistors for logic applications", *Electron Devices Meeting, IEDM '01 Technical Digest., International*, pp.159-162.

Mautry, p. G., and Trager, J., 1990, "Self-heating and temperature measurement in sub-μm-MOSFETs," *Proceedings of the IEEE International Conference on Microelectronic Test Structure,* Vol. 3, pp. 221- 226.

Maywald, M., Pylkki, R.J., and Balk, L.J., 1994, "Imaging or local thermal and electrical conductivity with scanning force microscopy," *Scanning Microscopy*, Vol. 8, No. 2, pp. 181-188.

Maloney, T.J. and Khurana, N., 1985, "Transmission line pulsing techniques for circuit modeling of ESD phenomena," *Proceedings of EOS/ESD Symposium,* pp. 49-54.

Miklos, A., and Lorincz, A., 1988, "Transient thermoreflectance of thin metal films in the picosecond regime," *Journal of Applied Physics*, Vol. 63, No. 7, pp. 2391-2395.

Mitsuhashi, Y., Shimada, J., and Mitsutsuka, S., 1981, "Voltage change across the self-coupled semiconductor laser," *IEEE Journal of Quantum Electronics*, Vol. QE-17, No. 7, pp. 1216-1225.

Nakabeppu, O., Chandrachood, M., Wu, Y., Lai, J., and Majumdar, A., 1994, "Scanning thermal imaging microscopy using composite cantilever probes," *Applied Physics Letters*, Vol. 66, No. 6, p.694-696.

Naoyuki, T., Tetsuya, B., and Akira, O., 1997, "Development of a thermal diffusivity measurement system with a picosecond thermoreflectance technique," *High Temperatures-High Pressures*, Vol. 29, pp. 59-66.

Negus, K.J., Franklin, R.W., and Yovanovich, M.M., 1989, "Thermal modeling and experimental techniques for microwave bipolar devices," *IEEE Transaction Component Hybrids Manufacturing Technology. (USA)*, Vol. 12, No. 4, pp. 680-689.

Nonnenmacher, M., and Wickramasinghe, H.K, 1992, "Scanning probe microscopy of thermal conductivity and subsurface properties," *Applied Physics Letters*, Vol. 61, No. 2, pp. 168-170.

Novotny, L., and Pohl, D.W., 1995, "Light propagation in scanning near-field optical microscopy," *Photons and Local Probes. Proceedings of the NATO Advanced Research Workshop* pp. 21-33.

Oesterschulze, E., Stopka, M., and Kassing, R., 1994, "Photo-thermal characterization of solids and thin films by optical and scanning probe techniques," *Microelectronic Engineering*, Vol. 24, No. 1-4, pp. 107-112.

Oesterschulze, E., Hadjiiski, L., Stopka, M., and Kassing, R., 1995, "Laser interferometry and SThM-techniques for thermal characterization of thin films," *Materials Science Forum*, Vol. 185-188, pp. 43-52.

Oesterschulze, E., Stopka,. M., Tochtrop-Mayr, M, Masseli, K., and Kassing, R., 1993, "Nondestructive evaluation of solids and deposited films by thermal-wave interferometry," *Applied Surface Science*, Vol. 69, No. 1-4, pp. 65-68.

Opsal, J., and Rosencwaig, A., 1985, "Thermal and plasma wave depth profiling in silicon," *Applied Physics Letters*, Vol. 47, No. 5, pp. 498-500.

Paddock, C.A., and Eesley, G.L., 1986, "Transient thermoreflectance from thin metal films," *Journal of Applied Physics*, Vol. 60, pp. 285-290.

Paesler, M.A., and Moyer, p. J., 1996, *Near-Field Optics,* Wiley, New York.

Partovi, A., Peale, D., Wuttig, M., Murray, C.A., Zydzik, G., Hopkins, L., Baldwin, K., Hobson, W.S., Wynn, J., Lopata, J., Dhar, L., Chichester, R., and Yeh, J.H.-J., 1999, "High-power laser light source for near-field optics and its application to high-density optical data storage," *Applied Physics Letters,* Vol. 75, No. 11, pp. 1515-1517.

Peters, L., 1993, "SOI takes over where silicon leaves off," *Semiconductor International*, Vol. 16, No. 3, pp. 48-51.

Picart, B., and Minguez, S.D., 1992, "Test method in voltage contrast mode using liquid crystals (VLSI)," *Microelectronics and Reliability*, Vol. 32, No. 11, pp. 1605-1613.

Picart, B., and Petit, O., 1990, "Internal noncontact testing method using ferroelectric liquid crystals (IC failure analysis)," *Microelectronic Engineering*, Vol. 12, No. 1-4, pp. 149-156.

Pylkki, R.J., Moyer, P.J., and West, P.E., 1994, "Scanning near-field optical microscopy and scanning thermal microscopy," *Japanese Journal of Applied Physics*, Vol. 33, No. 6, pp. 3785-3790.

Quintard, V., Deboy, G., Dilhaire, S., Lewis, D., Phan, T., and Claeys, W., 1996, "Laser beam thermography of circuits in the particular case of passivated semiconductors," *Microelectronic Engineering*, Vol. 24, pp. 291-298.

Radmacher, M., Hillner, A.P.E., and Hansma, P.K., 1994, "Scanning nearfield optical microscope using microfabricated probes," *Review of Scientific Instruments*, Vol. 65, No. 8, pp. 2737-2738.

Raha, P., Ramaswamy, S., and Rosenbaum, E., 1997, "Heat flow analysis for EOS/ESD protection device design in SOI technology," *IEEE Transactions on Electron Devices*, Vol. 44, pp. 464-471.

Ramo, S., Whinnery, J.R., and Van Duzer, T., 1984, *Fields and waves in communication electronics, 2nd edition*", Wiley; New York, NY, USA, pp. 817.

Rantala, J., Lanhua, W., Kuo, P.K., Jaarinen, J., Luukkala, M., and Thomas, R.L., 1993, "Determination of thermal diffusivity of low-diffusivity materials using the mirage method with multiparameter fitting," *Journal of Applied Physics*, Vol. 73, pp. 2714-2723.

Rausch, M., Kaltenbacher, M., Landes, H., and Lerch, R., 2001, "Numerical computation of the emitted noise of power transformers," *The International Journal for Computation and Mathematics in Electrical and Electronic Engineering*, Vol. 20, No. 2, pp. 636-648.

Roberts D. M. and Gustafson, T.L., 1986, "Time modulation techniques for picosecond to microsecond pump-probe experiments using synchronously pumped dye lasers," *Optics Communications*, Vol. 56, No. 5, pp. 334-338.

Roger, J.P., Lepoutre, F., Fournier, D., and Boccara, A.C., 1987, "Thermal diffusivity measurement of micron-thick semiconductor films by mirage detection," *Thin Solid Films*, Vol. 155, No. 1, pp. 165-174.

Schoenlein, R.W., Lin W. Z., Fujimoto, J.G., and Eesley G.L., 1987, "Femtosecond studies of nonequilibrium electronic process in metals", *Physical Review Letters*, Vol. 58, No. 16, pp. 2680-2683.

Skumanich, A., Dersch, H., Fathallah, M., and Amer, N.M., 1987, "A contactless method for investigating the thermal properties of thin films," *Applied Physics* A (Solids and Surfaces), Vol. A43, No. 4, pp. 297-300.

Sodnik, Z., Tiziani, Hj., Hess, P., and Pelzl, J. (eds.), 1988, *Photoacoustic and photothermal phenomena III*, Springer Verlag Berlin, pp. 400.

Solkner, G., Wolfgang, E., and Bohm, C., 1994, "Advanced diagnosis techniques for submicron integrated circuits," *ESSCIRC '94. Twentieth European Solid-State Circuits Conference. Proceedings,* pp. xvi+314, 11-17.

Soref, R.A., and Bennett, B.R., 1987, "Electrooptical effects in silicon," *IEEE Journal of Quantum Electronics*, Vol. QE-23, No. 1, pp. 123-129.

Soref, R.A., and Rafuse, M.J., 1972, "Electrically controlled birefringence of thin nematic films (Light values)," *Journal of Applied Physics*, Vol. 453, No. 5, pp. 2029-2037.

Su., L.T., Antoniadis, D.A., Arora, N.D., Doyle, B.S., and Krakauer, D.B., 1994, "SPICE model and parameters for fully-depleted SOI MOSFET'S including self-heating," *IEEE Electron Device Letters*, Vol. 15, No. 10, pp. 374-376.

Sverdrup, P.G., Ju, Y.S., and Goodson, K.E., 1998, "Sub-continuum simulations of heat conduction in silicon-on-insulator transistors," *Journal of Heat Transfer*, Vol. 120, pp. 30-36.

Sze, S.M., 1998, "VLSI technology," McGraw-Hill, New York.

Tang, A.P.S., and Cheng, K.S., 2001, "Thermal X-ray pulses resulting from pulsar glitches," *Astrophysical Journal*, Vol. 549, No. 2, p.1039-1049.

Tenbroek, B.M., Redman-White, W., Lee, M.S.L., and Uren, M.J., 1996, "Electrical measurement of silicon film and oxide thicknesses in partially depleted SOI technologies," *Solid-State Electronics*, Vol. 39, No. 7, pp. 1011-1014.

Terris, B.D., Mamin, H.J., and Rugar, D., 1996, "Near-field optical data storage," *Applied Physics Letters*, Vol. 68, No. 2, pp. 141-143.

Toigo, J.W., 2000, "Avoiding the data crunch," *Scientific America,* Vol. 282, No. 5, pp. 58-74.

Touzelbaev, M.N. and Goodson, K.E, 2001, "Impact of experimental timescale and geometry on thin-film thermal property measurements," *International Journal of Thermophysics*, Vol. 22, pp. 243-263.

Wallash, A.J., 2000, "ESD in magnetic recording: past, present and future," www.wallash.com.

Weaver, J.M.R., Walpita, L.M., and Wickramasinghe, H.K, 1989, "Optical absorption microscopy and spectroscopy with nanometer resolution," *Nature*, Vol. 342, No. 6251, pp. 783-785.

Williams, C.C., and Wickramasinghe, H.K., 1986, "Scanning thermal profiler," *Applied Physics Letters*, Vol. 49, No. 23, pp. 1587-1589.

Williams, C.C., and Wickramasinghe, H.K., 1988, "Thermal and photothermal imaging on a sub 100 nanometer scale," *Proc. SPIE*, Vol. 897, pp. 129-134.

5. Nanoscale Mechanical Characterization of Carbon Nanotubes

R.S. Ruoff and M.-F. Yu

5.1 Introduction

The discoveries of multi-walled carbon nanotubes in 1991[1] (MWCNT) and single wall carbon nanotubes (SWCNT) in 1993 [2, 3] ushered in a new era of research in nanomaterials, where the focus is the synthesis and study of materials having size in the nanometer scale. More than 4100 scientific publications on carbon nanotubes (CNTs) have appeared in the last decade. As a new member of the carbon family, which includes diamond, graphite and fullerenes, carbon nanotubes (CNT) have received significant attention as model system for fundamental researches related to low dimensionality. CNT can be described as a seamless cylinder (SWCNT), or nested cylinders (MWCNT), of rolled graphene sheet(s) that can have either capped or opened ends. Novel discoveries related to the mechanical and electronic properties of the rolled graphene sheet, of quantum confinement in small dimensions, and of particularly the chirality of the shell structure of CNTs as defined by the rolling direction and the longitudinal axis, have been made. Potential applications have been proposed or pursued in the area of materials reinforcement, [4, 5] electronic devices, [6-8] conductive nanowires, [9, 10] field emission panel display, [11-13] chemical sensors, [14] H_2 gas storage[15], scanning microscopy probes, [16, 17] super electrochemical capacitor, [18] drug delivery capillary and others.

Due to the highly graphitized structure of CNT, its mechanical properties have been expected to be comparable to or even better than both graphite and diamond. Indeed, modeling has predicted that CNT possesses mechanical properties superior to commercially available carbon fibers in wide current use. High Young's modulus (~ 1 TPa) similar to the in-plane modulus value for high quality graphite, and high tensile strength (in the range ~ 100 GPa) much greater than any other known materials are predicted, [19-22] and experimentally verified, [23-31] for CNT. For comparison, the highest strength commercially available carbon fiber has a breaking strength value of ~ 7GPa. [32]

CNTs made to date typically have a diameter of a few tens of nanometers (for multiwalled carbon nanotubes, MWCNT) about 1 nm (for singlewalled carbon nanotubes, SWCNT) and lengths of a few microns. Such small dimensions impose a tremendous challenge for experimental study. Many principles used for the mechanical study of bulk materials can still be applied for nanostructures, however some new technical obstacles need to be overcome first. Individual CNT need to be placed in an appropriate testing configuration. Sub-micron-sized clamps need to be fabricated for controlling the boundary conditions for loading.

Methods for controllably applying sub-mN force with nN resolution and nanometer displacement need to be developed, and finally, techniques for characterizing and measuring the mechanical deformation at the nanometer or perhaps even atomic scale need to be attained. High-resolution microscopes are indispensable instruments for the characterization of nanomaterials, and recent innovative developments in the new area of "nanomanipulation," based on inserting or adapting new tools for use in such high resolution microscopes, have enhanced our ability to probe nanoscale objects. In this chapter, we review some new developments in instrumentation and some new capabilities demonstrated from experiments. We then speculate about future directions for studies of the mechanics of individual nanostructures.

5.2 Instruments for Nanoscale Characterization

Electron microscopy (EM) and scanning probe microscopy (SPM) have been the most widely used methods for resolving and characterizing nanoscale objects. SPM's use extremely sharp probes (that can have 10 nm or smaller radius of curvature at the tip) controlled by sensitive sensing and actuation feedback electronics for obtaining nanoscale and even atomic scale mapping. In a typical imaging experiment the tip is rastered over the sample and the sample geometry is thereby mapped out, but SPM can also be used to nanomachine surfaces, to nanoindent samples, and to bend and manipulate nanostructures. EM's use high-energy electron beams (several keV up to several hundred keV) as a source for scattering and obtaining diffraction pattern from a sample, which allows the achievement of high resolving power down to sub-nanometer resolution because of the extremely short wavelength (a fraction of an Angstrom) of electrons at high kinetic energy. We and others have primarily used SPM and EM instruments to study nanotube mechanics. We give a brief review of the methods of operation of these types of microscopes.

5.2.1 Atomic Force Microscope (AFM)

The atomic force microscope (AFM) has been particularly useful for the mechanical studies of CNTs. Since its invention in 1986, [35] it has been used as a standard tool for many applications related to surface characterization. High-resolution mapping of surface morphology on either conductive or nonconductive material can be achieved with an AFM.

The principle of operation of an AFM is relatively simple. A probe having a force sensitive cantilever with a sharp tip is used as a sensor to physically scan the sample surface.

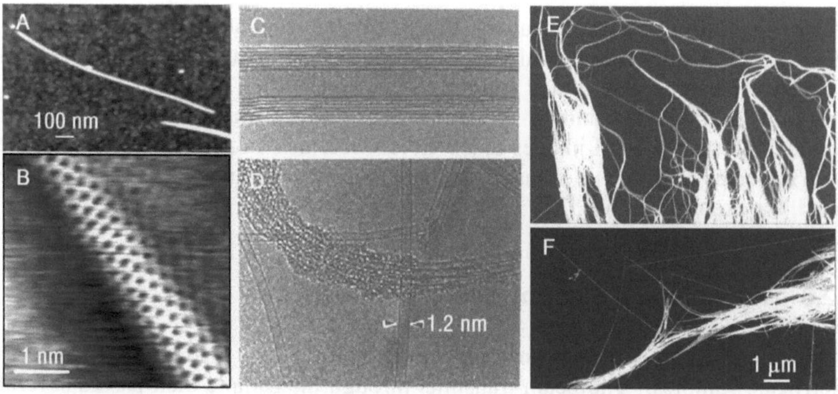

Fig. 5.1. (A) A representative AFM image of MWCNTs on a silicon substrate acquired in tapping mode. (B) An atomic resolution STM image of a SWCNT. From [33]. (C) Transmission electron microscope, TEM, images of a MWCNT and (D) of SWCNTs. From [34]. The interlayer distance in MWCNT is ~ 0.34 nm. (E) Typical SEM images of SWCNTs and (F) of MWCNTs. Individual MWCNTs can be seen sticking out from the bulk sample, while SWCNTs generally form ropes and exist in an entangled web structure.

A piezoelectric tube capable of nanometer resolution translation in the x, y and z directions is used to drive the probe and the tip of the probe normally has a radius of curvature on the order of 10 nm. The force interactions between tip and sample deflects the cantilever. While the sample surface is scanned in the x and y direction, the deflection of the cantilever is monitored by a simple optical method, or other approaches. A feedback electronic circuit that reads the deflection signal and controls the piezoelectric tube guarantees a constant force between the tip and the sample surface. A surface profile of the sample can thus be obtained.

Fig. 5.1A shows a typical image of MWCNTs on a substrate acquired by AFM. Depending on the type of interaction force involved for sensing, an SPM includes a family of microscopes such as the atomic force microscope (AFM), friction force microscope, magnetic force microscope, electric force microscope, and so on. Depending on the mechanism used for measuring the force interaction, the SPM also includes many modes of operation, such as contact mode, tapping mode, force modulation mode and so on. We refer to, for example, references. [35-37]

5.2.2 Scanning Tunneling Microscope (STM)

The detection mechanism of the scanning tunneling microscope (STM) is based on monitoring the tunneling current (on the order of nA and less) between a sharp conductive tip and a sample when in close proximity and under a constant bias. STM imaging thus requires a non-insulating sample. With appropriate imaging conditions atomic resolution can be obtained on many crystalline samples, due to the strong dependence of the tunneling current on the electronic density of states of the substrate and on the tip-sample distance. There is an exponential dependence of the current on this distance. Fig. 5.1B shows an atomically resolved image of a SWCNT by Odom et al.[33] The lattice structure and thus the chirality of the SWCNT can be determined from such images, as well as the electronic structure from additional scanning tunneling spectroscopy measurements. Similar atomically resolved STM images of SWCNTs were also obtained at the same time by Wildoer et al. [38] A detailed explanation on the principle of STM can be found, for example, in ref. [36]

5.2.3 Transmission Electron Microscope (TEM)

In TEM, an accelerated electron beam from a thermal or a field emitter is used to interrogate samples. The beam transmits through the sample then passes several stages of electromagnetic lenses, and projects the image of the studied sample region to a phosphor screen or other image recording media. A thin (typically several tens of nanometer or less in thickness) and small (no more than ~50mm^2) sample is a typical requirement since only a small sample chamber is available and a dedicated holder is typically used in these expensive instruments (which are thus typically time-shared among many users) for sample transfer. The spread in the electron beam energy and the quality of the ion optics are limiting factors in TEM, which can have a resolution on the order of 0.2 nm. Reference [39] is a suggested textbook on TEM. Figs. 5.1C and D shows typical high-resolution images of CNTs [34]. Fringes corresponding to individual shell(s) in each CNT are easily resolved.

An exciting new development in electron microscopy is the move towards adding aberration correction. We provide no extensive review of this topic here, but note for the reader that a coming "revolution" in electron microscopy could allow for image resolution of approximately 0.04 nm with TEM, and of about 0.2 nm for appropriately outfitted scanning electron microscopes (SEM). There are two types of corrective ion optics, the first corrects for spherical aberration (to correct for aberration in the lenses) and the second for achromatic aberration (for the spread in the wavelengths of the electrons emanating from the emitter). As newer instruments are installed in the next few years, for example, at national laboratories, improvement in the image resolution for mechanics studies of nano-sized specimens is an important goal.

5.2.4 Scanning Electron Microscope (SEM)

In SEM, a focused electron beam (nanometers in spot size) is rastered across the sample surface and the amplified image of the sample surface is formed by recording the secondary electron signal or the back scattering signal generated from the sample. In principle, there is no strict limit on sample size, and normally a large sample chamber is available such that samples can be surveyed over large areas. SEM is limited by the scattering volume of the electrons interacting with the sample material, and commercial high end instruments are capable of achieving a resolution of a few nanometers. Typical SEM images of a purified MWCNT sample, and of a SWCNT sample, are shown in Figs. 5.1E and F. Individual MWCNTs can be seen sticking out from the bundle, while only bundles of SWCNTs having diameters ~10 nm can be readily seen in the SWCNT sample.

5.2.5 New Tools for SEM

The high resolution and the relatively large available sample chamber space make SEM a good candidate for modification to include three dimensional nanomanipulation capabilities. A multiple degree-of-freedom manipulation device inside SEM was developed by Yu et al. to perform a variety of functions for handling, characterizing, and building with CNTs and other nanostructures. [40] The device possesses the capability and precision to probe a collection of CNTs, whether an ordered array or disordered bundle or aggregate, and then to isolate the CNT and extract it from the ensemble for individual study. Once a CNT has been isolated from the group, the manipulator can be used as a testing stage to allow measurement of the mechanics and transport properties, while the CNT is freely suspended in vacuum and thus free from contact with a surface.

Simultaneous mechanical and electrical measurement can be made with conductive force probes, or independent probes that are brought into contact with the CNT from the side. The device fits well inside the vacuum chamber of an SEM, and can be operated without interfering with the components of the microscope or disturbing the imaging quality. Similar devices were then also developed by Nishijima et al. for making CNT attached AFM tips and for mechanical measurement of CNTs. [41] In the following, we mainly focus on the design and the functions of our SEM nanomanipulation/testing tool.

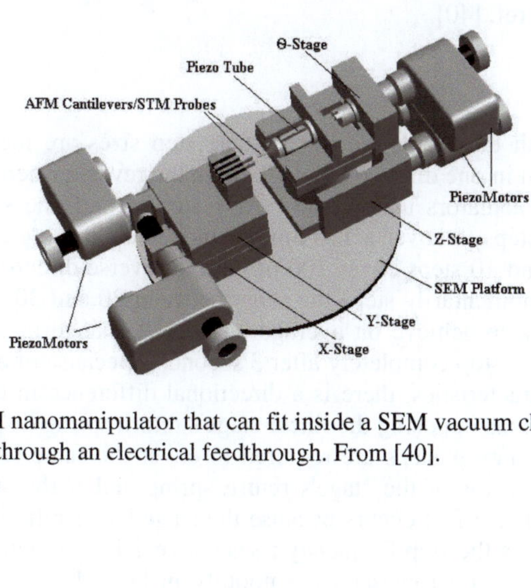

Fig. 5.2. The SEM nanomanipulator that can fit inside a SEM vacuum chamber and be controlled externally through an electrical feedthrough. From [40].

Design

The manipulator is shown in Fig. 5.2. For clarity, the electrical connections and grounded shields are removed and only the major components are shown. The manipulator was designed with wide translation range, reasonable precision, small size, low-cost, and rapid assembly in mind. To avoid interference with the SEM electron optics, the x-y and z-theta motions are grouped into two low profile, opposing stage sub-modules anchored symmetrically on the SEM platform around the axis of the electron beam column. Coarse 3-axis linear motions up to 6 mm and single-axis 360-degree rotational probe motion are provided by vacuum-prepared stainless steel stages driven by long travel piezo actuators. An integral x-y stage guides motion parallel to the plane of the SEM stage, and a separate z-axis stage is used for motion along the SEM beam axis. Rotational motion normal to the beam is accomplished using a continuous rotating piezo actuator mounted atop the z-stage. This actuator is attached mechanically to a tungsten wire with an electrically insulating Delrin coupling.

The length of the tip passes through a ceramic bushing bonded to the tip end of a piezo tube, which is mounted coaxial to the rotating actuator. The four-quadrant piezotube serves both as a support for the rotating tip and as a fine motion actuator in order to provide continuous motions. The SEM stage manipulator occupies roughly 50 cm^3. Actuator electrical control signals are conducted through isolated vacuum feedthroughs passing through the SEM main chamber wall. The translation stages share a common electrical circuit, which is often grounded, and the rotating tip and sample holder atop the z-stage and x-y stages, respectively, are all connected through the vacuum feedthrough so that the articulating elements can be electrically addressed separately from outside the vacuum. Finally, all insulated components and wires are shielded with grounded covers around the SEM observation region to minimize image distortion from charging effects. More details are given in ref. [40].

Performance

As observed with the SEM, the linear stage step sizes are measured to be approximately 4 nm in one direction and 10 nm in the reverse when driven slowly by the linear piezo actuators under load. At 1 step/second, the stages require approximately 25 steps to cover a 100 nm distance when driving against the stages' return springs, and 10 steps cover 100 nm in the reverse direction. A single step of the actuator momentarily steps the stage between 20 and 30 nm; however, the stage settles back to achieve on average an overall change in distance of 4 nm. Settling appears to stop completely after 3 seconds. Because of combined loading and actuator characteristics, there is a directional difference in the degree of settling, in that motions opposing the linear stage's return spring display a greater degree of settling. Fewer steps are required to cover the same territory if moving along the force vector of the stage's return spring and if the step period is decreased. This latter effect occurs because the stage has insufficient time to settle back completely as the step frequency rises above 1 Hz. When driven at 1 kHz, the stages travel 25 microns/second smoothly in both directions, thus giving a "dynamic" step resolution of 25 nm. The rotational actuator, which is useful for examining all sides of the tungsten tip and the attachments to it, gives angular step sizes of <0.02 degrees with a maximum rotation rate of ~20 degrees/sec.

The piezotube atop the z-stage is necessary for continuous motions after the linear stages are brought to within a micron or less of the final desired positions of a manipulation operation. Voltages to the piezotube supplied by a three-axis controller (Thorlabs) drive the tube to frequencies of up to 10 kHz with translation ranges of several microns. Although no minimum step resolution for the piezotube could be directly observed, according to noise figures from the piezo driver and accounting for piezo drift and nonlinearities, the spatial resolution of the piezotube can be estimated conservatively to be under 1 nm. For CNT experiments, well-controlled lateral and longitudinal motions are necessary for manipulation and in order to measure, for example, strain-induced conductance properties. More details are given in ref. [40]

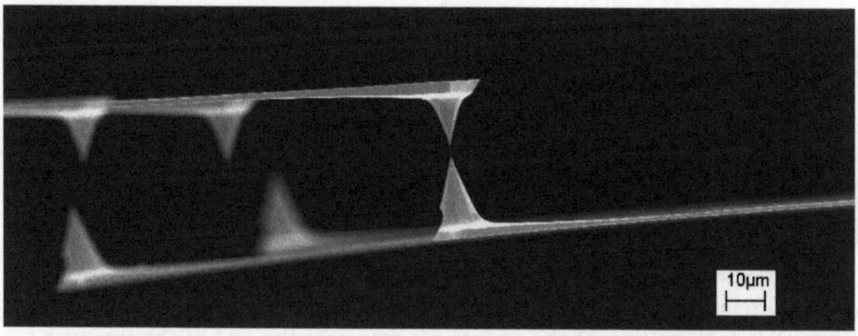

Fig. 5.3. An SEM image of AFM tips mounted on the nanomanipulator and used as sharp "fingers" for manipulation.

Manipulation "Finger" and Force probe

AFM tips with rigid cantilevers (TESP and FESP AFM cantilever from Digital Instruments) and soft cantilevers (CSCS12 AFM cantilever from NT-MDT) have been used (Fig. 5.3) by our group, along with electrochemically etched tungsten and mechanically sharpened gold and platinum-iridium tips. AFM tips were mounted opposite the rotating tungsten probe tip, which also served as a mount for an AFM cantilever when "dueling" AFM tips were used. Some AFM cantilevers were coated with gold to make them conductive.

Attachment of CNT

In using the tool as described above, picking up and attaching an individual CNT or CNT bundle to an AFM or STM tip is always the first step. It is done by a straightforward way. A visible quantity of purified CNT material is loaded onto the metal tip and the tip is placed into the tip holder on the x-y stage along with three to six other tips ready for CNT attachment. The AFM or STM tip on the piezotube can then be brought close to the raw material while the operation is directly viewed in the SEM and if desired simultaneously video-recorded. When the tip approaches close enough to a protruding CNT, it "jumps" to the tip and is held in place through the van der Waals attractive forces. The initial jump to the tip could be due to an electrostatic attraction as the elements could be unequally charged from the electron beam, or could simply be from van der Waals forces. A third and interesting possibility is that the difference in the work function of the nanostructure (in this case, a CNT) and the tip, can lead to an additional attractive force due to a slight charge buildup at the end of the CNT. [42]

After "jump to tip" the van der Waals forces are then sometimes enough to hold the tube and tip together as the CNT is pulled from the bunch. If not, a stronger bond can be made by using the electron beam to perform localized "electron impact-induced deposition," (EBID) of carbonaceous material due to the presence of some residual hydrocarbon contaminant in the SEM chamber, a process which we refer to as "nano-welding." (We note that this is not "welding" per se, so the analogy is not an exact one.)

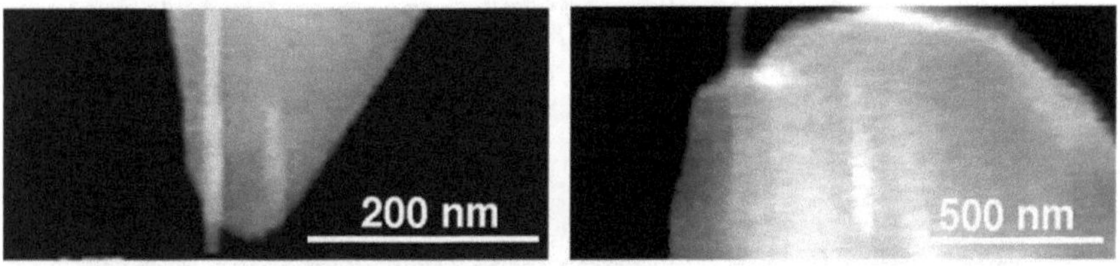

Fig. 5.4. High magnification SEM images showing the attachment of MWCNT onto AFM Si tips. Localized deposition of the square patches near the end of the tips was realized by electron beam induced deposition method inside SEM. From [29].

Attaching CNTs to AFM tips has been previously done by Dai et al. while observing with a light microscope, [16] and their work involved the first example of a CNT as a tip for AFM, and the first detailed studies of the mechanical performance of such a CNT AFM tip. Our technique, attachment with simultaneous viewing in the SEM, allows the CNT tip to be inspected at much higher spatial resolution, and immediately altered if desired. Fig. 5.4 shows images of MWCNT-attached AFM tips showing the attachment. Attachment of short-length nanotubes (particularly for a SWCNT because of its flexibility) which can be more rigid laterally and as a result more mechanically stable, is essential for use as a very high-resolution AFM or STM tip.

Of course, this general approach is not limited to CNTs, and we expect that a large number of different types of nanofilaments, such as metal nanowires, inorganic nanowhiskers, and nanoplatelets of various layered materials, will be "nano-clamped" in various types of testing stages configured to be in SEMs, TEMs, or SPMs, or adapted to various spectroscopic probes, such as Raman. Indeed, we describe the case of amorphous SiO_2 nanowires and our study of their mechanical resonance response, below. The method of making clamps, and the types of clamps, will likely be sample dependent.

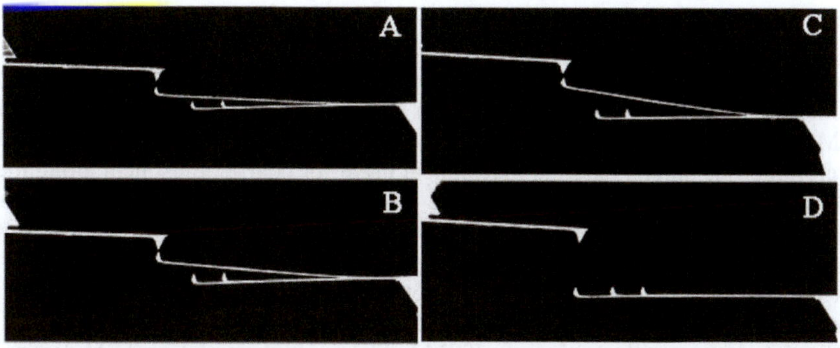

Fig. 5.5. An SEM image sequence showing the tensile loading experiment on MWCNTs (A MWCNT with both ends attached to the AFM tips is not resolved in this small magnification image). From [40].

Mechanical Measurement Capability

Fig. 5.5. shows the SEM images sequentially recorded in the process of the mechanical measurement of CNT. CNTs were attached to a stiff AFM cantilever on the left (spring constant 100N/m) and a soft AFM cantilever on the right (cantilever constant 0.03 N/m). The sequential images show the softer cantilever's increasing deflection as the stiff cantilever is moved in the upward direction. The return to zero deflection is shown in Fig. 5.5D after the tube has broken. The use of such AFM cantilevers allows the force to be measured as the tubes are tensile-loaded. For this set of images, the total deflection of the softer cantilever (45 μm) yielded a calculated breaking force of 1.3 μN.

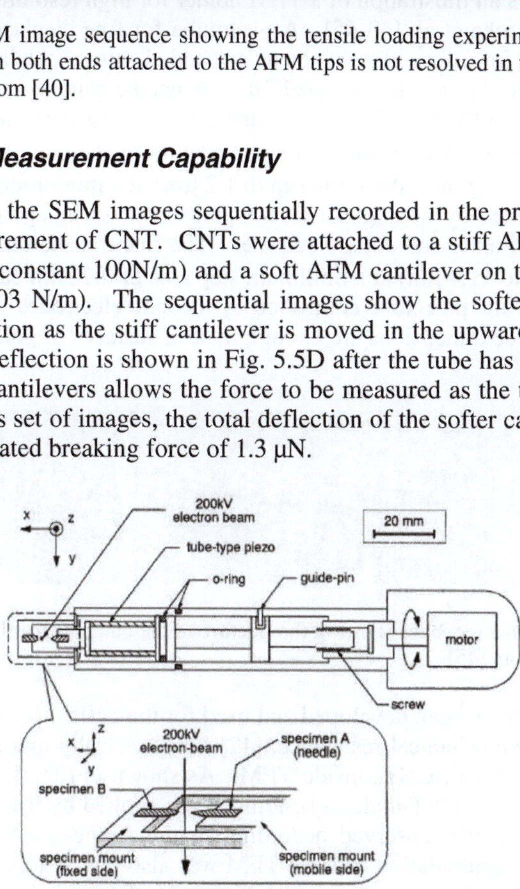

Fig. 5.6. Schematic of a TEM sample holder with mechanical translation adjustment and piezoelectric actuators for manipulation. From [44].

5.2.6 New Tools for TEM

Owing to the high resolving power of TEM, recent effort has also been devoted to the development of manipulation tools for TEM. Typical manipulation tools for TEM incorporate a single piezotube for fine motion in x, y and z in the range of several microns and an external mechanical drive for coarse adjustment along the axial direction of the TEM holder. The limited maneuverability is mostly constrained by the small sample space available in TEM and the design requirement for a standard-sized TEM holder that can fit into the general commercial TEM's that are typically time shared with a variety of users, most of whom want to do more standard imaging/analysis experiments, and not nanomanipulation studies.

Fig. 5.6 shows an illustration of a TEM holder for high resolution TEM demonstrated by T. Kizuka et al. [43-45]. A piezotube for fine displacement and a microscrew motor for coarse displacement are added into a standard TEM sample holder to provide the translation capability. A needle sample can be mounted at the mobile side on the tip of a lever connected with the piezotube. The mobile side can translate along the x direction up to ±1 mm by the microscrew motor. The fine translation along the x direction (up to 1.2 μm) at a minimum step size of 0.16 nm can be adjusted by homogeneous elongation and shrinkage of the piezotube controlled by the inner and outer electrodes. The fine translations along the y and z directions (up to 11.4 μm) at a minimum step size of 0.22 nm can be adjusted by the deflection of the piezotube controlled by the side electrodes. Such step resolutions along three dimensions are enough to scan surfaces of gold at atomic resolution.

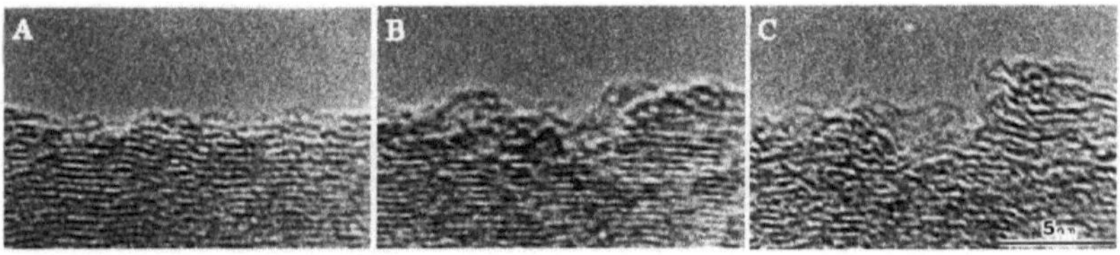

Fig. 5.7. TEM image sequence showing the fracture of the outer layers of a MWCNT under bending stress. From [45].

Similar tools have been developed and used for the deflection and bending, [42, 45] for inducing mechanical resonance, [42] for electrically modification [46]and for telescoping, [47] of CNTs inside TEM. As shown in Fig. 5.7, fracture of the outer layers of a MWCNT under a bending stress applied by the manipulation inside TEM was clearly observed according to the fringe-resolved images. [45] Similar bending manipulation inside a TEM was also realized by Ruoff et al. [48] using an unusual method of a thermally distortable Formvar film onto which the NTs were dispersed. The deformation through mechanical load was created by 2 different methods, either *in situ* in a TEM environment by the electron beam flux locally heating the thin film of Formvar, or *ex situ* by gentle heating of the thin polymer (Formvar) support film of a TEM grid onto which the nanotubes or whiskers had been, as mentioned, previously dispersed.

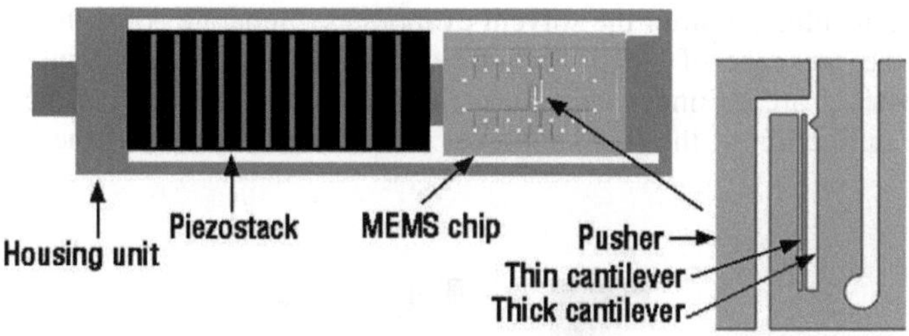

Fig. 5.8. Schematic showing the stressing stage unit for being incorporated into a TEM sample holder for in situ observation of the tensile measurement of carbon nanotubes. Designed by H. Rohrs and R. S. Ruoff.

Recently, Ruoff's group at Northwestern University has developed a TEM tensile loading tool that combines with microelectromechanical system (MEMS) technology to include the direct force load and sensing capabilities essential for a detailed mechanical property study of CNT. Shown in Fig. 5.8 is a schematic of this "TEM nano-stressing stage". The stage is designed as a separate unit that can fit into a TEM holder but is detachable. The central component in the stage is a MEMS-like chip fabricated in silicon wafer by a deep reactive ion (Bosch) etching process. It is composed of two main functional parts: a thin cantilever on a rigid fixture, and a linear pusher and a thick cantilever on a soft fixture. The pusher contacts a piezostack, which provides the fine linear translation as well as the load. This device can be placed inside a modified TEM holder and in operation was inserted into a TEM. The piezostack is connected to a power supply to control the moving stage position. Voltage supplied to the piezostack is regulated with an accuracy of 10mV, which allows the control of the movement of the pusher with sub-nanometer resolution.

When in operation, the unit is detached from the TEM holder, and the gap between two cantilevers is adjusted to ~0.5 μm and fixed in place by locking the fixed end of the piezostack. The preload is done using a linear piezo inchworm actuator while monitoring with a high magnification optical microscope. A liquid suspension of CNTs was drawn into a glass micropipette, which was then positioned above the gap between the cantilevers, to allow for deposition of nanowires such as CNT. The micropipette tip position was monitored with an optical microscope and controlled by an *x-y-z* stage. The micropipette was then lowered into contact with the cantilevers so that capillary action can draw a very small volume (10-100 femtoliter) of CNT suspension into the gap. The capillary force in the gap holds the liquid drop in between the cantilevers and typically makes the free end portion of the thin cantilever stick to the thick cantilever. When the droplet dries, the thin cantilever typically smoothly releases and returns to its original position, and a small number of CNTs can be found being placed directly across the gap between the cantilevers.

For the case of SWCNT suspension, such operation tends to gently draw the SWCNT nanorope or individual SWCNTs across the gap, leaving them slightly mechanically loaded by the deposition. The SWCNTs are at times held firmly in place by a residue left after the solvent evaporates. Separate AFM imaging indeed showed the presence of small amounts of residual organic material. SWCNTs thus deposited are so under an initial tension, and the preload can be calculated from the deflection of the thin cantilever if the force constant of the cantilever is known.

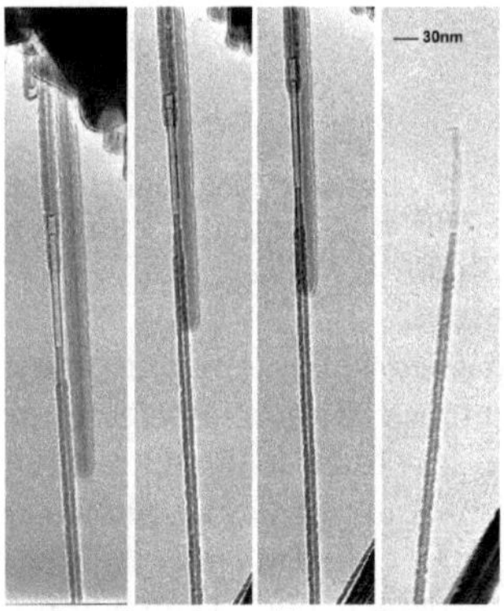

Fig. 5.9. TEM image sequence showing the pullout of the internal shells of a MWCNT using the stressing stage. Data taken by O. Lourie.

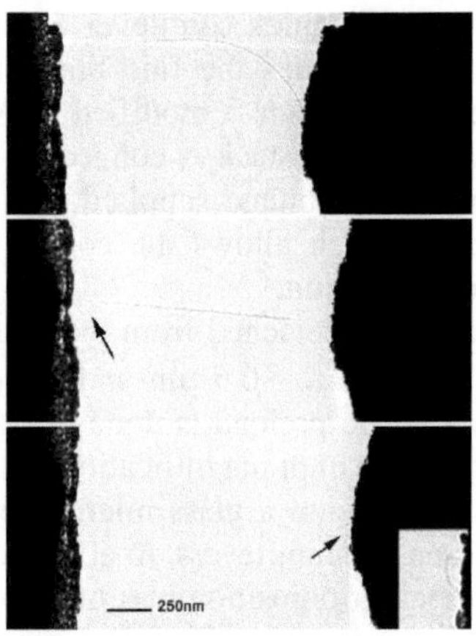

Fig. 5.10. TEM image sequence showing the stretching and the final break of a very thin SWCNT rope (consists of only several SWCNTs) mounted between two cantilevers in the stressing stage.

After the deposition, the device was inserted into the TEM. Load is applied by extending the piezostack to push the thick cantilever. The deflection of the thin cantilever was then measured during the loading process, which gives the applied load, and the length of CNTs can be obtained using a formula which includes the calibrated piezostack extension under different applied voltage and the initial gap distance and the deflection of the cantilever, or can be measured from the recorded

TEM images in some cases. Such a device was used to break SWCNT ropes having only several SWCNTs as shown in Fig. 5.9, [49] and also was used to directly observe the fracture process of CNTs under tensile load by Lourie et al [50] as shown in Fig. 5.10.

Two different methods were used to obtain the force constant of the force-sensing cantilever. The force constant was first calculated using the cantilever dimensions measured by SEM, and the standard cantilever beam-bending model. Second, AFM was used to calibrate the cantilever force constant (we carefully cleaved the central component wafer piece to expose the cantilever for such an AFM calibration) using a calibrated AFM probe. The two methods agreed within 10%.

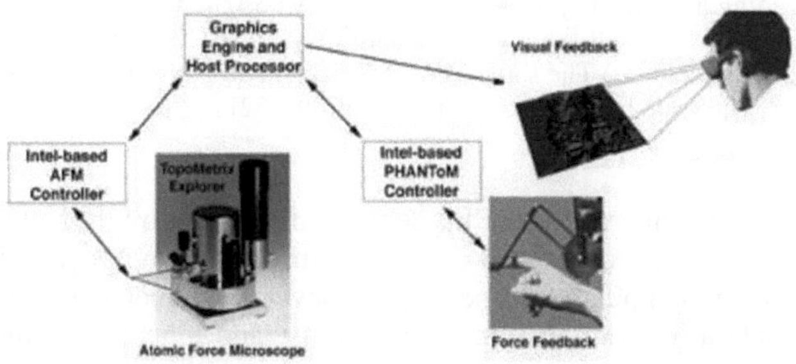

Fig. 5.11. Panel diagram showing the design and operation principle of the AFM nanomanipulator. From http://www.cs.unc.edu/Research/nano/.

5.2.7 New Tools for AFM

By interfacing with a force feedback controller and 3D computer graphic scheme, a modified Scanning Force Microscope with real time manipulation and visualization capability has been developed at the University of North Carolina at Chapel Hill (Fig. 5.11). [51] Using such a nanomanipulation system, the sample can be not only imaged but also manipulated in a controlled matter. Such control is realized by interfacing a hand-held force stylus with the scanning tip of the microscope. When the microscope is switched to manipulating mode, the scanning tip moves according to the motion of the hand-held stylus, thus enabling controlled manipulation of the sample. The manipulation force, speed, and direction of manipulation are under user control. Following manipulation, the microscope can be switched back to imaging mode to view the manipulation. This cycle can be repeated as desired.

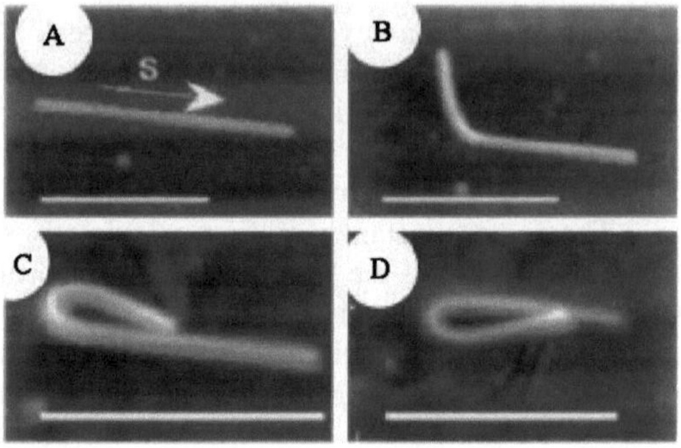

Fig. 5.12. Bending and buckling of MWCNTs. (A) An original straight MWCNT. (B) The MWCNT is bent upwards all the way back onto itself. (C) The same MWCNT is bent all the way back onto itself. (D) The same MWCNT is bend all the way back to itself from another direction. The scale bar represents 500 nm. From [52].

All features encountered by the tip can actually be felt by the user through the hand-held stylus, as it is connected to the scanning tip by an integrated force feedback loop. As the manipulation is performed, several parameters of interest (modifying force, lateral or friction force, topography, and others) are simultaneously recorded. The system has been used to manipulate CNTs as shown in Fig. 5.12 and study nanoscale tribology and electrical properties of CNTs. [52-54]

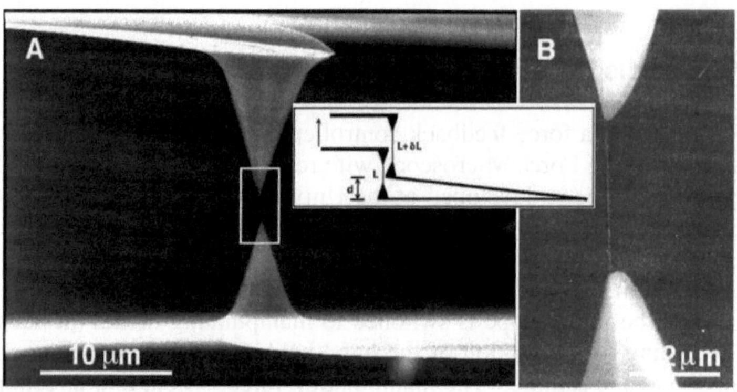

Fig. 5.13. (A) An SEM image showing the setup for the tensile mechanical measurement of an individual MWCNT mounted between two counter AFM probes. (B) A large magnification SEM image showing the MWCNT clamped between two counter AFM tips. Inset: Schematic of the tensile loading experiment. From [29].

5.3 Techniques for Nanoscale Mechanical Characterization of CNT

5.3.1 Tensile Testing Method

The axial tensile loading response of individual MWCNTs was realized by Ruoff and co-workers using a new testing stage based on a nanomanipulation tool operating inside an SEM described above. [29] The nanomanipulation stage allowed for the three-dimensional picking, positioning, and clamping of individual MWCNTs as demonstrated previously. [40] Individual MWCNTs were attached inside the SEM, by electron beam induced deposition (EBID) of carbonaceous material, to AFM probes having sharp tips. A MWCNT clamped in this way between two AFM probes was then tensile loaded by displacement of the rigid AFM probe, and the applied force was measured by the cantilever deflection of the other, more compliant, AFM probe (Fig. 5.13). The measured values of force vs. elongation were converted, from the geometry of the MWCNT measured in the SEM, to a stress-strain curve. The breaking strength of each MWCNT was obtained by measuring the maximum tensile loading force at break. The authors discovered that MWCNT's loaded in this manner normally break with a "sword-in-sheath" mechanism, where outermost layer in the MWCNT breaks followed by pull out of the inner shells.

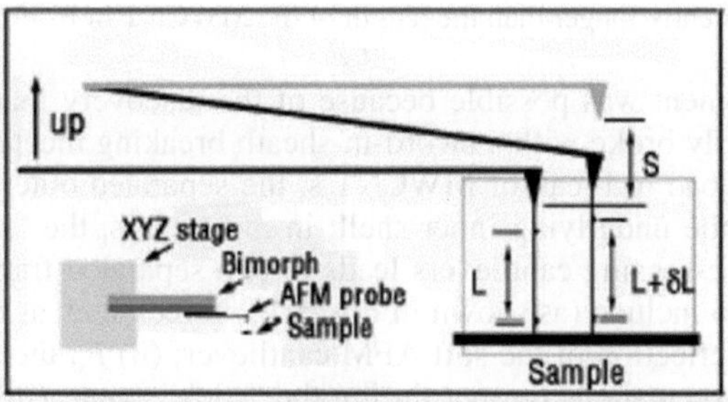

Fig. 5.14. Schematic showing the principle of the experiment for the measurement of the tensile strength of SWCNT nanoropes. The gray cantilever indicates where the cantilever would be if no rope were attached on the AFM tip after its displacement upward to achieve tensile loading. From [30].

A similar approach for measuring the tensile strength of small bundles of SWCNTs was implemented by Yu et al. [30] The entanglement in raw samples made it difficult to find an individual SWCNT and resolve it by SEM or to pick out individual SWCNT nanobundles, so a modified approach was used for the experiment. SWCNT bundles having a strong attachment at one end to the rest of the sample were selected for the measurement. The free end of such a SWCNT bundle was then attached to an AFM tip by the same approach and EBID clamp fabrication method outlined above. The AFM tip was used to stretch the bundle to the breaking point and in this implementation, the same AFM tip served the dual purpose of acting as the force sensor of the applied force (Fig. 5.14). Stress versus strain curves for SWCNT bundles were obtained as well as the breaking strength. [30]

A further interesting subject for experimental study is that of the shear strength between the shells of a MWCNT. Using the same apparatus for measuring the tensile strength of individual MWCNTs described above, Yu et al. were able to directly measure the friction force while pulling the inner shells out of the outer shells of a MWCNT, as shown in Fig. 5.15. [31]

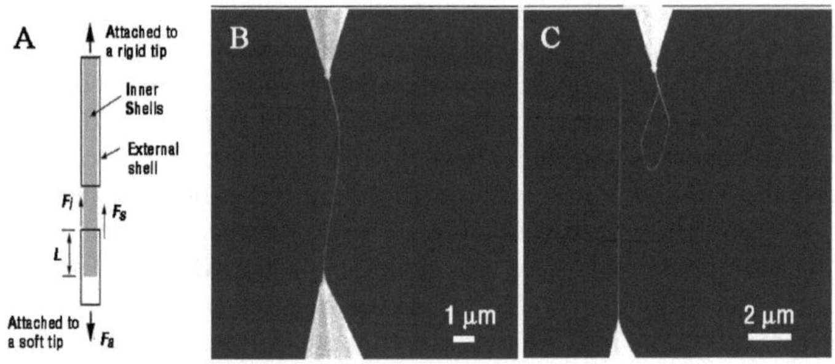

Fig. 5.15. (A) Schematic showing the sliding between the inner shells and outer shells of a MWCNT and the force diagram. (B-C) SEM images showing a MWCNT before and after the total pullout of the inner shells. Notice the total length of the MWCNT fragments after the pullout is apparently longer than the length of the MWCNT in B. From [31].

This measurement was possible because of the discovery that a tensile-loaded MWCNT normally broke with a sword-in-sheath breaking mechanism. In certain cases of tensile load to break of MWCNT's, the separated outer shell can still be in contact with the underlying inner shell; in most cases, the "snap back" of the loading and force-sensing cantilevers leads to two separated fragments. A model was developed to include (as shown in Fig. 5.15) forces such as (i) F_a, the applied force from the deflection of the soft AFM cantilever; (ii) F_s, the static shear interaction force between shells present during the "stick" event; (iii) F_d, the dynamic shear interaction force between shells in the "slip" event; (iv) F_c, the solid-solid interface force that is due to the creation of new surface area during pullout (thus due to the surface tension effect); (v) other forces, for example, a force F_e perhaps present due to the interaction of the dangling bonds on the edge of the fractured MWCNT cylinder with the internal shell surface.

The intershell shear strength was related to the shear interaction force as shown by the authors. The continuous measurement of force and "contact length" (the overlap length between the outer shell and its neighbor) in the pullout process provided the necessary data for obtaining the dynamic and static shear strength (0.08 MPa in one case and in another MWCNT case 0.30 MPa) between the shells. [31] Such measurement also allowed an estimation of the surface energy of graphite.

A similar shell-sliding experiment done in a TEM rather than an SEM, was that of Cummings et al. who used a holder having a piezoelectric-driven translation stage for approaching and opening the end of a MWCNT. [47] The MWCNT cap was "eroded" away using an electric discharge method inside the TEM. The end of the exposed core part was attached to the moving probe using a short electrical pulse and the MWCNT was then "telescoped" by drawing out the core part from the outer shell housing. It was then possible to disengage the core part from the attachment spot, and observe the retraction of the core part back into the housing by the surface-driven forces (Fig. 5.16). The authors used published parameters and modeling to estimate the upper limit values for the dynamic and static friction force between the shells. However, they did not experimentally measure these values, thus doing so in a TEM device remains a challenge.

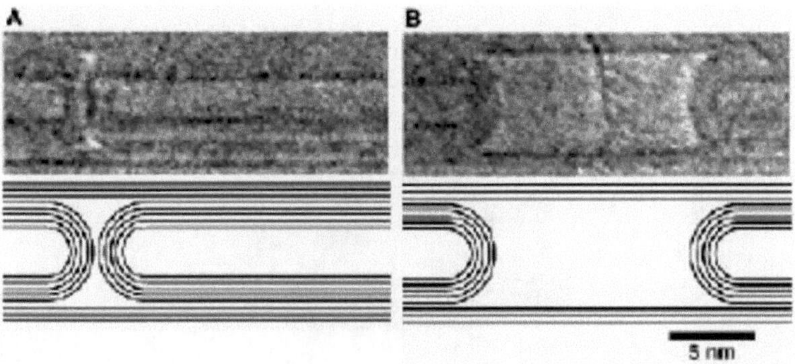

Fig 5.16. (A) An as-grown bamboo section. (B) The same area after the core tubes on the right have been telescoped outward. The line drawings beneath the images are schematic representations to guide the eye. From [47].

5.3.2 AFM Lateral Deflection and Indentation Method

The atomic force microscope (AFM) operated in either lateral force mode, contact mode, or tapping mode has been the main tool in studying the mechanical response of individual CNTs under static load, and when in contact with surfaces. Falvo et al. used a nanomanipulator and contact mode AFM to manually manipulate and bend MWCNTs deposited on a substrate surface. [52] The strong surface force between the MWCNTs and the substrate allowed such an operation to be performed. By intentionally creating large curvature bends in MWCNTs, buckles and periodic ripples were observed. These authors estimated that, based on the local curvature of the bend found, some MWCNTs could sustain up to 16% strain without obvious structural or mechanical failure.

Hertel et al. used a similar approach. [55, 56] In their experiment the deformation of MWCNTs while under the influence of the surface-CNT interaction, or additional CNT-CNT interactions, were studied. They were able to estimate the CNT-Si substrate binding energy and the shear stress responsible for pinning a bent CNT in place after manipulation. In one case, a thin MWCNT (~4 nm in diameter), strongly bonded to the substrate due to the presence of amorphous carbon contamination, was cut by the lateral AFM manipulation on surface.

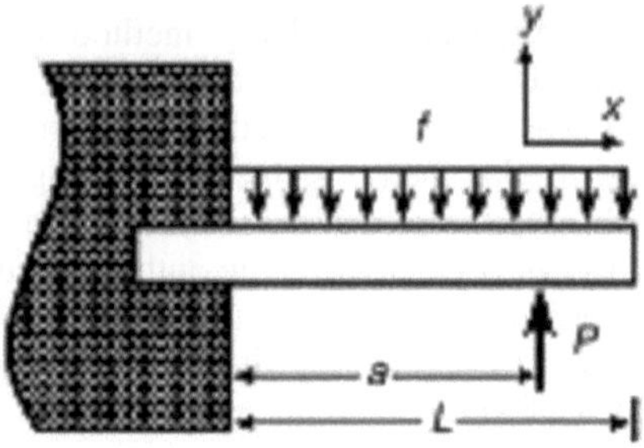

Fig. 5.17. Schematic of a pinned beam with a free end. The beam of length L is subjected to a point load P at x = a and to a distributed friction force f. From [24].

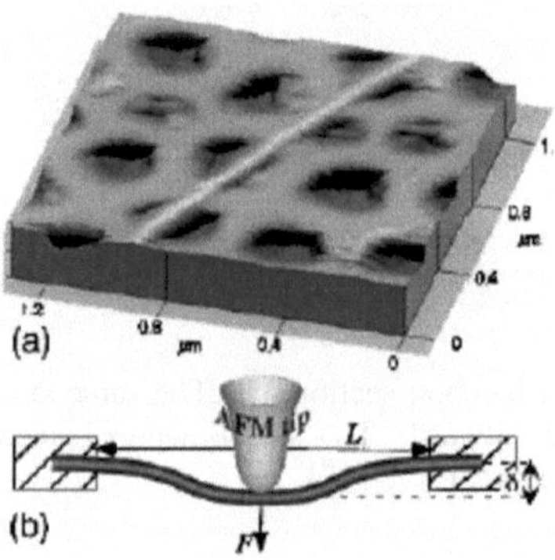

Fig. 5.18. (a) AFM image of a SWNT rope bridging a pore of the membrane. (b) Schematic of the measurement: the AFM is used to apply a load to the "nanobeam" and to determine directly the resulting deflection. From [26].

Wong et al. measured the bending modulus of individual MWCNTs using an atomic force microscope operated in lateral force mode as shown in Fig. 5.17. [24] The MWCNTs, deposited on a low friction MoS_2 surface, were pinned down at one end by an overlaying SiO pad using lithography. AFM was then used to locate and measure the dimension of the MWCNT, and lateral force was applied at the different contact points along the length of the MWCNT. By laterally pushing the MWCNT, lateral force versus deflection data were recorded. The data were then analyzed using a beam mechanics model that accounted for the friction force and the concentrated lateral force as well as the rigidity of the beam, $EI\, d^4y/dx^4 = -f + P\delta(x-a)$, and $k(x) = 3\pi r^4 E/4x^3$, where E is the bending modulus, I is the moment of inertia of the beam, f is the friction, and P is the force applied at point x from the fixed end, r is the radius of the beam, k is the force constant of the beam. By determining the force constant k at different point x along the beam, the bending modulus value (1.28±0.59 TPa) for the MWCNT was obtained by data fitting. Such a method also allowed the bending strength (Maximum: 28.5 GPa, average: 14.2±8 GPa) to be determined by deflecting the beam past the critical buckling point.

Salvetat et al. used another approach to deflect under load MWCNTs [26]and SWCNT ropes [27]by depositing them onto a membrane having 200 nm pores as shown in Fig. 5.18. By positioning the AFM tip directly on the midpoint of the CNT spanning the pore and applying an indentation force, force versus deflection curves were obtained and compared with theoretical modeling based on beam mechanics, which can be described as $\delta = \delta_B + \delta_S = FL^3/192EI + f_S FL/4GA$, where δ is the deflection of the beam which includes the contribution from bending and shear, *F* is the applied fore, *L* is the length of the suspended beam, *E* is the bending modulus, *I* is the moment of inertia, *G* is the shear modulus and *A* is the cross-sectional area of the beam. Elastic modulus for MWCNTs (Young's modulus: 810 GPa) and SWCNT ropes (Young's modulus: 1TPa, shear modulus: 1 GPa) were deduced. In principle, such a measurement requires a well-controlled and stable environment to eliminate the errors induced by unexpected tip-surface interactions and instrument instability, as well as a very sharp AFM tip for the experiment.

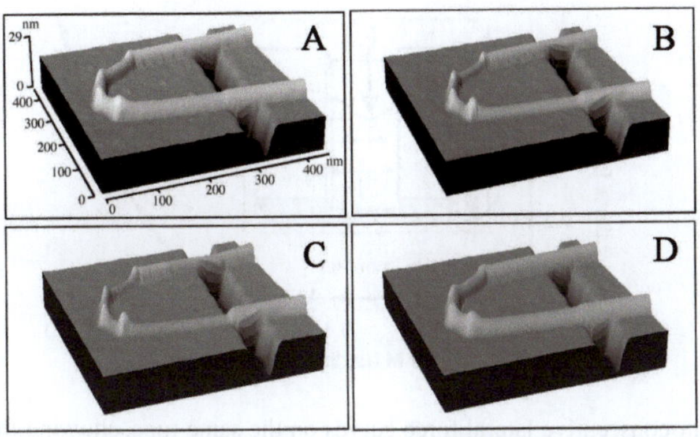

Fig. 5.19. (A-C) AFM image sequence of a MWCNT imaged in tapping mode with increasing tapping force. (D) The same MWCNT imaged with a small tapping force after the above tapping indentation experiment. From [58].

The radial deformability of individual MWCNTs was studied by Shen et al. using a static indentation method, [57] and Yu et al. using a tapping mode indentation method (Fig. 5.19) [58] in AFM, respectively. Load was applied along the radial direction (perpendicular to the axial direction that is defined as along the long-axis of the CNT) of MWCNTs deposited on surface, and the applied force versus indentation depth curve was measured. Using the classic Hertz theory, the deformability of a MWCNT perpendicular to the long axis direction was obtained. (The reader should please note that this is not the radial compressibility, because the force is not symmetrically applied in the radial direction and so is not isotropic. Thus one might think of this as "squashing" the MWCNT locally by indentation.)

The two approaches of Shen et al. and Yu et al. are technically different. In the static indentation method, the image scan is stopped and the AFM tip is held steady and used to apply a vertical force at a single location on the MWCNT through the extension and retraction of the piezoelectric tube along the z direction. A force versus indentation depth curve is obtained by monitoring the AFM cantilever deflection under the extension or retraction. In the tapping mode method, an off resonance tapping technique is used so that the tapping force can be quantitatively controlled by adjusting the free cantilever amplitude and the set point. The set point is a control parameter in tapping mode AFM for keeping the cantilever amplitude constant in imaging scan mode, thus maintaining the distance between the AFM tip and the sample surface constant. AFM images of each MWCNT are acquired using different set points, and a force versus indentation depth curve is obtained by plotting the curve of the set point versus MWCNT height. The advantage of using the tapping mode method is that the "squashing" deformability of the MWCNT along its whole length can be obtained through several image acquisitions, though care need be taken to choose the appropriate tapping mode imaging parameters for such experiment.

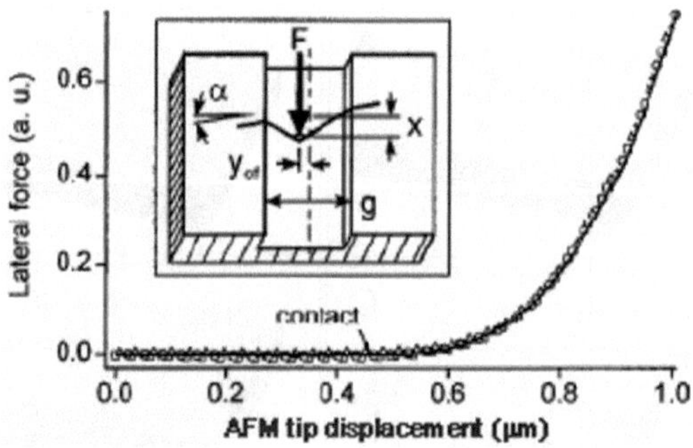

Fig. 5.20. Four consecutive lateral force curves on the same rope, showing that this rope is straining elastically with no plastic deformation. Inset. The AFM tip moves along the trench, in the plane of the surface, and displaces the rope as shown. From [28].

Walters et al. studied the elastic strain of SWCNT nanobundles by creating a suspended SWCNT rope that was clamped at both ends by metal pads over a trench created with standard lithographic methods. [28] Using an AFM operated in lateral force mode, they were able to repeatedly stretch and relax the nanobundles elastically as shown in Fig. 5.20 including finally stretching to the breaking point of four ropes to determine the maximum strain (5.8±0.9%). The SWCNT bundles were found to behave like elastic strings. The absolute force used to stretch the SWCNT rope was not measured and the breaking strength was estimated by assuming the theoretical value of ~1 TPa for Young's modulus for the SWCNTs in the rope.

5.3.3 Mechanical Resonance Method

The values for Young's modulus for a set of MWCNTs was measured by Treacy and co-workers by measuring the amplitude from recorded TEM images of the thermal vibration of each when naturally cantilevered. [23] Using a similar method, Krishnan et al. succeeded in measuring the Young's modulus of SWCNT's. [25] The amplitude is measured from the blurred spread of tip positions of the free end of the cantilevered CNT as compared to the clamped end. This tip blurring originates from thermal activation of vibrations (the CNT behaves classically because of the low frequency modes that are populated by the expected kT of thermal vibration energy). The amplitude can be modeled by considering the excitation of mechanical resonance of a cantilever:

$$\sigma^2 = \frac{16L^3kT}{\pi Y(a^4 - b^4)}\sum_n \beta_n^{-4} \approx 0.4243\frac{L^3kT}{Y(a^4 - b^4)}$$

where σ is the amplitude at the free end, L is the length of the cantilevered beam, k is the Boltzman constant, T is the temperature, a is the outer radius and b is the inner radius of the CNT, Y is the Young's modulus, and β_n is a constant for free vibration mode n. Because the frequency is high relative to the several second integration time needed for generating the TEM image the image is blurred. Since the geometry is directly determined by the TEM imaging and the resonance is a function of the cantilever stiffness, the Young's modulus values could be fit. This method is simple to implement without the need for additional instrument modification or development—only a variable temperature TEM holder is needed. As long as the tip blurring effect is obvious the principle can also be applied for the study of other nanowire type materials. The drawback is that a model fit is needed to determine the real cantilever length, and human error is inevitable in determining the "exact" amplitude of the blurred tip. The error for the Young's modulus estimation using such a method, as pointed out by the authors, is around ±60%.

Poncharal et al. introduced an electric field excitation method for the study of mechanical resonance of cantilevered MWCNTs, and measured the bending modulus. [42] In their experiment, a specially designed TEM holder that incorporated a piezo-driven translation stage and a mechanical driven translation stage, was developed. The translation stages allowed the accurate positioning of the MWCNT material inside the TEM relative to a counter electrode. Electrical connections were made to the electrode attaching the MWCNT materials and the counter electrode, so that DC bias as well as AC sinusoidal voltage could be applied between the counter electrode and the MWCNT. The generated AC electric field interacts with induced charges on the MWCNT, thus producing a periodic driving force. When the mechanical resonance frequency of the MWCNT matched the frequency of the input AC signal, obvious oscillation corresponding to the resonance mode of the cantilever MWCNT was observed, and the resonance frequency of the MWCNT thereby determined.

The bending modulus of the MWCNT was calculated, using continuum beam mechanics, from the measured resonance frequency and CNT geometry according to $f_i = \frac{\beta_i^2}{8\pi L^2}\sqrt{(D^2 + D_I^2)}\sqrt{\frac{E_b}{\rho}}$, where f_i and β_i is the resonance frequency and the constant for ith harmonic, D is the outer diameter and D_I is the inner diameter of the CNT, L is the cantilever length, ρ is the volume density, E_b is the bending modulus . The elastic bending modulus was found to decrease sharply (from about 1 to 0.1 terapascals) with increasing MWCNT diameter (from 8 to 40 nanometers). The authors speculated that this was a result of the "rippling effect" in large diameter MWCNTs caused by the bending in oscillation.

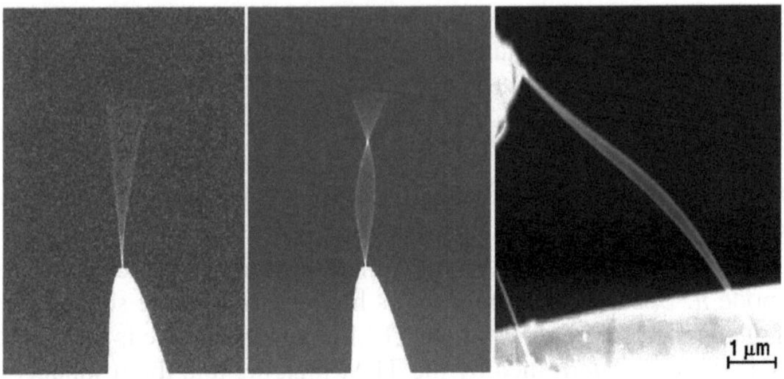

Fig. 5.21. SEM images showing the first harmonic and the second harmonic resonant oscillations of an individual MWCNT, and the resonant oscillation of a MWCNT bounded at both ends.

The benefits of such an approach are that various mechanical resonance modes can be selectively excited, and since the whole experiment is done inside a TEM, high aspect ratio nanostructures, such as CNTs, can be analyzed in detail.

Such a technique can also be easily applied inside an SEM. [59, 60] By combining the in situ manipulation and characterization capabilities provided by the SEM tools described previously, individual MWCNTs can be manipulated and excited to resonant oscillation as shown in Fig. 5.21. The different imaging mechanism of the SEM from TEM also allowed the automated acquisition of the mechanical resonance response curve from such nanoscale objects. In the acquisition, the SEM beam control is first set in line scan mode across the nanowire. The sine wave signal generator is programmed to tune the drive frequency at fixed step (10Hz to 10 kHz depending on the frequency resolution needed for the response curve), and at each step, the SEM line scan signal is acquired and processed to obtain the amplitude of the driven nanowire at that driving frequency (Fig. 5.22). Alternatively, by setting the beam control for the SEM in "spot mode" so that the beam scan is stopped, a periodic signal from the SEM detector output can be acquired (within the frequency response limit of the secondary electron detector electronics) when the laterally resonating nanowire traverses the stationary electron beam. This technique provides a direct measurement of the real oscillating frequency and phase of the nanowire.

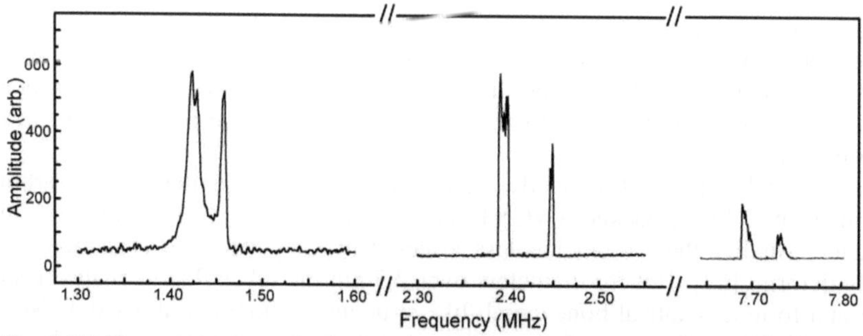

Fig. 5.22. The acquired amplitude versus drive frequency response curve from an individual cantilevered MWCNT.

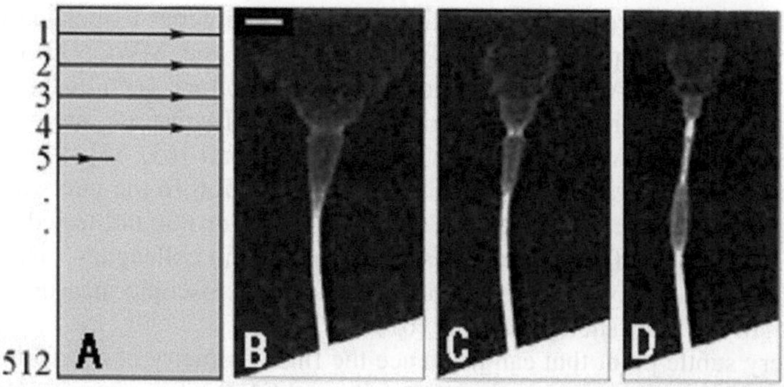

Fig. 5.23. "Strange" shapes of the vibrated NW obtained at three different scan modes of the SEM, together with a schematic representation of the scanning electron beam (A). Time interval between each closed scan-line inside of one frame is: (B) 4 ms, (C) 17 ms, (D) 50 ms.

A recent discovery is the study of the mechanical resonance of insulating SiO_2 nanowires inside SEM which revealed the effect of charge trapping. [61] Unevenly distributed charge along the SiO_2 nanowire can be introduced by controlling the exposed section length of the nanowire and the scan rate of the rastering SEM electron beam. There is a preferred charge trapping at the defect sites of the nanowire, and consequently the interactions (mostly charge-charge interaction) between the nanowire and the resonance driving mechanism are influenced. The resonance of the nanowire can then amplify such differences and demonstrate the presence of the nanoscale electronic or structural defects as shown in Fig. 5.23. Such a technique could in principle be further developed and applied to characterize other dielectric nanostructures.

5.3.4 Other Methods

Ruoff et al. first studied radial deformation between adjacent MWCNTs. [62] Partial flattening due to the van der Waals forces was observed in TEM images of two aligned and adjacent tubes along the contact region. This was the first observation that showed that CNTs were not necessarily perfectly cylindrical, and were readily deformable along its radial direction. Indeed, all CNTs in an anisotropic physical environment are likely to be not perfectly cylindrical due to mechanical deformation.

Tersoff and Ruoff subsequently studied the deformation pattern of carbon nanotubes in a closest-packed SWCNT crystal and concluded that rigid tubes with diameters smaller than 1 nm are less affected by the inter-tube attraction and hardly deform. [63] But for diameters over 2.5 nm the tubes flatten against each other and form a beautiful honeycomb-like structure. Chopra et al. used TEM to observe MWCNTs that were fully collapsed and showed that the collapsed state can be energetically favorable for nanotubes having a certain critical radius and wall thickness. [64] Yu et al. used AFM to find and examine a set of collapsed MWCNTs on surface to systematically study the energetics associated with stable or metastable collapse of MWCNT; structures of the MWCNTs were reconstructed from their AFM images and contributing factors, such as the mechanical deformation, van der Waals interaction, the MWCNT/substrate interaction and interface condensation meniscus, are analyzed in detail [65, 66]. Benedicts et al. proposed using the ratio of the mean curvature modulus to the interwall attraction of graphite to predict whether CNT would collapse or not and tested their model with TEM images of collapsed tubes from Chopra and colleagues. This combination of theory and experiment provided the first microscopic measurement of the strength of the inter-shell attraction. [67]

A very subtle point that can influence the final geometry of a deformed CNT is the effect of interlayer interactions for collapsed CNTs. For instance, Yu et al. observed collapsed and periodically twisted MWCNT ribbons with transmission electron microscopy. [68] One of the observed cantilevered MWCNT ribbons had a twist present in the freestanding segment. Such a configuration can not be accounted for by elastic theory since no external load is present to hold the MWCNT ribbon in place. A recent treatment of the interlayer binding energy of the AA and the AB stacking configurations of graphite yields a 0.012 eV/atom energy difference for two rigid graphitic layers spaced 0.344 nm apart (AB more stable). [69] Inclusion of the influence of this rather subtle energetics suggests that the elastic energy cost for the twist formation of this particular CNT ribbon can be partially compensated by achieving more favorable atomic registry between neighboring layers. The observation of the existence of this freestanding twist in the ribbon can only be explained by assuming that an energy barrier exists to keep the twisted ribbon from untwisting. The twisted structure of this particular MWCNT ribbon is probably metastable rather than stable, from the energetics treatment presented by Yu et al. [68].

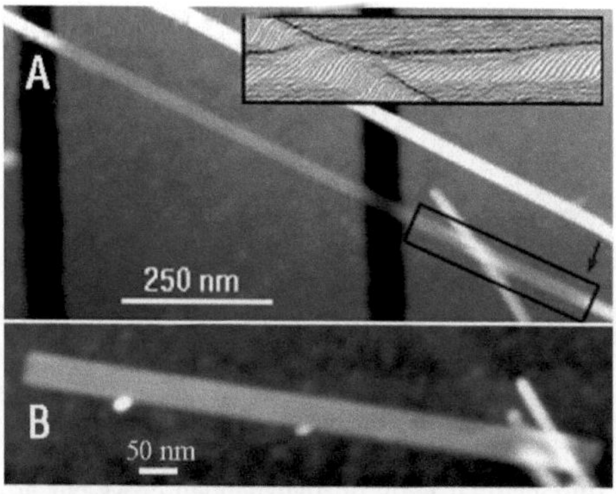

Fig. 5.24. (A) An AFM image of a MWCNT having a 1 μm long section collapsed on a trenched Si substrate. The inset shows the surface profile of a collapsed section indicated by arrow in (A) as a result of the further advancement of the collapse from the original collapsed section. (B) An AFM image showing the flexibility of a collapsed MWCNT. Noticing the collapsed MWCNT conforms closely to the underlying surface structures. From [65].

5.4 Mechanical Engineering Applications of Individual CNTs for Actuation and Electromechanics

Rueckes et al. suggested using the electrostatic force induced deflection of individual SWCNTs in a crossbar structure for nonvolatile random access memory application as shown in Fig. 5.24. [70] Bistable states exist in such suspended and crossed individual SWCNTs: the off state, where the SWCNTs are in an unstrained condition and separated by a certain distance so the van der Waals attraction forces are small; and the on state, where the SWCNTs are deflected so strained but stick together by the strong van der Waals forces at the contact point. The switch between the on and off states can be controlled by the applied static voltage between the SWCNTs, and the states can be addressed externally through SWCNT itself due to its excellent transport properties. A prototype device using two crossed SWCNT ropes was used to demonstrate such concept.

Tombler et al. demonstrated the conductivity modulation of an individual, suspended SWCNT reversibly deflected by an AFM probe tip. [71] Two orders of magnitude change in conductance were observed and were attributed to the formation of local sp3 bonds at the highly strained location. The study presented another example of utilizing individual CNTs for nanoscale electromechanical device and high-sensitivity sensor applications.

The potential merits of using nanostructures for device applications include, generally, high sensitivity, fast response time, and low power consumption. Indeed, a recent theory proposed another type of electromechanical CNT device, an intra-MWCNT oscillator, which has the potential of reaching mechanical resonance frequency up to 1 GHz. [72] Cantilevered oscillators using individual MWCNTs have been realized at resonance frequency up to 300 MHz, [59] and more interestingly, parametrically-driven nanowire and CNT oscillators have also been demonstrated, which has the potential of utilizing nanowire or CNT for ultrahigh-sensitivity sensor applications.

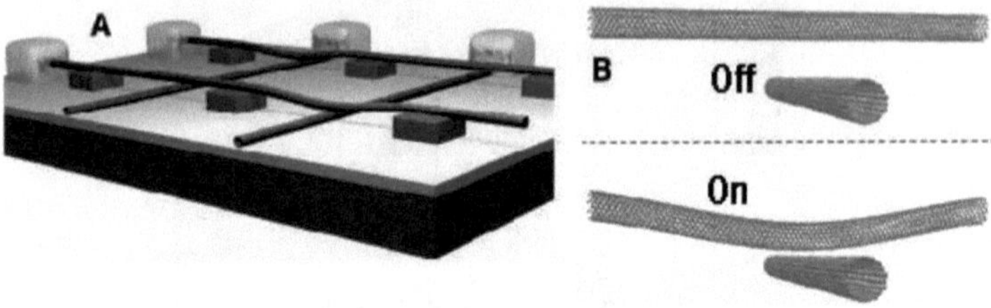

Fig. 5.25. (A) Three-dimensional view of a suspended cross-bar array showing four junctions with two elements in the ON (contact) state and two elements in the OFF (separated) state. (B) Calculated structures of the 20-nm (10, 10) SWNT device element in the OFF (top) and ON (bottom) states. The initial separation for this calculation was 2.0 nm. From [70].

5.5 Conclusion and Future Directions

New developments in instrumentation for nanoscale manipulation and measurement, as reflected in the studies presented in this chapter, have certainly helped our understanding of the mechanics of CNTs. Since CNTs possess unique structures that essentially maintain their conformation while being manipulated (in contrast, e.g., to biomolecules or certain polymer systems), they represent a kind of "tinker-toy" or "lego block" for manipulation on the nanoscale. Therefore, innovation leading to new tools capable of probing mechanics of nanostructures such as CNTs also provides a picture of current capabilities for exploring and exploiting the "nano-world," and for doing useful experiments related to nanotechnology. Perhaps more exciting is that the community, while achieving significant progress, has so much more to do. The tensile loading response of an individual SWCNT has still not been measured, nor have we applied a known torque or controllably twisted CNTs. SWCNT bundles have not been twisted into "nanoropes" and intricate analogs of textiles have not yet been made from CNTs, although the rich fields of twisted wire mechanics and textile mechanics suggest that doing so will be a rewarding endeavor. The influence of environment on NT mechanics has not yet been explored in any detail— the influence of parameters such as temperature, chemical environment, loading rate, and defect density, remain for future work. We do not have a clear and detailed picture of the road to failure resulting from nucleation and propagation of defects. From the experimental side, such advances will come with new approaches and new tools generated by innovative thinking. It is clear that focused effort in developing new measurement tools that can be integrated into high spatial resolution imaging instruments is necessary for further advances in nanostructure mechanics. We envision that future efforts will be dedicated to adapting such tools to other high resolution instruments in addition to the SEM and TEM, such as greater flexibility for nanomanipulation and probing that will be coupled to scanning probe microscopes, and also to test beds that allow for a variety of spectroscopic probing. As an example, Raman spectroscopy of individual CNTs under mechanical load is a promising approach to building a database that will find use in understanding the stress-strain state of CNTs in, e.g., CNT polymer composites under load.

References

1. Iijima S (1991) Helical microtubules of graphitic carbon. Nature (London) 354: 56-58
2. Iijima S and Ichihashi T (1993) Single-shell carbon nanotubes of 1-nm diameter. Nature (London) 363: 603-605
3. Bethune DS, Kiang CH, de Vries MS, Gorman G, Savoy R, Vazquez J and Beyers R (1993) Cobalt-catalyzed growth of carbon nanotubes with single-atomic-layer walls. Nature (London) 363: 605-607
4. Schadler LS, Giannaris SC and Ajayan PM (1998) Load transfer in carbon nanotube epoxy composites. Appl. Phys. Lett. 73: 3842-3844
5. Wagner HD, Lourie O, Feldman Y and Tenne R (1998) Stress-induced fragmentation of multiwall carbon nanotubes in a polymer matrix. Appl. Phys. Lett. 72: 188-190
6. Tans SJ, Verschueren ARM and Dekker C (1998) Room-temperature transistor based on a single carbon nanotube. Nature (London) 393: 49-52
7. Derycke V, Martel R, Appenzeller J and Avouris P (2001) Carbon Nanotube Inter- and Intramolecular Logic Gates. Nano Lett. 1: 453-456
8. Bachtold A, Hadley P, Nakanishi T and Dekker C (2001) Logic Circuits with Carbon Nanotube Transistors. Science (Washington, D. C.) 294: 1317-1321
9. Thess A, Lee R, Nikolaev P, Dai H, Petit P, Robert J, Xu C, Lee YH, Kim SG, Rinzler AG, Colbert DT, Scuseria GE, Tomanek D, Fisher JE and Smalley RE (1996) Crystalline ropes of metallic carbon nanotubes. Science (Washington, D. C.) 273: 483-487
10. Tans SJ, Devoret MH, Dal H, Thess A, Smalley RE, Geerligs LJ and Dekker C (1997) Individual single-wall carbon nanotubes as quantum wires. Nature (London) 386: 474-477
11. de Heer WA, Chatelain A and Ugarte D (1995) A carbon nanotube field-emission electron source. Science (Washington, D. C.) 270: 1179-1180
12. Wang QH, Setlur AA, Lauerhaas JM, Dai JY, Seelig EW and Chang RPH (1998) A nanotube-based field-emission flat panel display. Appl. Phys. Lett. 72: 2912-2913
13. Choi WB, Lee YH, Lee NS, Kang JH, Park SH, Kim HY, Chung DS, Lee SM, Chung SY and Kim JM (2000) Carbon-nanotubes for full-color field-emission displays. Jpn. J. Appl. Phys., Part 1 39: 2560-2564
14. Kong J, Franklin NR, Zhou C, Chapline MG, Peng S, Cho K and Dailt H (2000) Nanotube molecular wires as chemical sensors. Science (Washington, D. C.) 287: 622-625
15. Chen P, Wu X, Lin J and Tan KL (1999) High H2 uptake by alkali-doped carbon nanotubes under ambient pressure and moderate temperatures. Science (Washington, D. C.) 285: 91-93
16. Dai H, Hafner JH, Rinzler AG, Colbert DT and Smalley RE (1996) Nanotubes as nanoprobes in scanning probe microscopy. Nature (London) 384: 147-150
17. Wong SS, Harper JD, Lansbury PT, Jr. and Lieber CM (1998) Carbon Nanotube Tips: High-Resolution Probes for Imaging Biological Systems. J. Am. Chem. Soc. 120: 603-604

18. Gao B, Kleinhammes A, Tang XP, Bower C, Fleming L, Wu Y and Zhou O (1999) Electrochemical intercalation of single-walled carbon nanotubes with lithium. Chem. Phys. Lett. 307: 153-157
19. Overney G, Zhong W and Tomanek D (1993) Structure Rigidity and Low-Frequency Vibrational-Modes of Long Carbon Tubules. Zeitschrift Fur Physik D-Atoms Molecules and Clusters 27(1): 93-96
20. Ruoff RS and Lorents DC (1995) Mechanical and thermal properties of carbon nanotubes. Carbon 33: 925-930
21. Yakobson BI (1997) Dynamic topology and yield strength of carbon nanotubes. In: Ruoff, RS and Kadish, KM (eds.) Proceedings of the Symposium on Fullerenes, Electrochem. Soc. ECS, Pennington, pp 549-560.
22. Lu JP (1997) Elastic Properties of Carbon Nanotubes and Nanoropes. Phys. Rev. Lett. 79: 1297-1300
23. Treacy MMJ, Ebbesen TW and Gibson JM (1996) Exceptionally high Young's modulus observed for individual carbon nanotubes. Nature (London) 381: 678-680
24. Wong EW, Sheehan PE and Lieber CM (1997) Nanobeam mechanics: elasticity, strength, and toughness of nanorods and nanotubes. Phys. Rev. B: Condens. Matter 56: 6420-6423
25. Krishnan A, Dujardin E, Ebbesen TW, Yianilos PN and Treacy MMJ (1998) Young's modulus of single-walled nanotubes. Phys. Rev. B: Condens. Matter 58: 14031-14035
26. Salvetat J-P, Kulik AJ, Bonard J-M, Briggs GAD, Stoeckli T, Metenier K, Bonnamy S, Beguin F, Burnham NA and Forro L (1999) Elastic modulus of ordered and disordered multiwalled carbon nanotubes. Adv. Mater. (Weinheim, Ger.) 11: 161-165
27. Salvetat J-P, Briggs GAD, Bonard J-M, Bacsa RR, Kulik AJ, Stockli T, Burnham NA and Forro L (1999) Elastic and Shear Moduli of Single-Walled Carbon Nanotube Ropes. Phys. Rev. Lett. 82: 944-947
28. Walters DA, Ericson LM, Casavant MJ, Liu J, Colbert DT, Smith KA and Smalley RE (1999) Elastic strain of freely suspended single-wall carbon nanotube ropes. Appl. Phys. Lett. 74: 3803-3805
29. Yu M-F, Lourie O, Dyer MJ, Moloni K, Kelly TF and Ruoff RS (2000) Strength and breaking mechanism of multiwalled carbon nanotubes under tensile load. Science (Washington, D. C.) 287: 637-640
30. Yu M-F, Files BS, Arepalli S and Ruoff RS (2000) Tensile loading of ropes of single wall carbon nanotubes and their mechanical properties. Phys. Rev. Lett. 84: 5552-5555
31. Yu M-F, Yakobson BI and Ruoff RS (2000) Controlled Sliding and Pullout of Nested Shells in Individual Multiwalled Carbon Nanotubes. J. Phys. Chem. B8764-8767
32. Dresselhaus MS, Dresselhaus G, Sugihara K, Spain IL and Goldberg HA (1988) Graphite Fibers and Filaments. Springer-Verlag, New York.
33. Odom TW, Huang J-L, Kim P and Lieber CM (1998) Atomic structure and electronic properties of single-walled carbon nanotubes. Nature (London) 391: 62-64
34. Ajayan PM and Ebbesen TW (1997) Nanometer-size tubes of carbon. Appl. Phys. Lett. 71: 2620-2622
35. Binnig G and Quate CF (1986) Atomic force microscope. Phys. Rev. Lett. 56: 930-933
36. Wiesendanger R (1994) Scanning probe microscope: methods and applications. Cambridge University Press, Oxford.
37. See: http://www.thermomicro.com/Spmguide/contents.htm
38. Wildoer JWG, Venema LC, Rinzier AG, Smalley RE and Dekker C (1998) Electronic structure of atomically resolved carbon nanotubes. Nature (London) 391: 59-62
39. Williams DB and Carter CB (1996) Transmission electron microscopy. Plenum Press, New York.

40. Yu M-F, Dyer MJ, Skidmore GD, Rhors HW, Lu XK, Ausman KD, Ehr JRV and Ruoff RS (1999) 3-dimensional manipulation of carbon nanotubes under a scanning electron microscope. Nanotechnology 10: 244
41. Nishijima H, Kamo S, Akita S, Nakayama Y, Hohmura KI, Yoshimura SH and Takeyasu K (1999) Carbon-nanotube tips for scanning probe microscopy: Preparation by a controlled process and observation of deoxyribonucleic acid. Appl. Phys. Lett. 74: 4061-4063
42. Poncharal P, Wang L, Ugarte D and de Heer WA (1999) Electrostatic deflections and electromechanical resonances of carbon nanotubes. Science (Washington, D. C.) 283: 1513-1516
43. Kizuka T (1998) Atomic Process of Point Contact in Gold Studied by Time-Resolved High-Resolution Transmission Electron Microscopy. Phys. Rev. Lett. 81: 4448-4451
44. Kizuka T, Yamada K, Deguchi S, Naruse M and Tanaka N (1997) Cross-sectional time-resolved high-resolution transmission electron microscopy of atomic-scale contact and noncontact-type scannings on gold surfaces. Phys. Rev. B: Condens. Matter 55: R7398-7401
45. Kizuka T (1999) Direct atomistic observation of deformation in multiwalled carbon nanotubes. Phys. Rev. B: Condens. Matter 59: 4646-4649
46. Cumings J, Collins PG and Zettl A (2000) Peeling and sharpening multiwall nanotubes. Nature (London) 406: 586
47. Cumings J and Zettl A (2000) Low-friction nanoscale linear bearing realized from multiwall carbon nanotubes. Science (Washington, D. C.) 289: 602-604
48. Ruoff RS, Lorents DC, Laduca R, Awadalla S, Weathersby S, Parvin K and Subramoney S (1995) Nanotubes: bending and filling: Part I. In: Ruoff, RS and Kadish, KM (eds.) Proc. - Electrochem. Soc. ECS 557-562.
49. Lourie O, Rohrs H, Huang H, Ausman K, Piner R, Yu M-F, Dyer M, Gibbons P and Ruoff R (2001) Mechanics of single walled carbon nanotubes. unpublished result
50. Lourie O, Rohrs H, Huang H, Ausman K, Piner R, Yu M-F, Dyer M, Gibbons P and Ruoff R (2001) TEM/SEM nanostressing stage. unpublished result
51. See: http://www.cs.unc.edu/Research/nano/
52. Falvo MR, Clary GJ, Taylor RM, II, Chi V, Brooks FP, Jr., Washburn S and Superfine R (1997) Bending and buckling of carbon nanotubes under large strain. Nature (London) 389: 581-584
53. Falvo MR, Taylor RM, II, Helser A, Chi V, Brooks FP, Jr., Washburn S and Superfine R (1999) Nanometer-scale rolling and sliding of carbon nanotubes. Nature (London) 397: 236-238
54. Paulson S, Helser A, Nardelli MB, Taylor RM, Falvo M, Superfine R and Washburn S (2000) Tunable resistance of a carbon nanotube-graphite interface. Science (Washington, D. C.) 290: 1742-1744
55. Hertel T, Martel R and Avouris P (1998) Manipulation of Individual Carbon Nanotubes and Their Interaction with Surfaces. J. Phys. Chem. B 102: 910-915
56. Hertel T, Walkup RE and Avouris P (1998) Deformation of carbon nanotubes by surface van der Waals forces. Phys. Rev. B: Condens. Matter 58: 13870-13873
57. Shen W, Jiang B, Han BS and Xie S-S (2000) Investigation of the Radial Compression of Carbon Nanotubes with a Scanning Probe Microscope. Phys. Rev. Lett. 84: 3634-3637
58. Yu M-F, Kowalewski T and Ruoff RS (2000) Investigation of the Radial Deformability of Individual Carbon Nanotubes under Controlled Indentation Force. Phys. Rev. Lett. 85: 1456-1459
59. Yu M-F. 2001. Multiprobe Nanomanipulation and Functional Assembly of Nanomaterials Inside a Scanning Electron Microscope., *IEEE NANO2001.*: Maui, HI

60. Yu M-F, Wagner GJ, Ruoff RS and Dyer MJ (2002) Realization of parametric resonance in a nanowire mechanical system with nanomanipulation in a scanning electron microscope. Phys. Rev. B: accepted
61. Dikin DA, Chen X, Ding W, Wagner G and Ruoff RS (Submitted, 2002) Resonance vibration of amorphous SiO2 nanowires driven by mechanical or electrical field excitation.
62. Ruoff RS, Tersoff J, Lorents DC, Subramoney S and Chan B (1993) Radial deformation of carbon nanotubes by van der Waals forces. Nature (London) 48: 195-198
63. Tersoff J and Ruoff RS (1994) Structural properties of a carbon-nanotube crystal. Phys. Rev. Lett. 73: 676-679
64. Chopra NG, Benedict LX, Crespi VH, Cohen ML, Louie SG and Zettl A (1995) Fully collapsed carbon nanotubes. Nature (London) 377: 135-138
65. Yu M-F, Dyer MJ and Ruoff RS (2001) Structure and mechanical flexibility of carbon nanotube ribbons: An atomic-force microscopy study. Journal of Applied Physics 89: 4554-4557
66. Yu MF, Kowalewski T and Ruoff RS (2001) Structural analysis of collapsed, and twisted and collapsed, multiwalled carbon nanotubes by atomic force microscopy. Phys. Rev. Lett. 86: 87-90
67. Benedict LX, Chopra NG, Cohen ML, Zettl A, Louie SG and Crespi VH (1998) Microscopic determination of the interlayer binding energy in graphite. Chem. Phys. Lett. 286: 490-496
68. Yu M-F, Dyer MJ, Chen J, Qian D, Liu WK and Ruoff RS (2001) Locked twist in multiwalled carbon-nanotube ribbons. Phys. Rev. B: Condens. Matter 64: 241403R
69. Kolmogorov AN and Crespi VH (2000) Smoothest Bearings: Interlayer Sliding in Multiwalled Carbon Nanotubes. Phys. Rev. Lett. 85: 4727-4730
70. Rueckes T, Kim K, Joselevich E, Tseng GY, Cheung CL and Lieber CM (2000) Carbon nanotube-based nonvolatile random access memory for molecular computing. Science (Washington, D. C.) 289: 94-97
71. Tombler TW, Zhou C, Alexseyev L, Kong J, Dai H, Jayanthi CS, Tang M and Wu S-Y (2000) Reversible electromechanical characteristics of carbon nanotubes under local-probe manipulation. Nature (London) 405: 769-772
72. Zheng Q and Jiang Q (2002) Multiwalled carbon nanotubes as gigahertz oscillators. Phys. Rev. Lett. 88: 045503

6. Applications of the Piezoelectric Quartz Crystal Microbalance for Microdevice Development

J. W. Bender and J. Krim

6.1 Introduction

Because of their ability to detect changes in mass down to sub-monolayers of adsorbed gases, piezoelectric quartz crystal microbalances (QCM) have historically been key to the study of thin film deposition, molecular beam and ion bombardment processes, and surface chemical reaction kinetics. Thin film deposition techniques, including physical vapor deposition, sputtering, and ion plating, are widely used as coating techniques for optical, electrical, and mechanical applications. In these applications, the QCM is used to measure film thickness and the rate of mass deposition or removal [55]. Experiments elucidating the sticking coefficients of gases onto metals, the diffusion of gases into metals, the oxidation of metal films, and the kinetics of surface migration, adsorption, and desorption have also been performed with the aid of a QCM under ultra-high vacuum conditions. Examples include hydrogen diffusion into palladium [10], oxidation kinetics of zinc, iron, and chromium films [11, 47], and the adsorption kinetics of carbon dioxide [41]. The QCM has also been used to measure vapor pressures via outgassing studies [52] and to monitor polymerization reactions on surfaces [48]. It has very recently been employed to probe the kinetics of contaminant up-take on protective carbon overcoat films in magnetic media[110], to quantify the kinetics and chemical moieties present during corrosion [36, 95, 103, 1, 51], to measure the degree and strength of molecular adhesion [24], as a substitute for radiolabelling in mass transport experiments, and to monitor self-assembly of composite superlattices [31].

Clearly, the versatility of the QCM makes it an important tool for the development of microdevices. Advances in our need to measure and manipulate matter on an ever-decreasing scale has driven the development of diagnostic tools to either characterize or to be an integral part of the microdevice. The piezoelectric properties of quartz make it ideal for converting electrical inputs to mechanical motion (and vice versa), and thus quartz resonators can be viewed as microdevices themselves, as well as tools in microdevice testing.

The purpose of this chapter is to provide a thorough introduction to QCM techniques. We have organized the presentation as follows: Section 6.2 covers the properties of piezoelectric quartz, section 6.3 discusses the theoretical framework for interpreting QCM data, section 6.4 describes the equipment and experimental methods, and sections 6.5 through 6.8 sequentially discuss emerging applications of the QCM as a microdevice to examine slip and frictional energy dissipation at interfaces, to quantify viscoelastic properties of films and fluids, to perform nanotribological studies using combined QCM/surface probe techniques, and to aid in the development of medical diagnostics. Our intent is to provide a comprehensive overview both of the capabilities and limitations of QCM techniques.

6.2 Properties of Piezoelectric Quartz

When a piezoelectric material such as quartz is subjected to an electric field, up to three fundamental modes of deformation take place: transverse (shear), torsional (twist), and longitudinal. Different surface acoustical modes can be excited depending on the relative orientations of the crystalline axis with respect to the applied electric field. For the applications considered here, the mode of greatest utility is the thickness-shear mode (TSM), and for brevity, our focus will be on this mode (Fig. 6.1). Since the TSM mode is used in applications that are not exclusively for measuring mass uptake, and since other acoustic wave modes have been developed for microgravimetry, some in the research community prefer to use the acronym TSM rather than QCM. For historical reasons, however, we will refer to the TSM device as QCM regardless of the application. Other piezoelectric acoustic wave devices that generate specific surface waves are being researched for chemical sensing and thin film moduli measurements, including surface acoustic wave (SAW) resonators and delay lines [63, 64, 32, 80, 15], flexural plate wave (FPW) devices [33, 108], and acoustic plate mode (APW) devices [108]. All piezoelectric acoustic wave devices can be viewed as MEMS devices, as piezoelectric materials can be used both to characterize materials for MEMS applications and as an integral component in a MEMS device itself.

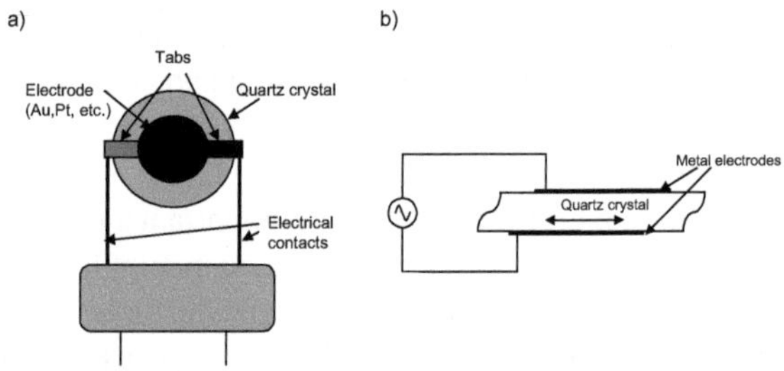

Fig. 6.1. Front (a) and side (b) views of a QCM. Under an AC electric field, the QCM is driven at resonance. In (a), there is one metal tab on each side of the crystal to permit electrical contact with driving electronics.

The AT- and BT-cuts of quartz (members of the TSM family) oscillate in the fundamental shear mode, and are 35° 15' and 49° from the primary crystalline axis, respectively. The 35° 15' AT-cut is generally preferred because its resonant frequency is relatively insensitive to temperature near room temperature, generally less than

±20 ppm change from -30°C to 90°C [55]. Frequency shifts can therefore be more easily be attributed to the deposited mass and not to changes in crystal temperature. The BT-cut has a higher mass sensitivity due to its higher node velocity (v_q = 5071 ms^{-1} versus 3322 ms^{-1} for AT-cut quartz), but has a quadratic frequency dependence on temperature. Thinner devices operate at higher frequencies and are thus more mass sensitive, but also more fragile. Typical fundamental mode oscillation frequencies are in the range of 3-10 MHz, with quality factors of the order of 10^5. At temperatures in excess of 573°C, quartz undergoes a phase transition to another solid phase, rendering the device inoperable.

6.3 Theoretical Models

In the basic QCM experiment, the frequency shift due to changes in the QCM environment is the measured quantity. Thus, relating the frequency shift to changes in mechanical character of the QCM depends on the equivalence of mechanical and electrical parameters. This can be readily seen through a comparison between the constitutive relations of mechanical and electrical damped oscillators (Eqs. 6.1a and 6.1b).

$$m\frac{d^2x}{dt^2} + b\frac{dx}{dt} + kx = F \tag{6.1a}$$

$$L\frac{d^2q}{dt^2} + R\frac{dq}{dt} + \frac{1}{C}q = V \tag{6.1b}$$

QCM analyses commonly begin with the (well-tested) assumption of equivalence between mechanical system parameters and their electrical analogues, e.g. the spring constant k and inverse capacitance $1/C$, mass m and inductance L, mechanical resistance b and electrical resistance R, position x and charge q, driving force F and voltage V, and particle velocity $v = dx/dt$ and current $j = dq/dt$. The solutions to Eqs. (6.1a) and (6.1b) are also analogous, as seen in the expressions for acoustic impedance Z^{ac} and electrical impedance Z^{el} (Eqs. 6.2a and 6.2b)

$$Z^{ac} = F/v = \sqrt{(m\omega - k/\omega)^2 + b^2} \tag{6.2a}$$

$$Z^{el} = V/j = \sqrt{(L\omega - 1/\omega C)^2 + R^2}, \tag{6.2b}$$

where ω is the angular frequency. The acoustic impedance Eq. (6.2a) is normalized to the QCM area, and is expressed in units of mass per second per unit area. The electromechanical constants needed to equate the measured Z^{el} to the acoustical impedance of the loaded QCM are obviated since in all experiments, frequency changes are measured in relation to the unloaded QCM, whose piezoelectric properties are inferred from the measured impedance at the beginning of the experiment.

An equivalent circuit that has been shown to be an appropriate description of the mechanically unloaded QCM is the Butterworth-Van Dyke (BVD) shown in Fig. 6.2 (from [55]). The two arms of the circuit are termed the motional branch, containing

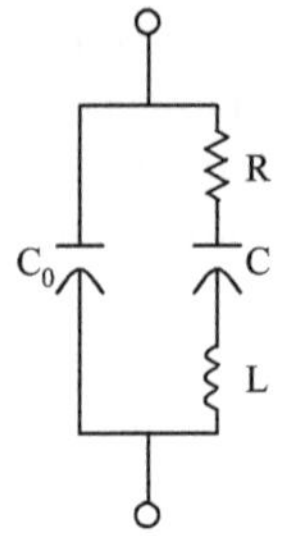

Fig. 6.2. The Butterworth-van Dyke equivalent circuit of a quartz crystal resonator. The resistance R corresponds to the total loss in mechanical energy, the motional inductance L is a measure of the vibrating inertial mass, and the capacitance C represents the mechanical elasticity. The shunt capacitance C_0 lumps the stray capacitance due to the supporting structure and that due to the electrodes.

the circuit equivalent of the quartz crystal motion itself, and the static branch, which accounts for the static capacitance of the electrical contacts. Thus, an increase in mass on the QCM acts as a perturbation on the inductance of the equivalent circuit, lowering the measured resonant frequency.

6.3.1 Theory for Thin Films and Purely Elastic Media

Sauerbrey pioneered the use of quartz crystals as mass measuring devices [88, 87]. From the knowledge that the wavelength of the fundamental shear-mode elastic wave equals twice the quartz crystal thickness at resonance, Sauerbrey derived an expression that linearly equates the mass per area m_f/A of a deposited layer to the shift in resonant frequency of the quartz crystal δf as

$$m_f/A = \rho_f d_f = \rho_q v_q \delta f/2f^2. \tag{6.3}$$

In Eq. (6.3), ρ_f and d_f are the density and thickness of the thin film, f is the resonant frequency before deposition, ρ_q and v_q are the quartz density and node (sound) velocity, respectively, assuming that the added mass acts equivalently to the underlying piezoelectric quartz. Subsequent perturbation analyses by Stockbridge [93], who assumed that the shear wave did *not* propagate through the added material, found that Eq. (6.3) holds to first order. Thus, in the thin film limit, Eq. (6.3) applies regardless of the detailed physical properties of the film.

For thicker films in which the added material must be accommodated, the relationship between the frequency shift and deposited mass depends on the dynamic mechanical characteristics of the film. For example, films that do not dissipate energy while oscillating are termed purely elastic. That is, they possess no viscous character. For purely elastic films, Lu and Lewis [56] derived an expression for a composite resonator which yields

$$m_f/A = \rho_f d_f = \frac{\rho_q v_q}{2\pi Z_r f_c} \tan^{-1}[Z_r \tan(\pi \delta f/f_q)] \tag{6.4}$$

where the dimensionless acoustic impedance ratio is given by

$$Z_r = Z_q/Z_f = \rho_q v_q/\rho_f v_f. \tag{6.5}$$

$Z_q = \rho_q v_q$ and $Z_f = \rho_f v_f$ are the quartz and film impedances, and ρ_f and v_f are the film density and velocity of sound, respectively. The use of Eq. (6.5) requires knowledge of the deposited film's acoustic impedance, which can be calculated using any two of three physical constants, v_f, ρ_f, and the shear modulus G_f, via the relation $v_f = (\rho_f/G_f)^{1/2}$. In practice, these constants may not be known for the film. However, Eq. (6.5) is not highly sensitive to the value of Z_r. Because the film is purely elastic, no changes in QCM amplitude or quality factor Q are expected because Q is proportional to the mechanical energy of the oscillator divided by the energy lost per cycle.

6.3.2 Example Calculation: Quartz Crystal Preparation

Gold is often used as an electrode for QCM measurements in liquids and as a substrate for self-assembled monolayers [92]. To promote adhesion and to produce an optically flat film, a layer of titanium is often deposited first on the polished quartz crystal. A rate monitor (commercial QCM) is used to determine the film thickness deposited on the crystal of interest (see Fig. 6.3). Allowance must be made for the difference between the rate monitor-source D_{rm} and the crystal-source separation distances D_q using $d_q = (D_{rm}/D_q)^2 d_{rm}$, where $d_{q,Au}$ and d_{rm} are the film thicknesses of gold on the quartz and rate monitor, respectively. Eq. (6.3) can be used to calculate the frequency shift on the rate monitor that would correspond to mass deposition. For

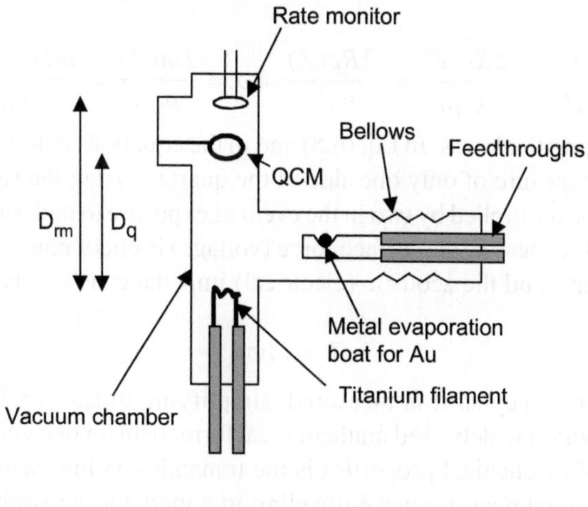

Fig. 6.3. Illustration of an vacuum chamber for depositing thin gold films on the quartz surface. The feedthroughs are for applying current to melt/evaporate the metals. The bellows allows retraction of the second metal, thus preventing contamination. Distances D_{rm} and D_q are described in Eq. 6.6. The titanium underlayer enhances the smoothness and adhesion of a gold electrode.

example, to deposit 50 nm of gold on one side of the crystal, a 9.15 kHz frequency shift is needed on an 8 MHz resonant frequency rate monitor, given that the rate monitor is one quarter more distant than the crystal (Eq. 6.6).

$$\begin{aligned}\delta f_{rm} &= 2f^2\frac{\rho_{Au}d_{q,Au}}{\rho_q v_q}(\frac{D_q}{D_{rm}})^2\\ &= 2(8\text{x}10^6\text{s}^{-1})^2\frac{(19.3\text{g/cm}^3)(50\text{x}10^{-7}\text{cm})}{(2.6\text{g/cm}^3)(3.322\text{x}10^5\text{cm/s})}\frac{1}{1.25^2}\\ &= 9.15\text{kHz}\end{aligned} \quad (6.6)$$

The vacuum conditions are of order 10^{-6} torr or below, and the deposition rate is kept below 1 nm s^{-1} (200 Hz/s) to promote a smooth film.

6.3.3 Transmission-Line Model

Extending the utility of the QCM to studies of mass adsorbtion in liquids, polymer shear moduli, and friction/interface slippage requires both more sophisticated models and more involved experimental procedures. Relationships between resonator *quality factor* changes and mechanisms of mechanical energy dissipation are becoming increasingly valuable, if not required, for these applications. These relationships can best be represented in terms of a complex acoustic impedance $Z(\omega)$, in which the shifts in both frequency $\omega = 2\pi f$ and quality factor Q can be expressed in terms of real (dissipative, $Re(Z)$) and imaginary (inertial, $Im(Z)$) components of a complex acoustic impedance Z as

$$Z(\omega) = Re[Z(\omega)] - iIm[Z(\omega)] \quad (6.7)$$

where

$$\delta(\frac{1}{Q}) = \frac{2Re(Z)}{\omega\rho_q t_q} = \frac{2Re(Z)}{\pi Z_q}, \delta\omega = \frac{Im(Z)}{\rho_q t_q} = \frac{\omega Im(Z)}{\pi Z_q}, \quad (6.8)$$

and t_q is the quartz thickness. In Eq. (6.8) and in the equations below, the expressions correspond to exposure of only one side of the quartz crystal; the right hand side of Eq. (6.8) must be multiplied by two in the event of exposure to both sides. For a purely elastic film of thickness d, the surface force (voltage) is out of phase with the particle velocity (current), and the acoustic (electrical) impedance is purely imaginary (Eq. 6.9).

$$Z = i\omega\rho d \quad (6.9)$$

Thus, only a frequency shift is measured, simplifying to Eqs. (6.3) and (6.4). For viscoelastic media, a widely used mathematical formalism for deriving the impedance as a function of mechanical properties is the transmission line model, which treats the one dimensional acoustic wave traveling in a media as an equivalent electrical circuit whose elements (segments of the wire) represent the action of the quartz and various attached layers. The transmission line model can then be used to construct generalized equations for impedance regardless of the details of the material, as detailed in the following subsections.

6.3.4 Theory for Purely Viscous Media

Immersing a QCM in a Newtonian fluid allows measurement of the quantity $\rho\eta$, where ρ is the density and η is the viscosity of the fluid [39]. Newtonian fluids have a constant viscosity irrespective of shear rate, and have no elastic character. As a starting point, Navier-Stokes equations can be used to calculate the transverse velocity profile $v_x(y)$ as a function of distance y from the quartz surface, where x is in a direction parallel to the surface. For one dimensional oscillatory flow, the Navier-Stokes equation reduces to the wave equation

$$\eta \frac{d^2 v_x}{dy^2} = \rho \frac{dv_x}{dt}, \tag{6.10}$$

whose solution is

$$v_x(y,t) = Ae^{-y/\lambda} cos(y/\lambda - \omega t). \tag{6.11}$$

A is the amplitude at $y = 0$, and the viscous penetration depth $\lambda = (2\eta/\rho\omega)^{1/2}$ marks the point where the velocity amplitude is $1/e$ of its value at the surface. The boundary conditions here assume no slip at the interface, i.e. that the shear stress and particle displacement are continuous. Noting that the acoustic impedance is defined as $Z = F/v$, where F is the driving force (calculated from known piezoelectric properties of quartz) and $v_x(0)$ is the surface velocity, one can proceed to calculate the impedance Z.

Utilizing the transmission line model, Filiatre [27] obtained Z for a quartz crystal in a semi-infinite viscous media as

$$Z = (1+i)\sqrt{\frac{\omega\rho\eta}{2}}. \tag{6.12}$$

which, according to Eq. (6.8) yields

$$\delta f = -\frac{f^{3/2}}{Z_q}\sqrt{\frac{\rho\eta}{\pi}}, \quad \delta(\frac{1}{Q}) = \frac{2}{Z_q}\sqrt{\frac{\rho\eta f}{\pi}} \tag{6.13}$$

for the frequency δf and inverse quality factor $\delta(1/Q)$ shifts. Since both the real and imaginary components of Z are proportional to the square root of the liquid viscosity-density product, simultaneous measurement of frequency and quality factor shifts provide a measure of the deviations from this model, e.g., due to surface roughness, slip at the interface, or non-Newtonian behavior (Fig. 6.4 after [99]).

Equation (6.12) assumes that the liquid is homogenous. For cases where van der Waals attractive forces between the liquid and quartz are large enough to cause variations in density over distances comparable to the viscous penetration depth λ (as in liquid helium), the equation for impedance must take on the more general form [50]

$$\frac{dZ(y)}{dx} = \frac{Z^2(y)}{\eta(y)} - i\omega\rho(y), \tag{6.14}$$

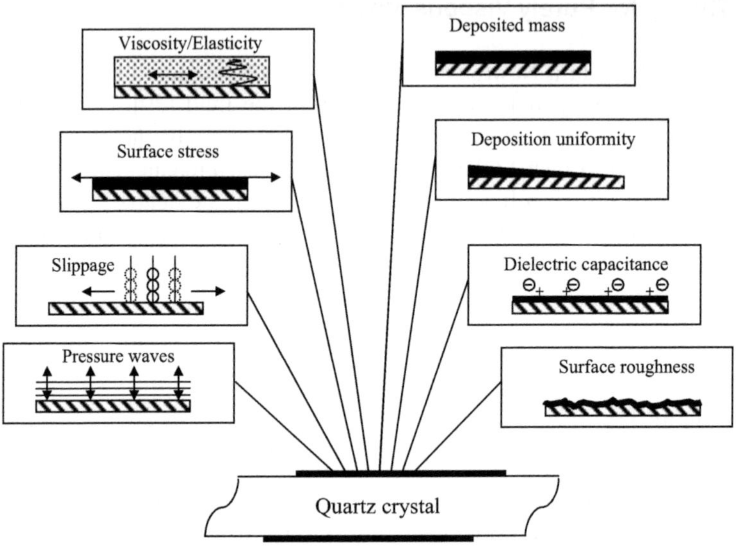

Fig. 6.4. Schematic of the interfacial factors which govern QCM behavior.

where $Z(y)$ is the acoustic impedance at a distance y from the surface. Only $Z(y)$ at the surface, namely $Z(0)$, has physical significance; it is the impedance experienced by the crystal. This first order inhomogeneous differential equation has no analytical solution. It can be solved numerically with the viscosity $\eta(y)$ and density $\rho(y)$ as inputs.

6.3.5 Theory for Viscoelastic Media

Polymeric and associated thin films are being developed for applications as biosensor substrates, membranes, optical devices, electroactive materials, and coatings. Thus, characterization of the mechanical attributes of the film is essential. Because thin films often possess both a viscous and elastic character, their dynamic mechanical properties are described by a frequency dependent complex modulus $G(\omega) = G'(\omega) + iG''(\omega)$ that relates the applied shear to the resultant stress. The complex modulus is composed of a real (elastic) component G', termed the storage modulus, and an imaginary (viscous) part G'', termed the loss modulus. Applying the transmission-line model to a single homogeneous viscoelastic film, Lucklum and Hauptmann [58] derived an expression for the acoustic impedance as

$$Z = i(\rho_p G)^{1/2}\tan(\omega d_p\sqrt{\frac{\rho_p}{G}}), \tag{6.15}$$

where ρ_p and d_p are the film density and thickness, respectively. In the thin film limit, Eq. (6.15) reduces to the purely imaginary impedance $Z = i\rho\omega d$, as it should.

Eq. (6.15) also reduces to $Z = (1 + i)(\rho_p \omega \eta_p / 2)^{1/2}$ for the semi-infinite, purely viscous case where $G = iG'' = i\omega\eta_p$.

In principle, a measurement of frequency and amplitude shifts can provide a complete description of the polymer moduli at that resonant frequency, provided that the film thickness and density are known. In practice, however, the QCM will cease to resonate when the $Re(Z) \approx 10^5$ kg m^{-2}s^{-1} [57].

6.3.6 Theory Including Gases at Low Pressures

The effect of a finite gas pressure on the QCM impedance must be considered in ultra-high vacuum experiments where a high degree of sensitivity is desired, such as measuring the slippage of a single monolayer of adsorbed gas [46]. At gas pressures above about 100 torr, the effect of the presence of the gas can be modeled as a viscous fluid using Eq. (6.12) above. However, at pressures below 100 torr, the time required for molecular momentum relaxation is $\approx$ 0.01 microsecond. This approaches the timescale probed by a QCM oscillating in the 3-10 MHz range. In fact, relaxation effects have been shown to be significant to 300 torr [93]. Since collision with other gas molecules is the only mechanism for velocity relaxation, a single relaxation time can be incorporated into the impedance equations by phenomenologically substituting the viscosity η with the complex viscosity

$$\eta^* = \frac{\eta}{1 + i\omega\tau_r} \tag{6.16}$$

to obtain

$$Re(Z) = \sqrt{\pi\rho\eta f}[\frac{\omega\tau_r}{1 + (\omega\tau_r)^2}[(1 + \frac{1}{(\omega\tau_r)^2})^{1/2} + 1)]]^{1/2} \tag{6.17}$$

$$Im(Z) = \sqrt{\pi\rho\eta f}[\frac{\omega\tau_r}{1 + (\omega\tau_r)^2}[(1 + \frac{1}{(\omega\tau_r)^2})^{1/2} - 1)]]^{1/2}. \tag{6.18}$$

To establish the importance of considering relaxation time τ_r, τ_r can be approximated by the collision time τ_c calculated from the mean free path of an ideal gas (Eq. 6.19),

$$\tau_c = \frac{\sqrt{mk_BT/6}}{\pi p D^2} \tag{6.19}$$

where m is the molecular mass, k_B is the Boltzmann constant, T is the temperature, p is the gas pressure, and D is the effective molecular diameter.

Note that the substitution of the real viscosity η with a complex viscosity η^* introduces an 'elastic-like' component to the gas motion under shear. In other words, the effect of momentum relaxations of dilute gases on acoustic impedance are analogous to conformational relaxations in polymers under shear. Thus, Eqs. (6.17) and (6.18) can be extended to describe the acoustical impedance of any semi-infinite viscoelastic material which is characterized by a single relaxation time τ_r.

6.3.7 Theory Combining Mass (Thin Film) and Semi-continuous Fluid Loading

The addition of a second interface adds considerable complexity to the solution of the equations for impedance by introducing two new boundary conditions. In instances in which the adsorbed film is thin compared to the acoustic wavelength in the fluid, the adsorbed layer can be assumed to be infinitesimally thin. Thus, only the acceleration of this thin mass layer needs to be considered, and the total frequency shift can be described as the simple addition of shifts due to mass and liquid loading as

$$\delta f = \frac{2f^2}{Z_q}\left(\frac{m_f}{A} + \sqrt{\frac{\rho\eta}{4\pi f}}\right), \tag{6.20}$$

where ρ and η are the density and viscosity of the semicontinuous fluid [65]. Again, this equation assumes that the combined mass and liquid loading are small compared to the mass of the quartz. Eq. (6.20) demonstrates that frequency information alone cannot distinguish between changes in mass from changes in viscous properties of the liquid. However, by assuming the mass is infinitesimally thin, the adsorbed layer is treated as a purely elastic layer. Thus, the quality factor shift will be a function only of the viscous liquid, which can be obtained via

$$Re(Z) = \frac{1}{\pi C_1}\sqrt{\frac{\rho\eta}{\pi f v_q \rho_q}} \tag{6.21}$$

ignoring the internal viscosity of the quartz. By comparing the frequency and quality factor shifts, the mass of the adsorbed layer can be determined [65].

6.3.8 Theory Incorporating Slip at the Interface

Until now, slip at the film-solid interface was either assumed not to occur, or was sufficiently small to be ignored. There are several theoretical frameworks for deriving the impedance for a system in which interfacial slip does in fact occur. Generalizing the impedance equations to allow for slip at the wall begins by relaxing the boundary condition that the transverse particle velocities across the interface are equal. All derivations employ the concept of a two-dimensional interfacial viscosity η_2, which relates the viscous force $\eta_2 v_r$ to the relative velocity between the film and substrate v_r. Krim and Widom [46] derived a purely quantum mechanical expression for the acoustic resistance $Re(Z)$ in terms of the correlation function of momentum fluctuations $M(t)$ in the film. Because $M(t)$ is proportional to the average particle surface velocity v_r, they could employ the two-dimensional equation of fluid motion to show that $M(t)$ is proportional to the average particle surface velocity v_r. They found that $M(t)$ exhibits an exponential decay as $M(t) = e^{-t/\tau}$, where the slip time τ is defined as $\tau = \rho_2/\eta_2$ and $\rho_2 = \rho d$ is the areal density.

Physically, the slip time can be viewed as the time required for a particle traveling at velocity v to slow to v/e in response to a step change in substrate velocity from v to zero. However, this picture does not imply that all particles are traveling at the same velocity. Strictly, it is the time required for the correlation of momentum fluctuations to relax to $1/e$ of the original value.

Using the expression for acoustic resistance, Widom and Krim [109] further showed that

$$\frac{1}{Z(\omega)} = \frac{1}{Z_{ns}(\omega)} + \frac{1}{Z_s(\omega)}, \tag{6.22}$$

where the slipping impedance $Z_s(\omega)$ is the frequency-dependent contribution of interfacial viscosity, and

$$Z_{ns}(\omega) = -\eta k_p \tan(k_p d), k_p^2 = i\omega\rho/\eta. \tag{6.23}$$

is the no slip case. $Z_s(\omega)$ can be approximated by the interfacial friction coefficient η_2 in the zero frequency limit, which is equivalent to assuming that η_2 does not vary with sliding velocity (Stoke's law). Eq. (6.22) implies that the impedance of the slipping film can be considered as a rigidly attached film in parallel with a purely resistive element that represents the slipping. In the thin film limit, $Z_{ns} = -i\omega\rho d$, and Z becomes

$$Z = \frac{-i\omega\rho_2}{1 - i\omega\tau}, \quad \tau = \frac{\rho_2}{\eta_2}. \tag{6.24}$$

In practice, most adsorbed films coexist with bulk vapor phases, and the impedance Z_{ns} should include contributions from the bulk phase. However, given the density - viscosity product mismatch between the film and bulk vapor, the no-slip impedance can be approximated as having contributions from the film alone. Thus, the slip time and friction can be obtained from impedance measurements using the relations

$$Re(Z) = \frac{\rho_2\omega^2\tau}{1+\omega^2\tau^2}, \quad Im(Z) = \frac{\rho_2\omega}{1+\omega^2\tau^2}, \quad \frac{Re(Z)}{Im(Z)} = \omega\tau, \quad \tau = \frac{\rho_2}{\eta_2}. \tag{6.25}$$

6.3.9 Theory for Combined Viscous Film, Slip, and Semicontinuous Vapor

By solving the Navier-Stokes equation for a film immersed in a vapor (including the slip boundary condition), Bruschi and Mistura [9] have recently derived a more general expression for Z as

$$Z = Z_f \frac{1 - \alpha e^{-2(1-i)d/\lambda}}{[1 + \alpha e^{-2(1-i)d/\lambda}] + \frac{Z_f}{\eta_2}[1 - \alpha e^{-2(1-i)d/\lambda}]}, \tag{6.26}$$

where $\alpha = (Z_f - Z_v)/(Z_f + Z_v)$ is the impedance mismatch between film and vapor, and $\lambda = \sqrt{\eta_f/\pi f \rho_f}$ is the viscous penetration depth in the liquid film. $Z_v = (1+i)\sqrt{\pi f \eta_v \rho_v}$ is the vapor acoustic impedance for a semi-continuous purely viscous fluid. Eq. (6.26) can be recast as

$$\frac{1}{Z} = \frac{1}{Z_{fv}} + \frac{1}{\eta_2} \tag{6.27}$$

where the impedance of the film and vapor Z_{fv} is given as

$$Z_{fv} = Z_f \frac{1 - \alpha e^{-2(1-i)d/\lambda}}{1 + \alpha e^{-2(1-i)d/\lambda}} \tag{6.28}$$

This set of equations reduce to Eq. (6.22) in the case of a small vapor impedance ($Z_{fv} = Z_f$), in which case Z_f is identical to Z_{ns}.

6.4 Equipment and Experimental Methods

6.4.1 Equipment

Figure 6.1b depicts a mounted quartz crystal. Typical dimensions are 1 *cm* diameter, and 0.2 *mm* thick. Quartz crystals of the type used for friction measurements are 'overtone polished' to reduce surface roughness. These crystals appear completely transparent. The surface area of typical commercial rate monitors are roughly twice that of polished crystals. Crystals can be purchased with or without electrodes, but as quartz is non-conductive, electrodes are necessary for operation. For highly exacting experiments where the electrode surface quality is crucial to the experiment, it is preferable to purchase bare crystals and deposit electrodes under high or ultra-high vacuum deposition conditions. Higher vacuums lead to cleaner, but not necessarily smoother films. QCM's can also be directly immersed; however, care must be taken not to short the electrical contacts, and electrode smoothness is particularly critical.

The simplest and most cost effective manner to drive a QCM at resonance is by an external circuit such as the Clapp circuit shown in Fig. 6.5. The crystal and electrical contacts are incorporated into a positive feedback oscillator circuit that tunes the applied frequency to the resonance frequency by minimizing the non-resistive impedance of the QCM. The drive amplitude is changed by varying the input voltage from a power supply, and a frequency counter is used to measure frequency shifts during an experiment. More sophisticated circuits have been invented for specific QCM applications that may provide a more cost effective approach [8]. Driving the resonator at other harmonic frequencies requires a function generator or a more specialized oscillator circuit.

Quality factor measurements can be obtained by using an oscilloscope to record the amplitude decay during an interruption in driving excitation [82]. The time constant associated with the amplitude decay τ_d is related to the quality factor by $Q = \omega\tau_d/2$. For a complete analysis of the resonance bandwidth and attenuation, an impedance analyzer can be used to measure the voltage and current supplied to the QCM as a function of applied frequency [97].

6.4.2 Experimental Considerations

There are a number of physical parameters other than mass loading that can affect the QCM resonant frequency and quality factor, including changes in temperature,

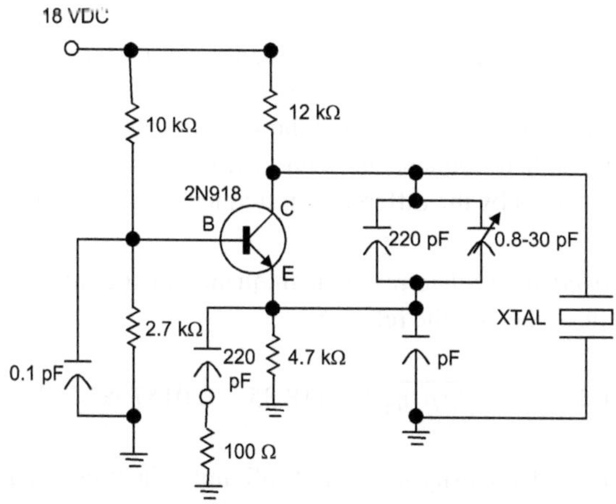

Fig. 6.5. Schematic of the Clapp oscillator circuit.

surface stress, hydrostatic pressure [56], motional resistance of the quartz itself, and surface roughness [17, 115] (Fig. 6.4). For measurements in liquid, stray capacitances generated at the electrode-liquid interface [90] and longitudinal pressure waves [69] can also introduce uncertainty in measurement.

Temperature variations: Most commercially available resonators are of AT-cut quartz and are designed to operate at room temperature. The mass measurements are relatively insensitive to modest changes in temperature. Departures from room temperature (say, during deposition) shift the resonant frequency, thus it is necessary either to compare frequency shifts at the same temperature, to regulate the temperature of the QCM, or to use a second QCM which responds only to changes in temperature. This is particularly true for transient measurements where thermal equilibrium is not achieved. Page 24, Fig. 5 of Ref. [55] contains a chart for evaluating frequency shifts for modest deviations from room temperature of AT-cut quartz.

Quartz viscosity: In most experiments, the motional resistance of the quartz itself (due to mode coupling and internal viscosity) is very low in comparison. Losses attributable to the mounting contacts can be significant; the baseline frequency for nearly all experiments is obtained on the secured crystal and mounting combined.

Surface stress: Stresses on the quartz generated by the deposited film can also affect a frequency shift that can be significant for thin films [55]. As the film grows, the relative effect of stress becomes small compared to the shift due to mass increase. To first order, treating the stress in the quartz as isotropic and biaxial, the frequency shift has been found to be proportional to the stress as

$$\delta f/f = K\delta s/t \tag{6.29}$$

where $K = -2.75\text{x}10^{-11} m^2/N$ ($K = 2.65\text{x}10^{-11} m^2/N$) for AT-cut (BT-cut) quartz, δs is the integral over the film thickness of the differential change of shearing stress (positive values indicate tension), and t is the crystal thickness [25]. Ion bombardment and surface chemical reactions can generate significant stress: in these applications, two crystals can be used in tandem. AT-cut and BT-cut crystals react in opposite manner with respect to stress, but the same manner with respect to thin film mass (at selected matched frequencies). Thus, the stress contribution to the calculated mass can be obtained by the difference in frequency between the AT- and BT-cut QCMs.

Gas pressure dependencies: The resonant frequency of the quartz depends on the fluid pressure as described by the relation

$$\frac{\delta f}{f} = -0.72\text{x}10^{-6}\sqrt{\pi \rho_g \eta_g f} + (18.35 - 0.015T)\text{x}10^{-10}P. \tag{6.30}$$

The gas density ρ_g and viscosity η_g are in CGS units, the pressure P is in torr, and the temperature T is in Kelvin. The first term arises from the viscous drag on the crystal, and is in the same form as Eq. (6.12), except that it accounts for exposure to both QCM faces. The second term reflects a change in the quartz crystal's elastic constants due to hydrostatic pressure. In total, the contribution to the frequency shift near monolayer completion for nitrogen gas at 150 torr is about 1-2 Hz for a 6 MHz crystal.

Longitudinal pressure waves: Although an AT-cut QCM acts primarily in a shear mode, longitudinal pressure waves have been reported [66, 69]. These pressure waves arise from the non-uniform amplitude distribution of the shear motion across the QCM surface, and propagate with little attenuation. Because they can be reflected by an opposing surface, constructive and destructive interferences can occur which can affect the damping of the QCM.

6.5 Experimental Observations of Slip at Interfaces

In the fluid dynamics analyses of most macroscale devices and equipment, velocity profiles of gases and liquids in contact with a solid are calculated assuming 'no slip' at the interface. That is, the gas or liquid molecules touching the solid surface are assumed not to move relative to the underlying solid surface. On this scale, slip has been primarily identified with the extrusion of high molecular weight polymers. However, there has been increasing experimental evidence that slip occurs at a multiplicity of surfaces, including monolayers of gases adsorbed on metal [105, 45, 19], water and aqueous solutions on hydrophilic and hydrophobic surfaces [14, 16, 118, 3, 84], and oligomers on mica surfaces [73, 72, 118]. The motivation for studying slip at interfaces arises from a need to understand lubrication mechanisms in confined geometries (e.g. for disk drive applications [67, 40] and MEMS devices [23, 2, 119]), hydrodynamic fluid flow at interfaces (e.g. microfluidics [74]), and the fundamental origins of friction [105, 45, 19]. The importance of understanding the nature of energy dissipation at sliding interfaces may become key to the design of MEMS which rely on sliding contacts. For example, electron transport during rubbing can generate significant Coulombic forces which, while largely inconsequential on the macroscale, may significantly affect device operation at the micro- and nanoscale. The QCM, with its ability to elucidate the nature of sliding contacts, is emerging as an important tool for studying slip at interfaces.

6.5.1 Slip of Adsorbed Monolayers of Gases

The QCM has the unique capability of directly measuring the frictional energy loss due to sliding interfaces. Krim and coworkers pioneered the use of the QCM in measuring the energy dissipation of gas monolayers sliding on metal surfaces, initiated by the unexpected experimentally observed shift in quality factor during film deposition [46, 105, 19, 81, 45]. By varying the gas pressure, they were able to vary the surface coverage and thickness of nitrogen and krypton layers physisorbed on gold, silver, or lead-coated QCMs. Since the experiments were performed in a regime satisfying $|k_p d| << 1$ (thin film), the film thickness and slip time could be calculated from the frequency and quality factor shifts using Eq. (6.25). For film thicknesses approaching macroscopic dimensions, the slip time monotonically decreased, which may validate the no-slip boundary assumption for such systems [105]. Other remarkable observations that elucidate the nature of friction include the increase in slip time during a film liquid to solid phase transition, and the experimental observation of phononic contributions to friction, which are discussed in greater detail below.

Effect of the Thermodynamic State of the Adsorbate

As gas pressure is increased, a monolayer film of physisorbed krypton on a gold-coated QCM at liquid nitrogen temperatures exhibits frequency shifts consistent with a 'liquid-solid' phase transition [45]. The lattice spacings calculated from these frequency shifts (10.4 and 12.5 Hz) corresponded to spacings of both bulk liquid and solid krypton, respectively. In passing from a liquid to a solid, the slip time increased by an order of magnitude. Since the frequency shift was relatively constant during this transition, the slip time increase can be interpreted as a reduction in friction. Denser layers slide more easily because they are more resistant to deformation by the moving substrate. Atomistic computer simulations revealed that the slip time increase could be modeled considering lattice vibrations alone [81]. Thus, these experiments were the first to clearly show the phononic origin of friction.

Experimental Studies of the Origins of Friction

Theoreticians have postulated that energy transfer away from a sliding contact occurs through a number of means. Lattice vibrations can be excited through localized variations in relative velocity (phonon generation), and can be affected by the degree of commensurability between the substrate lattice and the lattice of the adsorbed layer. Also, since adsorbates may exchange electronic charge with the underlying substrate, the motion of adsorbates on the surface can contribute an electronic friction which can be modeled as charges and dipoles moving through a 'viscous' medium [98]. For example, IR spectroscopy and near-edge x-ray absorption spectroscopy has been used to measure energy dissipation via vibrational relaxations in adsorbate molecules translationally fixed to the surface, and may be generalized to surfaces in motion [111]. While phononic contributions to the friction may be intuitive, electronic contributions to the overall friction have been evidenced both directly [19] and indirectly [70].

To experimentally distinguish between phononic and electronic contributions to the friction, Dayo et al. [19] performed QCM experiments of nitrogen on lead under UHV conditions. In these experiments, the film thickness was constant and the lead substrate temperature was varied. Since lead becomes superconducting at liquid helium temperatures, the electronic contributions to friction should decrease dramatically. That is, any charge exchanged with the substrate should exhibit no resistance to motion through the substrate. Dayo et al. found that both the quality factor and frequency shifts changed at the critical temperature. In passing from the superconducting state to the normal state, the quality factor increased, indicating a decreased energy loss. Similarly abruptly, the resonant frequency decreased, indicating an increase in *effective* mass. Taken together, the slip time was calculated to decrease by half (Eq. 6.25). For a constant film thickness, the friction is inversely proportional to the slip time; thus, the friction doubled in passing to a normal state. Since the magnitude of phononic contributions does not change abruptly when crossing the critical temperature, the contribution of electronic friction to the total friction was estimated to be about 40% of the total.

6.5.2 Liquid Phase Slip

There has also been a recent surge of research devoted to studying liquid slip at interfaces using the surface forces apparatus (SFA), the atomic force microscope (AFM), internal reflection-fluorescence, and the QCM. The SFA, pioneered by Israelachvili [116, 35, 79, 60], shears molecularly thin films between two crossed cylinders of mica. For example, Yoshizawa and Israelachvili [116] studied the 'stick-slip' behavior of hexadecane and isooctadecane confined between surfaces separated by only a few multiples of the molecular dimensions. A model based on a solid-liquid phase transition was supported by the data, in which the transitions between sticking and slipping were associated with a solid-liquid phase transition. There is nonetheless still considerable debate regarding whether these experiments are measuring 'true' slip, defined as a discontinuity in the rate of shear across an interface. For these highly confined fluids in which separation distances approach molecular dimensions, the molecules have lost their freedom of movement and exhibit strongly enhanced 'viscosities.' Zhu and Granick [118] studied the slip of tetradecane against both adsorbed surfactant and a methyl-terminated self-assembled monolayer (SAM), and water against the same SAM. In these experiments, the tetradecane (and water) molecules are much smaller than the surface spacing; thus, the fluid is expected to behave as a Newtonian fluid. They found that in some systems, notably where wetting is presumed partial or small, deviations from the classical no-slip boundary conditions are seen.

Further evidence for interfacial slip was reported by Craig et al. [14] using an atomic force microscope (AFM). They attached a silica sphere to a cantilever tip and coated it with gold and a mixture of hydroxy- and methyl-terminated thiols to produce a chemically bound SAM. The tip was brought toward a similarly coated mica surface at a constant velocity in the presence of a sucrose solution. The hydrodynamic drainage force deflected the tip during its approach to provide a measure of the force applied to the cantilever. In comparing experimentally obtained force versus distance curves to theory, Craig et al. found that their data could be modeled using a modified Stoke's law incorporating a correction factor for slip. Further, the slip length, defined here as the distance below the surface at which the liquid velocity extrapolates to zero, was found to increase monotonically with increasing velocity (see Fig. 6.6).

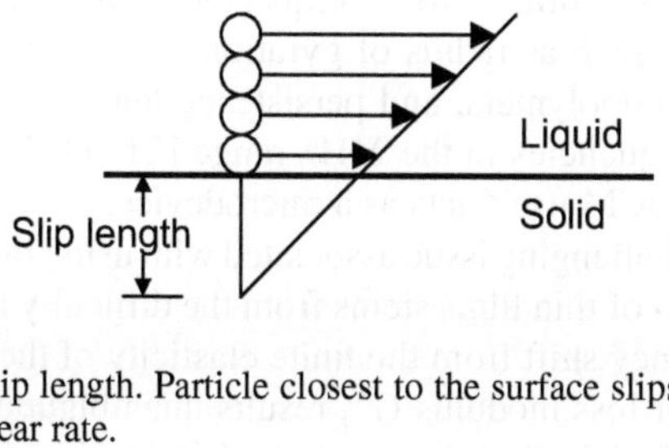

Fig. 6.6. Depiction of slip length. Particle closest to the surface slips along surface, creating a discontinuity in the shear rate.

Pit et al. [72, 73] used internal reflection-flouresence to monitor fluid flow close to the solid boundary. Evanescent waves extending about 80 nm from the solid surface excite fluorescent molecules dissolved in low concentration. Through a measure of fluorescence recovery after photobleaching, the velocity of the liquid can be calculated. Their data appeared consistent with a slip boundary condition for hexadecane on a lyophobic (non-wetting) surface. This method, while not providing direct measurement of forces, does allow considerable distancing of the second surface. Thus, anomalies due to finite confinement effects on slip were avoided.

The QCM, like the internal reflection-fluorescence technique, allows study of interfacial slip without finite confinement effects, and can quantify the frictional energy loss as well. Rodahl and Kasemo [84] monitored the quality factor and frequency shifts associated with water adsorption on gold at various relative humidities. Under the conditions of their experiment, the QCM impedance shift is a function of the mass of water adsorbed, the viscous dissipation of the water film, and any frictional slippage. They observed slip only for molecularly thin films: Submerging the QCM in water gave an impedance shift consistent with the no-slip boundary condition.

6.6 Measurement of Viscoelastic Properties of Films

6.6.1 Moduli Measurements

Considerable research has focused on developing acoustical techniques for the dynamical mechanical characterization of thin films. This work has been motivated by the need to develop shock-resistant organic coatings, disk drive lubricants, nanostructured electroactive films and electrical insulators, and optical devices such as waveguides. The development of the QCM as an in-situ biosensor has received particular attention, and will be discussed separately in section 6.8. In addition, the measurement of viscoelastic properties of thin films using QCM has been applied to fundamental studies of solvent molecule relaxation dynamics [42], plastification [20], polymer glass transitions [58, 57], surfactant phase transitions [30, 96] and viscoelasticity [91], wetting rates [54], polymer complex moduli [58, 57, 21, 38], and interfacial slippage [46]. The MHz resonant frequency associated with the QCM allows probing of the dynamics of molecular motion on fractions of a microsecond timescale. In addition, the thickness of many films is roughly equivalent to the wavelength of sound in the film at MHz frequencies. Thus, many of the dynamical properties of the film, such as radius of gyration, hydrodynamic screening length, domain size in block copolymers, and persistence length of stiff main chains will have characteristic frequencies in the MHz range [21, 112]. In all of these studies and applications, the QCM itself acts as a microdevice.

One particularly challenging issue associated with using the QCM to characterize the dynamic properties of thin films stems from the difficulty in separating the effect of mass on the frequency shift from the finite elasticity of the film. (In contrast, the viscous component, or loss modulus G'', results unambiguously in a quality factor shift, excluding interfacial slip.) As mentioned in section 6.3.5, measurement of the complex moduli depends on an independent measurement of film thickness and density. Since the elastic contribution scales as the second power of mass, accurate measurement of the film thickness is crucial especially for thin films. Wolff et al.[112] describe and experimentally test a method to circumvent this difficulty by measuring the quadratic frequency dependence of the normalized frequency shift using (in our notation)

$$Z = i\omega\rho d[1 + \frac{\rho d^2 \omega^2}{3G}]. \tag{6.31}$$

Eq. (6.31) is Taylor series expansion of Eq. (6.15) about $d = 0$ for the thin film limit. Since this method requires the measurement of Z at multiple resonances, an impedance analyzer was used instead of including the resonator in an oscillator circuit. Using this technique, Wolff et al. were able to measure elastic moduli of the order 50 MPa for polyglutamate Langmuir-Blodgett films.

6.6.2 Solvent Dynamics

There is fundamental interest in understanding polymer-solvent interactions. Katz and Ward [42] were able to measure the orientation relaxation time of solvent toluene in polystyrene. In their experiment, polystyrene dissolved in toluene was spin-coated on one side of the QCM metal electrode. As the polymer film dried, the time associated with toluene orientation relaxation could be quantified. Because the thickness of the polymer film was small, and because the segmental relaxation times of the polymer were significantly longer than those probed at the resonant frequency, changes in the moduli were associated with changes in solvent dynamics alone. In analogy with time-temperature superposition principles, in which changes in oscillation frequency and changes in temperature can elicit the same viscoelastic response, changes in solvent concentration were equivalent to changes in frequency. A single relaxation time described the dynamics of solvent reorientation.

6.7 Tribology and Tribochemistry of Surfaces

6.7.1 Friction and Wear in MEMS

A fundamental issue in the development of many microelectromechanical devices (MEMS) is their limited mechanical durability in sliding or rotary contact. The majority of MEMS are constructed of silicon, which permits the use of fabrication techniques common to the semiconductor industry. However, silicon has a low cohesive energy, giving it poor strength [75, 23]. Efforts to protect the surface from wear include diamond-like carbon (DLC) [104, 4, 61] and SiC coatings [77] to improve hardness, and self-assembled monolayers to reduce friction and water condensation at junctures [2, 89]. Ion bombardment has been attempted [34], as has low pressure gas phase lubricants, but both suffer from near line-of-sight coverage [75]. At low pressures, molecules impact surfaces much more frequently than they encounter other lubricant molecules, and thus are hindered from penetrating gaps $<1\ \mu m$. Finally, MEMS have also been made from more wear resistant materials such as transition metals [62], diamond [13] and Si_3N_4 [94], but fabrication techniques need to be developed for large-scale manufacture.

Our lack of a comprehensive understanding of the relative importance of various environmental and material factors requires that tribological studies be performed under conditions that mimic actual operating conditions of the device. Because the friction depends so highly on surface properties, interfacial distances, operating conditions, and details of the MEMS preparation technique, the range of static and dynamic friction coefficients reported in the literature vary by too great an extent to be useful for MEMS designers. In addition, given the large surface area to volume ratio of these devices compared to macroscopic machines, forces that could be neglected in the macroscale, such as electrostatic and capillary forces, can be important if not dominant at the microscale [107]. Finally, frictional energy dissipation mechanisms involve not only excitations of atomic lattice vibrations (phonons), but electronic charge transfer between insulating rubbing surfaces. The latter, while generally inconsequential at the macroscale, may have an impact on the operation of a microdevice. For these reasons, developing tribological capabilities that elucidate the physical processes occurring during tribological contact on a microscale become imperative.

Perhaps the most obvious method is to use a MEMS device itself for frictional studies. Dugger [22] designed a MEMS device that combines sliding, tapping and rotating contacts in the same device to evaluate the effects of surface treatments on a wide variety of contact conditions. A quantitative measure of the friction coefficient can be obtained through a knowledge of the applied voltage, the degree of motion, and the mechanical deflection spring constants of the comb drive elements. The time and expense required to produce MEMS devices for testing, however, has driven the need for alternate methods for obtaining tribological data, such as combined QCM/surface probe instruments.

6.7.2 Combined QCM/Surface Probe Instruments

The evolution of the QCM into a tribological device follows from its successful use in measuring interfacial slip (see section 6.5). In comparison to the atomic force microscope and the surface forces apparatus, the QCM is uniquely suited as a micro- and nanotribological medium by virtue of the high linear velocities it can attain, up to 2 ms^{-1}. Moreover, these velocities and contact pressures overlap those of a typical microdevice (Fig. 6.7, from [22]). Extending the use of the QCM to applications of engineering importance to microdevices has been accomplished with the development of combined QCM/scanning tunneling microscope (STM) [18, 86, 6], QCM/AFM [43, 114], and QCM/indenter instruments [28, 7, 49] (Figs. 6.8–6.10, from [5], [114], and [7], respectively).

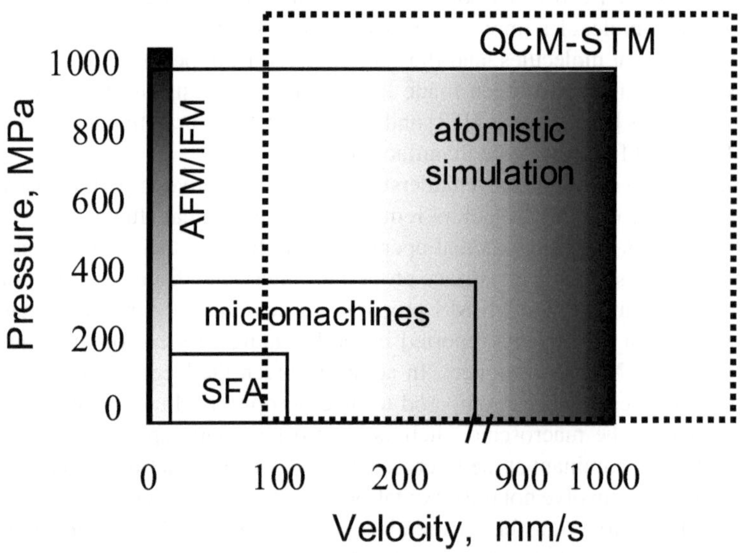

Fig. 6.7. Comparison of the pressure-velocity ranges of the surface forces apparatus (SFA), atomic force microscope (AFM), and QCM/STM to the ranges seen in microdevices.

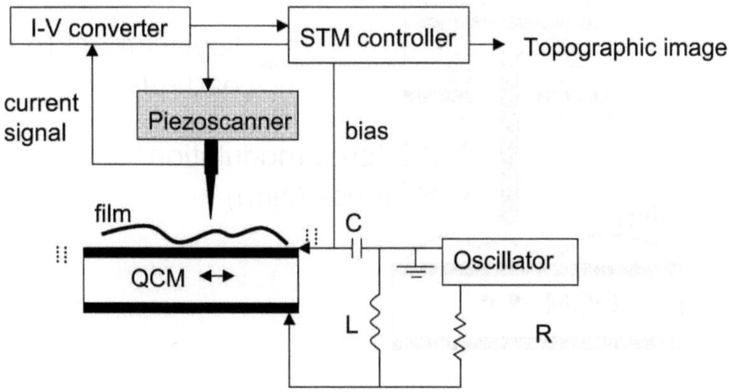

Fig. 6.8. Schematic of QCM/STM instrument. The oscillator consisted of a function generator whose drive signal cycled on an off every 5 sec to enable quality factor measurements using the 'ring-down' approach. Resistor R = 220 Ω, C = 0.5 μ F, L = 2 μ H.

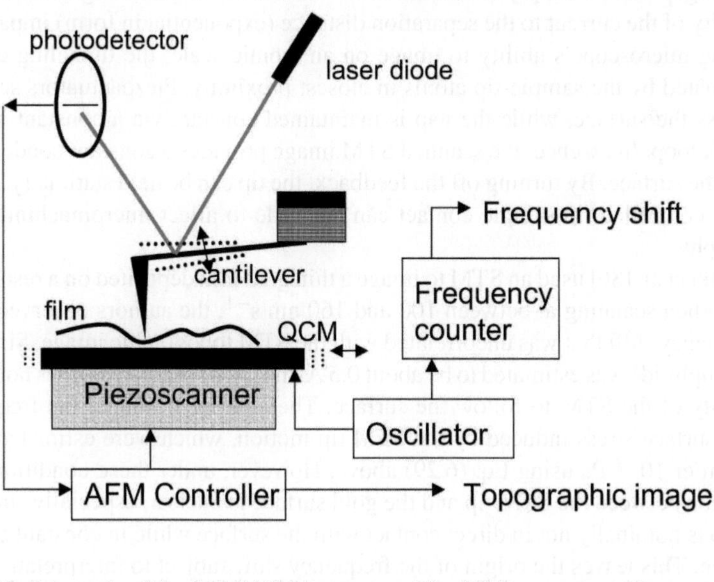

Fig. 6.9. Schematic of the QCM/AFM instrument. The AFM was operated in contact mode.

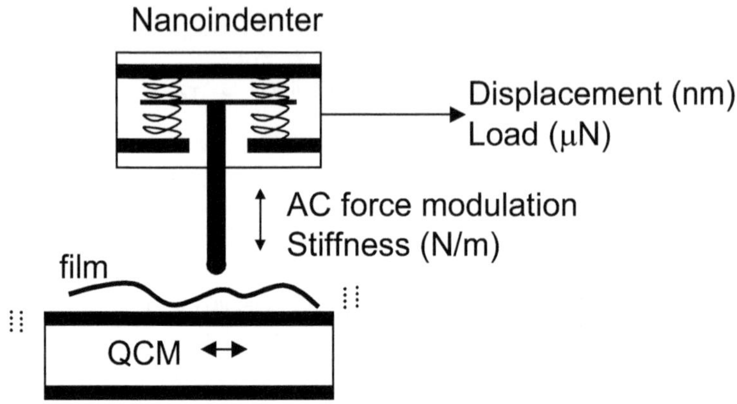

Fig. 6.10. Schematic of QCM/indenter instrument.

QCM/STM Experiments

The STM is a surface probe instrument in which a sharp PtIr or W tip is brought to close proximity to a conducting or semiconducting surface. The sample is voltage biased relative to the tip to generate a current on the order of 0.1 to 10 nA. As the sample and tip are not in contact, electrons 'tunnel' across the nanometer-wide gap. The gap can be simply a vacuum or be filled with an insulating material. The sensitivity of the current to the separation distance (exponential in form) imparts the tunneling microscope's ability to image on an atomic scale; the tunneling current is dominated by the sample-tip atoms in closest proximity. Piezoactuators scan the tip across the surface, while the gap is maintained constant via a constant current feedback loop. In essence, the scanned STM image provides a constant conductivity map of the surface. By turning off the feedback, the tip can be held stationary. In this manner, controlled tip-sample contact can be made to affect micromachining and lithography.

Sasaki et al. [86] used an STM to image a thin gold film deposited on a resonating QCM. When scanning at between 100 and 160 nm s^{-1}, the authors observed a 3-4 Hz frequency shift that was uncorrelated with the STM topographic image. Since the QCM amplitude was estimated to be about 0.5 Å, the QCM oscillation does not affect the ability of the STM to follow the surface. The authors attributed the frequency shift to surface stress induced by the STM tip motion, which were estimated to be of the order 10^{-7} Pa using Eq. (6.29) above. However, under these conditions, the interaction between the STM tip and the gold surface is unclear, especially since the STM tip is nominally not in direct contact with the surface while in constant current operation. This leaves the origin of the frequency shift subject to interpretation.

Borovsky et al. [5, 6] more clearly demonstrated the potential of a QCM/STM combination as a micro- to nanoscale friction tester. In controlled current mode, the STM was used to measure the amplitude of an oscillating quartz crystal up to 80 nm by varying the drive voltage [5]. At 5 MHz resonant frequency, the QCM achieved ms^{-1} surface velocities. Borovsky et al. [6] further used the QCM/STM in high vacuum to study the lubricating properties of tertiary-butyl phenyl phosphate (TBPP) on a tungsten tip/platinum electrode contact. The probe tip was used to micromachine the platinum by rastering the tip sufficiently faster than the current feedback response time. In the absence of lubricant, the machining process was accompanied by a negative frequency shift. Under room temperature lubricated conditions, however, the frequency shift was *positive*. After annealing TBPP at 100°C, at which the TBPP chemically reacts, the positive frequency shift was reduced by an order of magnitude. The changes between unlubricated, lubricated, and lubricated and annealed conditions are indicative of a fundamental change in the tip-electrode interaction, and illustrates the potential of the QCM/STM instrument in elucidating mechanisms of lubrication.

QCM/AFM Experiments

The QCM has also been used in conjunction with an AFM to measure a localized elasticity. Yamada et al. [114] brought a silicon AFM cantilever tip into contact with a resonating QCM having bare gold and polymer coated gold regions, and monitored both the applied force (through deflection cantilever deflection) and the QCM frequency shift as a function of position. For both the gold and polymer regions, they observed a positive frequency shift that increased in magnitude as the apply force was increased. The authors surmised that when the tip comes in contact with the QCM surface, the cantilever acts as an additional spring to the acoustic impedance, resulting in an increase in the resonant frequency. Further, in scanning the AFM tip across the oscillating gold/polymer surface, the frequency image distinguished between the gold and polymer regions and matched the AFM image.

In a similar experiment, Kim et al. [43] observed *negative* frequency shifts when a silicon nitride AFM tip was brought into contact with both bare gold and polystyrene. While these results seem contradictory, improvements in modeling will relate the nature of the mechanical contact to its acoustic response. For example, Laschitsch and Johannsmann [49] developed a model describing the acoustic impedance as a function of the tip-QCM contact radius r_c as

$$Z = \frac{1}{r_e^2}\frac{G' r_c}{i\omega}(1 + ikr_c) \tag{6.32}$$

where k is the wave number, r_e is the electrode area, and G' is the elastic modulus of the contact material. This equation assumes both that no slip occurs at the interface and that the contact radius is small compared to the acoustic wavelength, termed the near-field region. It predicts that the frequency shift and 'loss tangent' Λ (given by $\Lambda = Re(Z)/Im(Z)$) are both proportional to the contact radius. The authors' model predicts an increasing positive frequency shift with increasing contact area, in agreement with the data of Yamada et al.

QCM Indenter Experiments

Using a QCM/indenter instrument, Borovsky et al. [7] tested the Laschitsch model by contacting alternately a silicon sphere and tungsten tip to a chrome or silver coated QCM. Assuming Hertzian contact, the contact area was found to be linearly proportional to the applied load, consistent with a multi-contact or plastically deformed interface. However, the frequency shift was found to increase linearly with contact area, rather than radius as predicted by the Laschitsch model. This result is corroborated by that of Flannigan et al. [28] in their study of the contact of a low modulus elastomer with a gold electrode, except that the frequency shift was negative. Although Borovsky et al. noticed a wear transfer film of silver from the electrode surface, implying fretting or slip at the interface, the no-slip model described their data well.

In summary, the combined operation of a QCM with a surface probe allows sensitive measurements of the nature of the tip-substrate contact. As improved models relating acoustical impedance to the physics of the tribological contact are developed, combined QCM/surface probe instruments will prove very helpful in elucidating lubrication and wear phenomena in MEMS applications.

6.8 QCM Uses in Physiological Processes

There is significant interest in employing the quartz crystal microbalance both as a sensing device for biomolecules and as a tool to characterize physiological processes. The goals include developing improved in-situ techniques in medical diagnoses, such as immunoassays, and to create new models for the development of innovative drug delivery systems, such as through the study of liposome adhesion [53]. The process of biofouling has also been the subject of studies using the QCM [71]. Key to the development of these applications (which rely on the QCM itself to act as a microdevice) is the functionalization of the QCM electrode surface.

6.8.1 Detection and Characterization of Cell Adhesion

One focus of QCM studies has been to characterize living cells during the process of adhesion. For example, Wegener et al. [106] demonstrated through a comparative study of the adsorption of cells of different types to polystyrene-coated QCMs that only specific cell adhesion leads to observed frequency shifts; the sole presence of the cell in proximity to the electrode is barely detectable. Thus, qualitatively, the QCM is sensitive to the nature of cell adhesion. Quantitative measurement of cell behavior and mechanical properties is the focus of current experimental and modeling research, and relies on both frequency and quality factor shift information [117, 37]. For example, in a study of monolayers of epithelial cells on bare gold electrodes, Janshoff et al. [37] confirmed that the presence of a cell-layer mainly increases damping of the shear wave and does not exhibit a pure mass-load behavior. The explanation for this behavior may arise from the fact that the decay length of a shear wave is of order 0.25 μm, which is significantly smaller than the typical cell size of 10 μm[29]. Thus, only the mechanical behavior of the cell components closest to the surface is probed.

As an example of how the QCM can be used to *characterize* cell adhesion, Dultsev et al. [24] developed a technique to distinguish between biomolecular interactions with surfaces. By increasing the amplitude of QCM oscillation, they showed the feasibility of monitoring bacteriophage (virus) detachment from the surface. In contrast with typical QCM measurements which monitor frequency and amplitude shifts at the resonant frequency, they monitored the acoustic emission resulting from the amplitude-induced detachment of bacteriophages. The mechanical stresses generated while the bacteriophage is attached to the oscillating surface are suddenly released during detachment. This energy excites other acoustical modes of the QCM, which can be monitored via higher harmonics of the resonant frequency. This harmonic motion is converted to an electrical signal by the QCM itself, which acts as a microphone. By estimating the amplitude of oscillation at detachment, Dultsev et al. were able to calculate and compare the binding force associated with specifically-bonded bacteriophages to those that were non-specifically bonded. These force values are comparable to those obtained from similar systems using different techniques.

Currently, theoretical models to describe the complex behavior of attached cells is still lacking [106]. This complex adsorption behavior includes (i) the initial binding contact, (ii) secretion of microexudates, (iii) spreading of the cell on the surface, (iv) modification of the adhesion properties, the number or type of binding proteins, and strength of adhesion, and (v) changes in the cytoskeleton of the cells which impacts their rigidity [29]. These factors, together with solvent entrainment, affect the acoustic impedance. Nonetheless, experiments performed on large, solvated macromolecules of a size intermediate to that of cells and proteins are aiding our understanding of the coupling between viscoelastic and mass contributions to the acoustic impedance [26, 53, 83].

6.8.2 Protein and Lipid Adsorption

Conventional immunoassays require radioisotopic, fluorescence, or enzymatic methods, which require significant washings, incubations, and separation steps. In contrast, techniques that are able to directly measure the presence of biomolecules via adsorption, such as surface plasmon resonance (SPR) and QCM, have the potential to substantially reduce the time and effort required. Because the surface of the bare electrode QCM permits non-specific binding to the surface, which can confound interpretation of impedance measurements, finding suitable functionalized coatings and methods of reproducibly applying them are currently subjects of intense research.

QCM Surface Preparation

QCM surface preparation for bioassay studies typically involves covering one surface of the electrode with molecules possessing complementary binding sites for the analyte of interest, such as an antigen-specific antibody. Functionalizing the surface can be accomplished in a number of ways. While immobilization of a binding agent via solution evaporation is the most expedient method, the proportion of available binding sites is limited by the lack of control of their molecular orientation. Thus, the sensitivity and selectivity of the assay is compromised. Other approaches to functionalize monolayers are designed to improve orientation control, including biotin/avidin chemistry [113], embedding binding sites in phospholipid monolayers using Langmuir-Blodgett methods [102], direct deposition of molecular binding sites on a protein sublayer [99, 12], and using lipids capable of linking the membrane to the analyte of interest [100]. Figure 6.11 illustrates an example biosensor. In this example, a self-assembled monolayer possessing a high degree of orientation is deposited on a gold QCM electrode. Since proteins are generally water soluble, considerable effort has focused on developing films based on Langmuir-Blodgett (LB) and Langmuir-Schaeffer (LS) methods. The Langmuir-Blodgett film can be largely composed of phospholipids to mimic biological membranes. The phospholipid layer aids in the proper orientation of the binding molecules and is deposited directly on the lipophilic surfaces created by SAMs on gold.

Quantitative Measurements of Binding

As a microdevice, the QCM has been indispensable for measuring binding affinities and kinetics of biofilm-analyte interaction [85, 101, 99, 100, 12]. A typical experiment involves measuring the transient and absolute frequency shifts during deposition. The removal of non-specifically bond molecules can be accomplished by subsequent rinsing, or by the addition of other reagents. For quantitative mass measurements, the interfacial reactions are performed in liquid, but the definitive frequency measurements are made on the dry QCM both before and after deposition [12]. The QCM analysis equipment involved in these experiments is typically simply a frequency counter.

Challenges to Quantitative Measurements in Liquid

The utility of the QCM as an immunosensor would be greatly enhanced provided quantitative measurements could be performed in the liquid phase. However, the degree to which the QCM acts truly as a microbalance depends on the acoustical properties of the functionalizing layers deposited on the electrode. To first order, the experimental data can be modeled as a thin, purely elastic film in a semi-infinite viscous medium (see section 6.3.7). However, the complex nature of these films creates challenges beyond binding site orientation control, including phase separation and unspecific binding, which hinder the reproducibility of film formation. Further, incomplete surface coverage, film compliance, and interfacial slip make the interpretation of the frequency shift data using the mass plus viscous medium model questionable (see Fig. 6.11). Examples of how the quartz crystal microbalance is being used to improve our understanding of these complexities and to evaluate potential solutions follow.

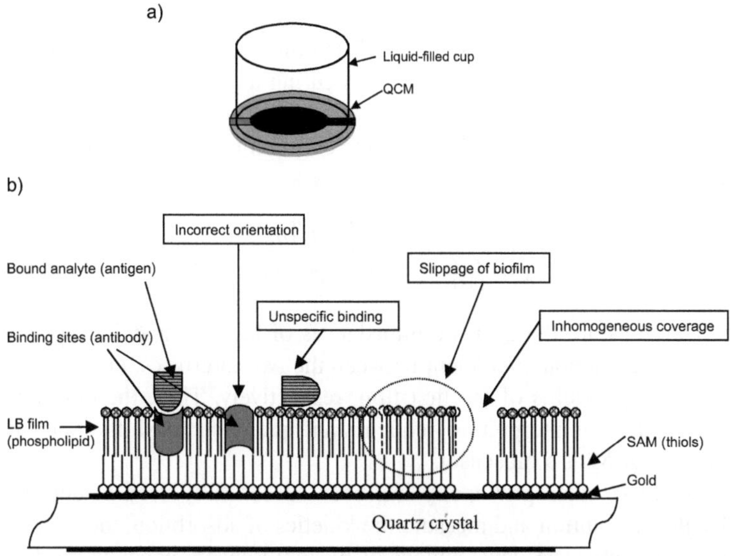

Fig. 6.11. Illustration of a liquid cell QCM apparatus (a) and example immunosensor structure (b). In (a), the cup/tube can be made of glass, polyacrylate, or other material and affixed to the QCM using non-cytotoxic silicone glue. In (b), the binding agent is incorporated into the Langmuir-Blodgett film. Two effects not illustrated are the influence of viscoelasticity of the film and the degree of phase separation, in which the multiple components comprising the SAM and LB film do not form an ordered, planar structure on the electrode surface.

Because a Langmuir-Blodgett film is comprised of multiple components possessing surfactant-like qualities, phase separation during monolayer compression is common, as is disruption during deposition. These may cause considerable loss in activity of the final film [102]. To help overcome this obstacle, Viitala et al. [100] have investigated the use of a polymerizable monolayer to stabilize the LB matrix against phase separation or disruption. Using a combination of QCM frequency measurements and atomic force microscopy, they showed that the cross-linked monolayer appeared as a two-dimensional planar film compared to the monomeric monolayer, which possessed large holes. In comparing the QCM-derived mass adsorption to that of surface plasmon resonance, Viitala et al. also suggested that accounting for the viscoelasticity of the film is necessary for the correct interpretation of the frequency shift. Protein hydration experiments confirm this [78].

McHale et al. [68] argued that at least some of the anomalous acoustic impedance results from surface wettability experiments may arise from interfacial slippage. The authors anticipate that slip may have a large impact on acoustic impedance measurements in biological sensor applications where large regions of hydrophilicity and hydrophobicity exist in the film. One of the most difficult aspects of modeling slip behavior is the introduction of additional parameters in the impedance equations (see section 6.3.8). McHale et al. show that introducing slip to the acoustic impedance of a single (non-slipping) layer Z_{ns} can be obtained by defining $Z_s = Z_{ns}/(1 + Z_{ns}/\eta_2)$, which is identical to Eq. (6.22). They further suggest a physical viewpoint for understanding the impact of slippage occuring at a successive interface, which introduces two more complex boundary conditions. The impedance equation for the case where slippage occurs at the interface between two layers of a bilayered film (like the film shown in Fig. 14) was derived as

$$Z = \left(\frac{Z_1 + Z_2}{1 + \frac{Z_1 Z_2}{\rho_1 G_1}}\right)\left(\frac{1 + Z_1 Z_2/[\eta_2(Z_1 + Z_2)]}{1 + Z_2/[\eta_2(1 + \frac{Z_1 Z_2}{\rho_1 G_1})]}\right), \tag{6.33}$$

where Z_1 and Z_2 are the acoustic impedances of layers 1 and 2, respectively, η_2 is the interfacial friction coefficient between the two interfaces, and ρ_1 and G_1 are the density and modulus of the first film, respectively. Thus, the development of applicable models for interpreting frequency and quality factor shifts should progress the use of the QCM as a biosensor.

In conclusion, microgravimetry has been successfully used to detect specific biomolecules in solution and measure the kinetics of adsorbtion, much as it has for inorganic materials. The development of piezobiosensors depends on developing processes that ensure film orientational homogeneity and reproducibility, and on the correct modeling of the acoustic properties of the functionalizing films.

This work has been supported by the NSF, AFOSR, and DOE.

References

[1] Aastrup T, Wadsak M, Leygraf C, et al.(2000) In situ studies of the initial atmospheric corrosion of copper influence of humidity, sulfur dioxide, ozone, and nitrogen dioxide. J Electrochem Soc 147 (7): 2543-2551

[2] Ashurst W, et al. (2001) Dichlorodimethylsilane as an anti-stiction monolayer for MEMS: A comparison to the octadecyltrichlorosilane self-assembled monolayer. J Microelectromechanical systems 10(1): 41-49

[3] Baudry J, Charlaix E, et al. (2001) Experimental evidence for a large slip effect at a nonwetting fluid-solid interface. Langmuir 17: 5232-5236

[4] Beerschwinger U, Albrecht T, Mathieson D (1995) Wear at microscopic scales and light loads for MEMS applications. Wear 181: 426-435

[5] Borovsky B, Mason BL, Krim J (2000) Scanning tunneling microscope measurements of the amplitude of vibration of a quartz crystal oscillator. J Appl Phys 88(7): 4017-4021

[6] In preparation.

[7] Borovsky B, Krim J, Syed Asif SA, Wahl KJ (2001) Measuring nanomechanical properties of a dynamic contact using an indenter probe and quartz crystal microbalance. Accepted J Appl Phys

[8] Bruschi L, Delfitto G, Mistura G (1999) Inexpensive but accurate driving circuits for quartz crystal microbalances. Rev Sci Instrum 70(1): 153-157

[9] Bruschi L, Mistura G (2001)Measurement of friction of thin films by means of a quartz microbalance in the presence of a finite vapor pressure. Phys Rev B 63 (23): 235411

[10] Bucur R, Mecea V (1980) Surf Technol 11: 305

[11] Buczek D, Sastri S (1980) J Appl Phys 51: 5013

[12] Caruso F, Rodda E, Furlong DN (1996) Orientational aspects of antibody immobilization and immunological activity on quartz crystal microbalance electrodes. J Coll Interf Sci 178: 104-115

[13] Chandrashekar S, Bhushan B (1992) Wear 153: 79

[14] Craig VSJ, Neto C, Williams DRM (2001) Shear-dependent boundary slip in an aqueous Newtonian liquid. Phys Rev Lett 87(5): 054504

[15] Crooks R, et al.(1997) Interactions between self-assembled monolayers and an organophosphate. Faraday Discuss 107: 285-305

[16] Daikhin L, Gileadi E, et al. (2000) Slippage at adsorbate-electrolyte interface. Response of electrochemical quartz crystal microbalance to adsorption. Electrochim Acta 45: 3615-3621

[17] Daikhin L, Urbakh M (1997) Influence of surface roughness on the quartz crystal microbalance response in a solution. Faraday Discuss 107: 27-38

[18] Daly C, Krim J (1994) Applications of a combined scanning tunneling microscope and quartz microbalance. In: Cohen SH, et al. (eds) Atomic Force Microscopy/Scanning Tunneling Microscopy. Plenum Press, New York, pp

[19] Dayo A, Alnasrallah W, Krim J (1998) Superconductivity-dependent sliding friction. Phys Rev Lett 80(8): 1690-1693

[20] Domack A, Johannsmann D (1996) Plastification during sorption of polymeric thin films: a quartz resonator study. J Appl Phys 80(5): 2599-2604

[21] Domack A, Johannsmann D (1998) Shear birefringence measurements on polymer thin films deposited on quartz resonators. J Appl Phys 83(3): 1286-1295

[22] Dugger MT (in press) Quantification of Friction in Microsystem Contacts. In: Nanotribology: Critical Assessment and Future Research Needs.

[23] Dugger M, Senft D, Nelson G (1999) Friction and durability of chemisorbed organic lubricants for MEMS. In: Tsukruk VV and Wahl KJ (ed) Microstructure and Tribology of Polymer Surfaces. American Chemical Society, Washington, pp. 455-473

[24] Dultsev FN, et al. (2001) Direct and Quantitative detection of bacteriophage by 'hearing' surface detachment using a QCM. Anal Chem 73: 3935-3939

[25] EerNisse EP (1972) J Appl Phys 43: 1330

[26] Fawcett NC, Craven RD, Zhang P, Evans JA (1998) QCM response to solvated, tethered macromolecules. Anal Chem 70: 2876-2880

[27] Filiatre C, et al. (1994) Transmission-line model for immersed quartz-crystal sensors. Sensors and Actuators A44: 137-144

[28] Flanigan CM, Desai M, Shull KR, (2000) Contact mechanics studies with the quartz crystal microbalance. Langmuir 16: 9825-9829

[29] Fredriksson C, Kihlman S, Rodahl M, Kasemo B (1998) The piezoelectric quartz crystal mass and dissipation sensor: a means of studying cell adhesion. Langmuir 14: 248-251

[30] Garrell RL , Chadwick JE (1994) Structure, reactivity and microrheology in self-assembled monolayers. Colloids Surf A 93: 59-72

[31] Ginzburg M, et al. (2000) Layer-by-layer self-assembly of organic-organometallic polymer electrostatic superlattices using poly(ferrocenylsilanes). Langmuir 16: 9609-9614

[32] Grate J, et al.(1993) Acoustic wave microsensors. Anal Chem 65(22): A987-A996

[33] Grate J, Wenzel SW, White RM (1991) Flexural plate wave devices for chemical analysis. Anal Chem 63: 1552-1561

[34] Gupta BK, Bhushan B, Chevallier J (1994) Modification of tribological properties of silicon by boron ion-implantation. Tribol Trans 37(3): 601-607

[35] Idziak S, et al.(1994) The X-ray surface forces apparatus: structure of a thin smectic liquid crystal film under confinement. Science 264: 1915-1918

[36] Itoh J, Sasaki T, et al. (1997) In situ simultaneous measurement with IR-RAS and QCM for investigation of corrosion of copper in a gaseous environment. Corros Sci 39(1): 193-197

[37] Janshoff A, Wegener J, Sieber M, Galla H-J (1996) Double-mode impedance analysis of epithelial cell monolayers cultures on shear wave resonators. Eur Biophys J 25: 93-103

[38] Johannsmann D, Mathauer K, Wegner G, Knoll W (1992) Viscoelastic properties of thin films probed with a quartz-crystal resonator. Phys Rev B 46(12): 7808-7815

[39] Kanazawa K, Gordon II J (1985) Frequency of a quartz microbalance in contact with liquid. Anal Chem 57: 1770-1771

[40] Karis T (2001) Tribochemistry in contact recording. Trib Lett 10(3): 149-162

[41] Kasemo B, Tornqvist E (1978) Surf Sci 77: 209

[42] Katz A, Ward D (1996) Probing solvent dynamics in concentrated polymer films sith a high frequency shear mode quartz resonator. J Appl Phys 80(7): 4153-4163

[43] Kim JM, Chang SM , Muramatsu H (1999) Scanning localized viscoelastic image using a quartz crystal resonator combined with an atomic force microscopy. Appl Phys Lett 74(3): 466-468

[44] Kobatake E, et al. (2000) Immunoassay systems based on immunoliposomes consisting of genetically engineered single-chain antibody. Sens Actuat B 65: 42-45

[45] Krim J, Solina H, Chiarello R (1991) Nanotribology of a Kr monolayer: A quartz crystal microbalance study of atomic-scale friction. Phys Rev Lett 66(2): 181-184

[46] Krim J, Widom A (1988) Damping of a crystal oscillator by an adsorbed monolayer and its relation to interfacial viscosity. Phys Rev B 38(17): 12184-12189

[47] Krozer R, Kasemo B (1980)Surf. Sci. 97: L339

[48] Kunze D, Peters O, Sauerbrey G, Angew (1967) Z Phys 22: 69

[49] Laschitsch A, Johannsmann D (1999) High frequency tribological investigations on quartz resonator surfaces. J Appl Phys 85(7): 3759-3765

[50] Lea M, Fozooni P (1985) The transverse acoustic impedance of an inhomogeneous viscous liquid. Ultrasonics 23: 133-137

[51] Lee SY, Staehle RW (1997) Adsorbtion studies of water on copper, nickel, and iron: Assessment of the polarization model. Z Metallkd 88 (10): 824-831

[52] Levenson L (1967) C R Acad Sci, Paris, 263: 1217

[53] Liebau M, Hildebrand A, Neubert RHH (2001) Bioadhesion of supramolecular structures at supported planar bilayers as studied by the quartz crystal microbalance. Eur Biophys J 30: 42-52

[54] Lin Z, Hill RM, Davis HT, Ward MD (1994) Determination of wetting velocities of surfactant superspreaders with the quartz-crystal microbalance. Langmuir 10(11): 4060-4068

[55] Lu C, Czanderna AW (1984) Methods and Phenomena 7: Applications of Piezoelectric Quartz Crystal Microbalances (eds) Elsevier Press, New York, pp

[56] Lu C, Lewis O (1972) J Appl Phys 43: 4385

[57] Lucklum R, et al. (1997) Determination of complex shear modulus with thickness shear mode resonators. J Phys D 30: 346-356

[58] Lucklum R, Hauptmann P (1997) Determination of polymer shear modulus with quartz crystal microbalance. Faraday Discuss 107: 123-140

[59] Lucklum R, Hauptmann P (2000) The QCM: mass sensitivity, viscoelasticity and acoustic amplification. Sensors and Actuators B 70: 30-36

[60] Luengo G , et al.(1997) Thin film rheology and tribology of confined polymer melts: contrasts with bulk properties. Macromolecules 30(8): 2482-2494

[61] Maboudian R, Howe RT (1997) J Vac Sci Technol B15: 1

[62] Majumder S, McGruer NE, Adams GG, et al. (2001) Study of contacts in an electrostatically actuated microswitch. Sensor Actuat A93(1): 19-26

[63] Martin SJ, Frye GC (1990) Surface acoustic wave response to changes in viscoelastic film properties. Appl Phys Lett 57(18): 1867-1869

[64] Martin SJ, Frye GC, Senturia SD (1994) Dynamics and response of polymer-coated surface acoustic wave devices: Effect of viscoelastic properties and film resonance. Anal Chem 66(14): 2201-2219

[65] Martin S, Granstaff V, Frye G (1991) Characterization of a quartz crystal microbalance with simultaneous mass and liquid loading. Anal Chem 63: 2272-2281

[66] Martin BA, Hager HE, (1989)J Appl Phys 65: 2637 ; ibid (1989) J Appl Phys 65: 2630

[67] Mate C, Marchon B (2000) Shear response of molecularly thin liquid films to an applied air stress. Phys Rev Lett 85(18): 3902-3905

[68] McHale G, Lucklum R, Newton MI, Cohen JA (2000) Influence of viscoelasticity and interfacial slip on acoustic wave sensors. J Appl Phys 88(12): 7304-7312

[69] McKenna L, Newton MI, et al. (2001) Compressional acoustic wave generation in microdroplets of water in contact with quartz crystal resonators. J Appl Phys 89(1): 676-680

[70] Merrill PB, Perry SS (1998) Fundamental measurements of the friction of clean and oxygen-covered VC(100) with ultrahigh vacuum atomic force microscopy: evidence for electronic contributions to interfacial friction. Surf Sci 418: 342-351

[71] Murray B, Deshaires C, (2000) Monitoring protein fouling of metal surfaces via a quartz crystal microbalance. J Coll Interf Sci 227: 32-41

[72] Pit R, Hervet H, Leger L (2000) Direct experimental evidence of slip in hexadecane: solid interfaces. Phys Rev Lett 85(5): 980-983

[73] Pit R, Hervet H, Leger L (1999) Friction and slip of a simple liquid at a solid surface. Tribology Lett 7: 147-152

[74] Polson N, Hayes M (2001) Microfluidics: Controlling fluids in small places. Anal Chem 73(11): 312A-319A

[75] Radhakrishnan G, Adams PM, Robertson R, Cole R (2000) Integration of wear-resistant titanium carbide coatings into MEMS fabrication process. Trib Lett 8: 133-137

[76] Reed CE, Kanazawa KK, Kaufman JH (1990) Physical description of a viscoelastically loaded AT-cut quartz resonator. J Appl Phys 68(5): 1993-2001

[77] Rajan N, et al.(1998) Surf Coat Technol 108-109: 391

[78] Reinisch L, Kaiser RD, Krim J (1989) Measurement of protein hydration shells using a quartz microbalance. Phys Rev Lett 63(16): 1743-1746

[79] Reiter G, Demirel A, Granick S (1994) From static to kinetic friction in confined liquid films. Science 263: 1741-1744

[80] Ricco A, et al.(1997) Single-monolayer in-situ modulus measurements using a SAW device. Faraday Discuss 107: 247-258

[81] Robbins RO, Krim J (1998) Energy dissipation in interfacial friction. MRS Bulletin: 23-26

[82] Rodahl M et al. (1995) Quartz crystal microbalance setup for frequency and Q-factor measurements in gaseous and liquid environments. Rev Sci Instrum 66(7): 3924

[83] Rodahl M, Hook F, Fredriksson C, et al.(1997) Simultaneous frequency and dissipation factor QCM measurements of biomolecular adsorption and cell adhesion. Faraday Discuss 107: 229-246

[84] Rodahl M , Kasemo B (1996) On the measurement of thin liquid overlayers with the quartz crystal microbalance. Sens Actuat A 54: 448-456

[85] Sakai G, Saiki T, Uda T, Miura N, Yamazoe N (1997) Evaluation of binding of human serum albumin (HSA) to monoclonal and polyclonal antibody by means of piezoelectric immunosensing technique. Sens Actuat B 42: 89-94

[86] Sasaki A, Katsumata A, Iwata F , Aoyama H (1994)Scanning shearing-stress microscopy of gold thin films. Jpn J Appl Phys 33: L547-L549 ; (1994) Scanning shearing-stress microscope. Appl Phys Lett 64(1): 124-125

[87] Sauerbrey GZ (1957) Phys Verhandl 8: 113
[88] Sauerbrey GZ (1959) Z Phys 115: 206
[89] Scherge M, Li X, Schaefer JA (1999) The effect of water on friction of MEMS. Trib Lett 6: 215-220
[90] Schmitt RF, et al.(2001) Bulk acoustic wave modes in quartz for sensing measurand-induced mechanical and electrical property changes. Sens Actuat B 76: 95-102
[91] Shinn ND, Mayer TM, Michalske TA (1999) Structure-dependent properties of C9-alkanethiol monolayers. Trib Lett 7(2-3): 67-71
[92] Skaife JJ, Abbott NL (1999) Quantitative characterization of obliquely deposited substrates of gold by atomic force microscopy:influence of substrate topography on anchoring of liquid crystals. Chem Mater 11: 612-623
[93] Stockbridge CD (1966) In: Vacuum Microbalance Techniques. Behrndt KH (eds) Vol 5, Plenum Press, New York, p 163
[94] Tai Y-C, Muller RS (1989) Sens Actuators 20: 41
[95] Telegdi J, et al. (2000) EQCM study of copper and iron corrosion inhibition in the presence of organic inhibitors and biocides. Electrochim Acta 45 (22-23): 3639-3647
[96] Teuscher JH, et al. (1997) Phase transitions in thin alkane films and alkanethiolate monolayers on gold detected with a thickness shear mode device. Faraday Discuss 107: 399-416
[97] Thompson M, et al.(1991) Thickness-shear mode acoustic wave sensors in the liquid phase, a review. Analyst 116: 881-889
[98] Tomassone MS, Widom A (1997) Electronic friction forces on molecules moving near metals. Phys Rev B 56(8): 4938-4943
[99] Tronin A, Dubrovsky T, Radicchi G, Nicolini C (1996) Optimization of IgG Langmuir film deposition for application as sensing elements. Sens Actuat B 34: 276-282
[100] Viitala T, et al. (2000) Protein immobilization to a partially cross-linked organic monolayer. Langmuir 16: 4953-4961
[101] Vikholm I, Albers WM, (1998) Oriented immobilization of antibodies for immunosensing. Langmuir 14: 3865-3872
[102] Vikholm I, Gyorvary E, Peltonen J (1996) Incorporation of lipid-tagged single-chain antibodies into lipid monolayers and the interaction with antigen. Langmuir 12: 3276-3281
[103] Wadsak M, et al. (2000) Combined in-situ investigations of atmospheric corrosion of copper with SFM and IRAS coupled with QCM. Surf Sci 454-456: 246-250
[104] Wang DF, Kato K (2001) Tribological evaluation of carbon coatings with and without nitrogen incorporation applicable to MicroElectroMechanical systems. Sensor Actuat A 93(3): 251-257
[105] Watts ET, Krim J , Widom A (1990) Experimental observation of interfacial slippage at the boundary of molecularly thin films with gold substrates. Phys Rev B41(6): 3466-3472
[106] Wegener J, Janshoff A, Galla HJ (1998) Cell adhesion monitoring using a quartz crystal microbalance: comparative analysis of different mammalian cell lines. Eur Biophys J 28: 26-37
[107] Weiss P (2000) The little engines that couldn't. Science News 158(4): 56-58
[108] White R (1997) Acoustic interactions from Faraday's crispations to MEMS. Faraday Discuss 107: 1-13
[109] Widom A, Krim J (1994) Spreading diffusion and its relation to sliding friction in molecularly thin adsorbed films. Phys Rev E 49(5): 4154-4156
[110] Windeln J et al. (2001) Applied surface analysis in magnetic storage technology. Appl Surf Sci 179: 167-180
[111] Witte G, Weiss K, Jakob P, Braun J, Kostov KL, Woll CH (1998) Damping of molecular motion on a solid substrate: evidence for electron-hole pair creation. Phys Rev Lett 80(1): 121-124

[112] Wolff O, Seydel E, Johannsmann D (1997) Viscoelastic properties of thin films studied with quartz crystal resonators. Faraday Discuss 107: 91-104

[113] Xiao C, Yang M, Sui S (1998) DNA-containing organized molecular structure based on controlled assembly on supported monolayers. Thin Solid Films 327-329: 647-651

[114] Yamada R, Ye S, Uosaki K (1996) Novel scanning probe microscope for local elasticity measurement. Jpn J Appl Phys 35: L846-L848

[115] Yang M, Thompson M, Duncan-Hewitt W (1993) Interfacial properties and the response of the thickness-shear-mode acoustic wave sensor in liquids. Langmuir 9: 802-811

[116] Yoshizawa H, Israelachvili J (1993) Fundamental mechanisms of interfacial friction. 2. Stick-slip friction of spherical and chain molecules. J Phys Chem 97: 11300-11313

[117] Zhou T, Marx KA, Warren M, Schulze H, Braunhut S (2000) The quartz crystal microbalance as a continuous monitoring tool for the study of endothelial cell surface attachment and growth. Biotechnol Prog 16: 268-277

[118] Zhu Y, Granick S (2001) Rate-dependent slip of Newtonian liquid at smooth surfaces. Phys Rev Lett 87(9): 096105

[119] Zhu XY, Houston JE (1999) Molecular lubricants for silicon-based microelectromechanical systems (MEMS): a novel strategy. Trib Lett 7: 87-90